Learning Experience Guides for Nursing Students

■ Volume II

5th Edition Revised by Mary Helen Patterson Ortega

R.N., C., C.S., B.S., M.S., Oklahoma Baptist University, Shawnee, Oklahoma; M.S., University of California, San Francisco. Formerly staff/head nurse, in-service coordinator in hospitals in Oklahoma, Michigan, California, and England; Coordinator, ADN program, Napa Valley College; currently, professor of nursing, Assistant Director, ADN program, Napa Valley College, Napa, California

Original Series Concept by Anne K. Roe

R.N., B.S., Stanford University; M.Ed., Florida Atlantic University. Formerly instructor, Broward Community College, ADN program and Broward County LPN program, Fort Lauderdale, Florida; office nurse, school nurse, and LVN instructor in California and Colorado

Mary C. Sherwood

R.N., St. Luke's Hospital, Cleveland, Ohio; B.S.N., M.Ed., University of Florida. Formerly in-service director at Everglades Memorial Hospital, Pahokee, Florida; instructor, Broward Community College ADN program, Fort Lauderdale, Florida; staff nurse and private-duty nurse in California, Ohio, New York, and Florida; school nurse in Florida

Contributor to LEGs VIII-A and VIII-B

Bonnie MacMaster Andersen

R.N., B.S.N., Pacific Lutheran University, Tacoma, Washington; M.N., University of Washington, Seattle. Formerly staff nurse at University Hospital, Seattle; Stanford University Hospital, Stanford; Prince George's General Hospital, Maryland; Instructor of Nursing, Pacific Lutheran University, Tacoma; and The Catholic University of America, Washington, D.C.; presently associate professor of nursing, Napa Valley College, Napa, California

Learning Experience Guides for Nursing Students

■ Volume II, 5th Edition

Mary Helen Patterson Ortega, R.N., C., C.S., B.S., M.S.

Anne K. Roe, R.N., B.S., M.Ed.

Mary C. Sherwood, R.N., B.S.N., M.Ed.

Maternity Consultant:

Bonnie MacMaster Andersen, R.N., B.S.N., M.N.
Associate Professor of Nursing
Napa Valley College
Napa, California

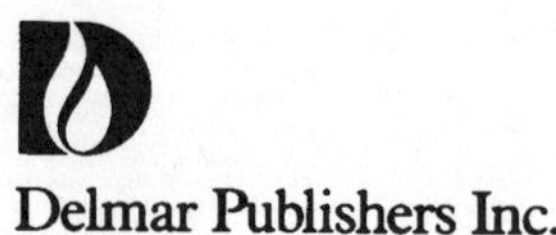

Notice to the Reader

Publisher does not warrant or guarantee any of the products described herein or perform any independent analysis in connection with any of the product information contained herein. Publisher and author do not assume, and expressly disclaim, any obligation to obtain and include information other than that provided to them by the manufacturer.

The reader is expressly warned to consider and adopt all safety precautions that might be indicated by the activities described herein and to avoid all potential hazards. By following the instructions contained herein, the reader willingly assumes all risks in connection with such instructions.

The publisher makes no representations or warranties of any kind, including but not limited to, the warranties of fitness for particular purpose or merchantability, nor are any such representations implied with respect to the material set forth herein, and the publisher and author take no responsibility with respect to such material. The publisher shall not be liable for any special, consequential or exemplary damages resulting, in whole or in part, from the readers' use of, or reliance upon, this material.

Cover design by Megan DeSantis
Delmar Staff
Sponsoring Editor: Patricia Casey
Associate Editor: Elisabeth F. Williams
Project Editor: Mary P. Robinson
Production Supervisor: Wendy Troeger
Art/Design Coordinator: Megan DeSantis

For information, address Delmar Publishers Inc.
3 Columbia Circle
Box 15015
Albany, NY 12212-5015

Printed in the United States of America
Published simultaneously in Canada
by Nelson Canada,
a Division of the Thomson Corporation

10 9 8 7 6 5 4 3 2 1 xxx 99 98 97 96 95 94 93

ISBN 0-8273-6047-9

Ortega, M. Helen.
Learning experience guides for nursing students / M. Helen Ortega, Anne K. Roe, Mary C. Sherwood. — 5th ed.
p. cm.
Roe's name appears first on earlier editions.
Includes index.
ISBN 0-8273-6108-4 (v. 4). — ISBN 0-8273-6046-0 (v. 1). — ISBN 0-8273-6047-9 (v. 2). —
ISBN 0-8273-6062-2 (v. 3)
1. Nursing. 2. Nursing—Problems, exercises, etc. I. Roe. Anne K. II. Sherwood, Mary C. III. Title.
[DNLM: 1. Nursing—programmed instruction. WY 18 077L 1993]
RT41.067 1993
610.73'07—dc20
DNLM/DLC
for Library of Congress 93-351
CIP

Contents

To the Student xv

Level Six

LEG VI-A: Crisis, Grief, and Psychoneurotic Disorders

Therapeutic Relationship and Psychosocial Assessment

Therapeutic Relationship (1)* 7

Psychosocial Assessment (2) 7

Crisis Intervention

Crisis Events and Nursing Interventions (3, 4) 10

Healthy Response to Crisis (5) 10

Using Nursing Process in Crisis Intervention (6) 10

Assisting the Patient in Coping with Grief and Death; Providing Postmortem Care

Normal Grieving Process (7) 14

Helping People Express Grief (8) 14

Helping Adapt to Loss (9) 14

Coping with a Fatal Illness (10) 14

Caring for a Dying Patient (11) 14

Postmortem Care (12) 14

Depression

Differences between Grief and Depression (13) 21

Behaviors in Depression (14, 17) 21

Nursing Interventions for Depressed Patients (15) 21

Therapeutic Communication with Depressed Patients (16) 21

Antidepressant drugs (18) 21

Numbers in parentheses refer to Objectives.

Disturbed Coping Patterns: Anxiety and Psychophysiologic Disorders

Neurotic Disorders (19, 20) 25

Nursing Interventions for Patients with Neurotic Disorders (21) 25

Psychophysiologic Disorders (22) 25

Antianxiety Agents (Minor Tranquilizers) (23) 25

LEG VI-B: Stress, Adaptation, and Diabetes

Stress and Charting

Adaptation to Stress (1, 2) 42

Charting (3) 42

Living with Diabetes

Actions of Insulin and Glucagon (4) 49

Comparing Types of Diabetes (5) 49

Signs, Symptoms, and Lifestyles (6, 7) 49

Diet History, Planning, and Teaching (8, 9) 49

Testing Blood and Urine

Testing Blood and Urine (10, 11) 55

Diagnostic Testing (12) 55

Pharmacology

Antidiabetic Drugs (13–15) 57

Teaching Insulin Administration (16) 57

Preventing Acute and Long-Term Complications

Hypo- and Hyperglycemia (17) 62

Preventing Long-Term Complications of Diabetes (18, 19) 62

Altered Sexual Function (20) 62

Community Resources

Community Resources for Diabetics (21) 69

LEG VI-C: Respiratory Problems

Assessing and Preventing Respiratory Problems

Factors Predisposing to Respiratory Problems (1) 81
Recognizing Hypoxemia and Hypercapnea (2) 81
Respiratory Assessment (3) 81
Analyzing Data and Making a Nursing Diagnosis (4) 81
Respiratory Infection Control (5) 81

Diagnostic Tests and Nursing Responsibilities

Diagnostic Tests and Nursing Responsibilities (6–8) 90
Arterial Blood Gases Related to Respiratory Acidosis and Alkalosis (9) 90

Relieving Respiratory Distress

Rationales for Medical Treatment of Respiratory Problems (10) 95
Aerosol Medication and Nose Drops (11) 95
Drugs Used for Respiratory Problems (12) 95

Respiratory Alterations

Nursing Process with Respiratory Problems (13) 98
Understanding and Intervening in Respiratory Alterations (14) 98
Effects of Aging (15) 98
Taking Action in Respiratory Distress (16) 98

Using the Nursing Process for Common Problems Occurring with Respiratory Alterations

Emotions Involved in Respiratory Distress (17) 104
Cough and Control (18) 104
Abnormal Sputum (19) 104
Hostility Related to Respiratory Distress (20) 104
Causes of Fatigue and Nursing Interventions (21) 104
Dealing with Anorexia (22) 104

Table of Contents

Table of Contents

Patients Receiving Oxygen and Humidity

Oxygen and Humidity (23) 111

Child in a Croupette (24) 111

Observations for Obstructed Airway

Observations for an Obstructed Airway (25) 115

Report on a Child with Croup (26) 115

Tracheostomy Care (EAO)

Tracheostomy Care (27, 28) 117

Intradermal Injections (EAO)

Intradermal Injection (29) 119

Level Seven

LEG VII-A: Surgery

Emotional Preparation for Surgery

Emotional Preoperative Preparation (1, 2) 134

Preparing for Change in Body Image (3) 134

Preoperative Teaching

Factors Influencing Perioperative Experience (4) 138

Preoperative Teaching (5, 6) 138

Physical Preparation for Surgery

Assessing Risks and Providing Nutritional Support (7, 8) 141

Preoperative Lab Tests (9) 141

Skin Preparation (10) 141

Preparing a Patient for Surgery Using a Checklist (11) 141

Preparing a Room for a Postoperative Patient (12) 141

Preoperative Medications

Preoperative Medications (13, 14) 147

Pediatric Calculations (15) 147

Immediate Postoperative Period

Early Postoperative Assessments and Actions (16, 17, 19) 151

Suctioning Mouth and Nose (18) 151

Using the Nursing Process for Postoperative Care

Preventing Postoperative Complications (20) 156

Using Drugs for Postoperative Problems (21) 156

Using the Nursing Process to Care for Postoperative Patients (22, 23) 156

Wound Care (24) 156

Planning Care for Two to Four Patients

Organizing Preoperative Care for Two to Four Patients (25) 161

Involving a Relative in Care of a Surgical Patient (26) 161

LEG VII-B: Fluid and Electrolyte Balance during Illness

Fluid Balance and Imbalance

Regulation of Fluid and Electrolyte Balance (1) 176

Dehydration in All Ages (2) 176

Fluid and Electrolyte Imbalances

Nursing Care for Fluid Volume Deficit (3) 180

Assessment of Fluid and Electrolyte Balance (4) 180

Sodium, Potassium, and Magnesium Imbalances (5) 180

Nursing Interventions for Nausea, Vomiting, and Diarrhea (6) 180

Acid-Base Imbalances

Causes of Respiratory and Metabolic Acid-Base Imbalances (7, 8) 188

Recognizing When Metabolic Alkalosis Might Occur (9) 188

Table of Contents

Parenteral Solutions

Using Parenteral Solutions (10) 195
Using a Microdrip Set (11) 195
Adding IV Solutions to Existing Infusion (12) 195
Caring for a Venipuncture Site (13) 195
Intervening When IV Equipment Fails to Function Properly 195

Gastric and Intestinal Tubes and Feedings

Insertion and Use of Gastrointestinal Tubes (15, 16) 199
Enteral Feedings (17) 199
Inserting a Nasogastric Tube (18) 199

LEG VII-C: Cardiac and Hypertensive Problems

Alterations in Cardiac Function

Lifestyles Leading to Alterations in Cardiac Function (1) 213
Pathophysiology, Causes, and Symptoms of Heart Problems (2, 3) 213
Effects of Stress (4) 213

Diagnostic Tests and Nursing Assessment

Diagnostic Tests (5, 6) 217
Physical Assessment (7) 217
Apical-Radial Pulse (8) 217

Planning Nursing Care

Rationales for Medical Orders and Nursing Goals (9, 10) 221
Pharmacology (11) 221
Discharge Planning for the Hypertensive Patient (12) 221
Community Resources (13) 221

Basic Needs after a Myocardial Infarction

Meeting the Basic Needs of a Convalescing MI Patient (14) 229
Approaches to Uncooperative Behavior (15) 229
Assessing Tolerance to Activity (16, 17) 229

Acute Care Requirements Related to Fluid Excess

Problems Related to Fluid Excess (18) 233

Planning Nursing Care for Patients with Acute CHF (19) 233

Level Eight

LEG VIII-A: Labor and Delivery

Growth and Development of the Fetus

Fetal Development (1) 248

Admission and Assessment of a Patient in Labor

Admission and Assessment of a Patient in Labor (2) 251

Nursing Interventions to Decrease Fear, Pain, Discomfort (3) 251

Observing Attitudes about Pregnancy and Childbirth (4) 251

Stages of Labor (5, 6) 251

Assessments and Interventions in Stages I and II (7) 251

Monitoring a Patient in Labor

Monitoring (Assessing) Fetal Heart Rate (8–10) 259

Assessing Cervical Dilatation (11) 259

Assessing Uterine Contractions (12) 259

Nursing Care during Labor (13) 259

Anesthesia and Analgesia

Types of Anesthesia and Analgesia (14, 15) 264

Nurse's Role in Giving Analgesia (16) 264

Drugs Used during Labor (17) 264

Second and Third Stages of Labor

Physiologic and Psychologic Changes in the Second Stage of Labor (18) 269

Teaching and Assisting with Breathing Patterns (19) 269

Mechanisms of Labor (20) 269

Nursing Care in Stages I and II (21) 269

Third Stage of Labor (22) 269

Table of Contents

Table of Contents

Signs of Placental Separation

Observing for Placental Separation (23) 272

Fourth Stage of Labor and Immediate Care of Newborn

Nursing Care during the Fourth Stage of Labor (24) 273

Assessing the Fundus (25) 273

Immediate Care and Assessment of the Newborn (26) 273

LEG VIII-B: Postpartum and Neonatal Care

Postpartum Assessment and Care

Postpartum Physiologic Changes (1) 289

Nursing Care Plan for a Normal Postpartum Patient (2) 289

Nursing Actions for Postpartum Problems (3) 289

Postpartum Checks and Perineum Care (4) 289

Oxytocics in Postpartum

Oxytocics (5) 293

Characteristics of the Normal Newborn

Characteristics of a Normal Newborn (6) 295

Breast and Bottle Feeding

Breast and Bottle Feeding (7, 8) 298

Methods to Suppress Lactation (9) 298

Caring for the Normal Newborn

Use of Apgar Scoring (10) 302

Admitting, Assessing, and Caring for a Normal Newborn (11, 12) 302

Teaching Newborn Care to a Mother (13) 302

Assessing a New Parent's Feelings and Attitudes

Mothering and Attainment of Maternal Role (14) 308

Assessing Attitudes and Emotional Needs of the New Mother (15, 16, 18) 308

Assessment for Blues and Psychoses (17) 308

Helping a Mother Have Success with Her Infant (19) 308

Using Positive Nursing Diagnoses in Nursing Care Planning (20) 308

Teenage Pregnancy, Single Mother, Nontraditional Childbearing Couples, and Birth Control

Nursing Care for Single Mothers and Nontraditional Childbearing Couples (21) 314

Teenage Pregnancy (22) 314

Contraception Methods (23) 314

Helping a Family Deal with Loss of Health or Life of Infant (EAO)

Helping a Family Deal with Loss of Health or Life of Infant (24) 317

LEG VIII-C: Gastrointestinal Problems

Admission and Assessment

Admitting Patients with Alterations in Gastrointestinal Function (1) 331

Physical Assessment of Patients with Gastrointestinal Problems (2) 331

Gastrointestinal Diagnostic Tests (3) 331

Nutritional Needs and GI Problems

Diet Therapy in Gastrointestinal Problems (4) 339

Caring for a Patient Receiving Hyperalimentation Therapy (5) 339

Pharmacology

Pharmacology (6, 7) 343

Nursing Care of GI Patients Receiving Conservative Medical Therapy

Using the Nursing Process with Patients Receiving Conservative Medical Therapy (8) 346

Teaching and Discharge Planning for Patients with Gastrointestinal Problems (9) 346

Hepatitis and Infection Control Measures

Nursing Care for Patients with Hepatitis (10, 11) 351

The Nursing Process and GI Surgical Patients

Caring for Patients with Gastrointestinal Surgery (12, 13) 355

Assessing for Complications Following Gastrointestinal Surgery (14) 355

Wound Care

Changing Surgical Dressings (15) 362

Irrigating a Wound (16) 362

Ostomy Care

Emotional Needs before a Colostomy (17) 366

Caring for a Patient with a Colostomy (18) 366

Index 375

To the Student

The LEGs curriculum centers around identified Objectives and planned Learning Experiences based on a *problem-solving approach.* You are continually encouraged to solve patient care problems in your own unique way for individual patients, on the basis of the patient's behavior, your knowledge of science and nursing, the medical treatment ordered, and the nursing process. This problem-solving approach carries through the LEGs concept of responsibility and the individuality of the patient and the nurse.

What's New in Volume II?

■ Content Organization (Conceptual Framework)

There are nine LEGs in this Volume. Each of them is longer and contains more Objectives and Learning Experiences than the LEGs in Volume I, and therefore may take longer to complete.

There are various ways of organizing the traditional medical-surgical, maternal-child, and psychiatric nursing content. We have chosen to group this nursing knowledge into three basic components of care: **Crisis, Regulatory,** and **Body Systems.** These *components of care* represent three ways of viewing a patient's problems:

(1) as a physical or emotional **crisis** event in the life of the patient,

(2) as a **regulatory** or homeostatic problem, and

(3) as an alteration in the function of a **body system.**

■ A **crisis** may or may not be recognized as such by the person experiencing it. Many people have a misconception that a crisis is not a crisis unless it is so labeled by public consensus. Not so! A crisis involves a loss, whether it be a life, limb, job, or childbirth. A nurse must recognize and understand a crisis event and be able to help patients resolve their turmoil. A healing process must follow the initial shock and disbelief of the crisis event. The **crisis** component will be the major content of the A LEG in each level, with reference and follow-through in the B and C LEGs.

■ The **regulatory** functions of the body are essential to life and function as a self-regulating system, with many "backup" systems available in case of emergency. In illness, (for example, in diabetes mellitus) certain regulatory functions fail, but medicine and treatment along with patient teaching and care by the nurse can reverse the pendulum. It is frequently the nurse who recognizes the first signs and symptoms of imbalance, and with immediate action, whether it be independent (based on nursing principles) or dependent (in response to a direct medical order), can help the patient regain the equilibrium lost because of the stressors of illness. *Regulatory* problems are introduced in the B LEG of each Level.

■ At first the **body systems** appear related only in that they all exist in the human body and are all necessary to life. But more than that, they depend on each other to transport nutrients and oxygen to the cells. Oxygenation, required by all body cells, could not occur if the lungs could not take in oxygen and give off carbon dioxide; the cells would not grow and multiply without nutrients and fluid prepared for absorption in the gastrointestinal system. Neither oxygenation nor cell growth would have any value without the heart and circulatory system to pump the particles throughout the body. **Body systems** are introduced in LEG C of each Level and are related to other *components of care* in the other LEGs.

In actuality, every health problem contains aspects of each of these three viewpoints. For example, a patient having suffered a myocardial infarction presents these challenges to the nurse or nursing student:

A. Crisis: What does this illness mean to the patient and to the family? How does the patient react to it emotionally, and how will that reaction affect the recovery period and the patient's future life? How can nursing care assist the patient to cope with crisis?

B. Regulatory: How does the body attempt to correct imbalance? Does pain force a patient to limit activity? Do blood cells and enzymes attack the damaged heart tissue to repair and replace it? Is nursing care planned to facilitate the body's ability to heal itself?

C. Body Systems: How do the anatomy and physiology of the body change with illness? How do the medications and treatments help return the organs to normal functioning? What signs and symptoms signal dysfunction of some part of the body?

By organizing the nursing content in this fashion, you can readily identify each *component* with all patients. You must recognize and understand that each *component of care* is equally important in giving good nursing care. As you study the problems of myocardial infarction in LEG VII-C **(body systems),** you will find aspects of the **regulatory** and **crisis** components. As you move to LEG VIII-A **(crisis),** you will be able to relate the aspects of the **regulatory** and **body systems** components to the obstetrical patient's problems.

Your instructors will relate your school's individual conceptual framework to this organizational framework.

■ Flow Chart

The flow chart for Volume II identifies the placement of content and indicates the relationships of the *components of care.* Note that as in Volume I, each Level must be completed before progressing to the next Level. Whether you begin the LEG with A, B, or C is between you and your instructor.

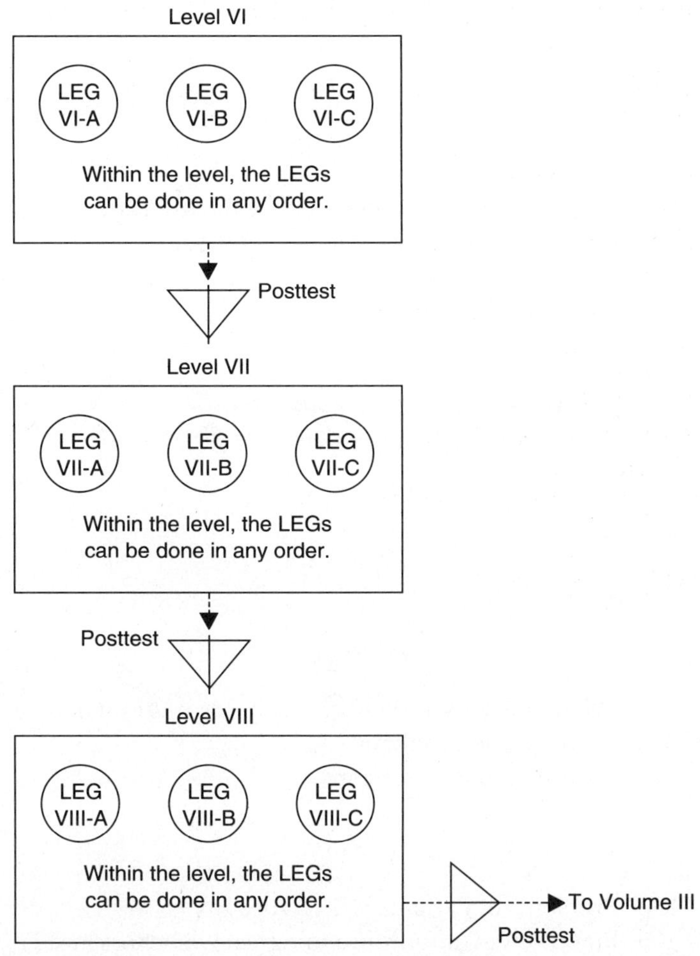

Levels and Content in Volumes II, III, IV

Descriptions of LEGs Content for Nursing Care of People of All Ages:

Volume II

Level Six

LEG VI-A Crisis, Grief, and Psychoneurotic Disorders
LEG VI-B Stress, Adaptation, and Diabetes
LEG VI-C Respiratory Problems

Level Seven

LEG VII-A Surgery
LEG VII-B Fluid and Electrolyte Balance during Illness
LEG VII-C Cardiac and Hypertensive Problems

Level Eight

LEG VIII-A Labor and Delivery
LEG VIII-B Postpartum and Neonatal Care
LEG VIII-C Gastrointestinal Problems

What's Ahead in Volumes III and IV:

Volume III

Level Nine

LEG IX-A Mental Illness and Other Long-Term Problems
LEG IX-B Orthopedic Problems
LEG IX-C Genitourinary Problems

Level Ten

LEG X-A Problems of Patients with Cancer
LEG X-B Blood, Liver, and Immunological Disorders and IV Therapy
LEG X-C Neurological Problems

Level Eleven

LEG XI-A High-Risk Pregnancy, Childbirth, and Newborn
LEG XI-B Genitourinary and Gynecological Problems
LEG XI-C Acute Cardiac Care
LEG PN/VN Transition to Employment

Volume IV

Level Twelve

LEG XII-A RN Transition to Employment
LEG XII-B Neurosurgical Problems
LEG XII-C Acute Surgical Care Including Cardiovascular Surgery

Level Thirteen

LEG XIII-A Emergency and Burn Care
LEG XIII-B Acute Pediatric Care
LEG XIII-C Acute Medical Care Including Endocrine Problems

Level Fourteen

LEG XIV-A What Do I Need to Know to Graduate?
LEG XIV-B Influencing, Regulating, and Extending Nursing Practice
LEG XIV-C How to Work within the System

Career Ladder Mobility (PN/VN Curriculum)

The Objectives in this volume that have the ladder symbol may be omitted from the PN/VN curriculum at your instructor's discretion, or they may be reworded for your use.

Clinical Performance Expectations

As you proceed from Level Six to Level Seven to Level Eight, you will be expected to gain an increasing amount of knowledge and skill. Read through all the Why Should I Study? sections at the beginning of the three Levels before you actually begin Volume II. The *clinical performance expectations* for each Level are stated there; they will give you an overview of the progress you must strive for as you study the LEGs in that Level. Review each past Level's *clinical performance expectations* before you start the next Level. At first reading, you may feel that the clinical focuses lack opportunity to improve on skills learned in Volume I. We intend for you to identify your own needs for those experiences and combine them with the new focuses in Volume II so that you are giving **total patient care.**

Postconference

You will not find guidelines for postconferences in Volume II, but only a few specific questions or comments when appropriate. You must assume that all postconferences follow each day of lab and require your *active* participation. Postconference should be a melting pot of shared experiences gained from the laboratory experiences suggested in each LEG of each Level. You must learn from other students, and they must learn from you.

Extra Added Objectives

Extra Added Objectives are included for your use only if you are ready and have the time, inclination, or opportunity. Some of these Objectives will be required Objectives at a later Level. Some of the Objectives in this group are included because it may be difficult to find some types of clinical experiences, and you need to take advantage of them whenever available (for example, tracheostomy care). See Objectives 27 and 28 in LEG VI-C. Ask your instructor which ones will be required.

To the Student

■ References

You will be reading about patient problems in medical-surgical, maternity, pediatrics, and psychiatric nursing textbooks. If you buy them now you will be able to use them for Volumes II, III, and IV. We have listed only a few of these books by name; your instructor will choose those that are preferred for your school.

■ Ideas on How to Use the LEGs in Volume II

When beginning a LEG, spend about 10 to 15 minutes reading the What page and all the Objectives. Then look at the Overview sheet. Use it to help you plan your week. Which Objectives must you study before attending each group discussion, each clinical lab, and so forth? When you can begin to visualize the work involved, write out your plan for the next few days. Set realistic goals for library time, and fill in the dates when each group of Objectives will be completed.

Then, begin using the audiovisual materials and readings for the first group of Objectives. Limit yourself to two or three different readings if possible. You do not have to answer every write-in question immediately. Look ahead to see if your articles and audiovisuals will help you with later Objectives. If convenient, work with one or two other students. Reading different articles and sharing answers saves time and improves critical thinking. Ask others to explain answers that are not clear. This exercise will train you to read more carefully and to question what you read. Tell each other of outstanding articles that should not be missed.

■ Group Discussions

Group discussions are very effective for learning. In order to benefit from a group discussion, you must come prepared. Preparation includes:

1. Finding out what group members should do. (See LEG; check with instructor.)

2. Finding out why the group is meeting. (Read Objectives.)

3. Signing up for a particular group. This may include indicating what you will do to prepare for the meeting. (See sign-up sheet.)

4. Attending the group, then evaluating how it went: that is, the degree of success or failure in accomplishing the task, and how you feel about your own performance and that of other group members.

Group discussions can be used for many purposes:

1. *Sharing information.* Sharing minimizes the time spent by an individual in studying the material and maximizes what you can learn in a limited time.

2. *Problem solving.* Input from several prepared people is usually very effective in leading to decisions and actions to improve a problem situation. Problem solving is frequently the purpose of group meetings of the nursing staff.

3. *Oral testing.* A quick way to find out what you know and what you still need to learn. A tense situation, but a very good way to stimulate group members to be quick with challenges and to defend their actions and those of their peers.

4. *Venting feelings.* Have you ever done this in an impromptu way after an emotionally charged clinical experience? The first few minutes of postconference sometimes serve this function. Venting feelings can make you feel better; realize that others have similar or very different feelings; clear the way for problem solving and changes that may make a situation better.

5. *Brainstorming.* Create and share ideas. Consider a subject from as many angles as there are group members. Come up with ideas of how to approach a problem or activity. "Two heads are better than one."

Think about group work. It is not fast. It involves compromise. How do you feel about group versus individual study, work, and play? Sometimes a decision must be made and an action taken without waiting for the group process. Later the group process may modify, change, or uphold the decision. You may compare group work to a democracy versus a dictatorship; cumbersome, but worthwhile for the good of each individual.

Think about group discussions as they are now. Are you taking an active role in both preparing for and participating in at least one a week? Are you satisfied with your own efforts and the efforts of other group members? Is it time well spent? Or is it time wasted? You can make groups effective. But you need to work at it.

■ Review "How Do I Use a LEG" and "How Do I Use My Instructor"

More will be expected of you this term. To perfect your learning skills, review "To the Student" in Volume I. Find out what you missed as a beginning student and get ideas for Volume II.

Test Yourself: See if you can answer these questions. If you can't, reread the appropriate paragraph.

1. Where are the clinical performance expectations found in the LEG?

2. Why are they included?

3. What are the three components of care that direct the content in A, B, and C LEGs?

4. How many LEGs are included in this Volume?

5. What should you do when beginning a LEG?

6. How do you use your instructor?

7. What does NCP stand for? Where is it found?

8. How do you prepare for a group discussion?

9. How can you reduce the time spent in the library?

10. What can the Overview page do for you? Where is it found?

■ Review How to Use the Steps of the Nursing Process to Write a Nursing Care Plan

Steps of the Nursing Process	Writing a Nursing Care Plan

In Volume I, you learned about the nursing process—a way of thinking and a way of caring for patients. Although you may not yet understand it completely or see what difference it can make in giving care, you will find as you study about patients in Volume II that it suddenly makes sense and is useful. If you do not feel totally familiar with all of the steps of the nursing process, review them now. Review the total process one more time before you use it in Level Six. Use the data base form and nursing care plan (NCP) format you used in Volume I. Review the format in its entirety and plan to use it with each LEG on each patient problem as you explore how best to care for your patients.

In order to meet the needs of patients, nursing must be problem oriented. The needs of individuals and groups change, and nursing care and nurse relationships vary. The nursing process must also be applicable in a variety of settings and with a variety of patients. You need to learn to think critically and to be able to organize knowledge in such a way that it can be used to plan patient care and make decisions.

The nursing process includes the problem-solving skills of assessment, analysis, planning, implementation, and evaluation to provide care according to the needs of individuals and groups of patients and their families. It gives organization and direction to the various and distinct elements of nursing practice. *It focuses the nurse's thinking on the individual rather than on the tasks* involved in giving care. Thus, patients' needs are thoroughly assessed, and effective plans can be made to meet the needs.

Decision making in nursing involves anticipation of a variety of consequences arising from any nursing intervention and individual acceptance of accountability and responsibility for nursing actions. Nursing within this framework of problem solving and decision making uses technical, communication, teaching, and leadership skills for patient care.

Assessment

Illness threatens one or more basic needs, producing consequences that are beyond the individual's ability to adapt. The nurse must look at the total person and make judgments regarding the satisfaction of or threats to each basic need.

Assessment is the systematic collection and appraisal of data about an individual, the family, or the community leading to identification of the problem and a nursing diagnosis that is used to give nursing care. It begins with the collection of data. Methods of data collection include observation and physical assessment ("observing" and "looking"), interviewing, and history taking ("listening" and "questioning"). Data may be either objective or subjective.

Patients are the primary resource for information. If they are reliable historians, they can best tell you what their current health status is, what their needs and problems are, and what their goals are. The information given you by a patient can be confirmed by secondary resources that include the patient's family, the doctor and other health care team members, a data base, the patient's record, your own knowledge, your instructors, and books and journals.

There are two phases of assessment. The first is the initial assessment and includes an interview and an examination. It provides a baseline by which to measure change. The second phase is an ongoing (continuous) assessment that gives current information. The time required for assessment depends on the amount of information to be collected and probably on how many previous assessments have been performed. The nurse should use every opportunity to make accurate, complete observations of symptoms without unduly inconveniencing the patient. Remember that you have previous knowledge and that it is useful to you in assessing your patients.

Normal psychology will help you evaluate behavior, emotion, and intellect, perceptions of self, and problem-solving abilities. Normal developmental stages help identify factors that hinder or promote progression through those stages.

Analysis

Do you know what analysis means? The dictionary describes it as "separation into parts." It is a mental activity that is both hard to teach and hard to learn. The best way to learn is to think out loud with an experienced person (your instructor). Learn how to evaluate information, keep what is valuable, discard what is irrelevant, see the relationships, and arrive at a conclusion—a nursing diagnosis.

Note: Analysis requires that you ask yourself the following questions: (1) Do I have enough of the right kind of data? (2) Are the facts correct? (3) Have I clarified words and concepts? (4) How reliable is my source of information? (5) Have I been objective?

Some data may require validation. Can you think of examples? Suppose you collect the following data by observation and listening to your patient.

She states she feels warm.
You see that she is flushed, that her skin feels warm and dry.

You form an impression or opinion that your patient has a fever. What further data could you collect to validate your opinion or impression? Right! You could take your patient's temperature.

You are now ready to identify the problems and make a nursing diagnosis.

Nursing Diagnosis

Data collection, analysis, and interpretation must be accurate, for they are the basis for your conclusions, or your nursing diagnosis. Errors or omissions can result in an incorrect nursing diagnosis.

A nursing diagnosis is a two-part statement that describes a person's (patient's) response or behavior and the factors that contribute to the response or behavior, and the signs and symptoms (defining characteristics) of the response. The response or behavior is determined by a nursing assessment, and a nurse can intervene to decrease, modify, or eliminate the response or behavior. The factors that contribute to the response can be etiologic, pathophysiologic, psychologic, environmental, developmental, cultural, age-related, treatment-related, or situational. The signs and symptoms validate the diagnosis.

Most textbooks use examples from a list of nursing diagnoses published by the North American Nursing Diagnosis Association (NANDA). Discuss nursing diagnoses with your instructors and use the guidelines they give you.

Problems versus Needs

Problems are different from needs. A need is a requirement that an individual must have to maintain balance. For example: elimination is a need; constipation or diarrhea may be a problem.

Actual versus Potential

Patients can have actual or potential problems. Actual problems are those the patient is experiencing at the present time. Potential problems are those that may occur because of the nature of the patient's actual health problems. They are suspected and written in order to gather more data or to prevent occurrence. What happens to one patient may not necessarily happen to another.

Potential problem statements include the potential problem and the risk factors. They do not have signs or symptoms.

Collaborative Problems

When patients are ill or receiving treatment, complications can occur. The nurse must know when they are most likely to occur and prevent them if possible, or assess the patient to identify them early enough to intervene to decrease the patient problems. When complications arise, they generally require both medical and nursing intervention and are therefore called collaborative problems. For example: potential complication: hemorrhage.

Nursing Diagnosis versus Medical Diagnosis

Nursing diagnosis is different from medical diagnosis. Remember that the nursing diagnosis must be derived from nursing assessment and must require interventions in the domain of nursing. A nurse may be able to prescribe treatment for limited ROM, constipation, or a lack of knowledge, but cannot prescribe for emphysema, diabetes, or anemia. Those diagnoses require medical intervention for control.

Planning

Information obtained by assessment is useful only if it is used. An organized, written nursing care plan is a means of making a patient's care individualized and patient-centered. The plan must be written, so that it can be communicated to other health care team members, to provide continuity and individuality. It should be simple to understand and easy to read.

Ranking

Physiologic problems generally take priority over other types of problems, especially in the critically ill patient. Once the physical condition has been stabilized, then the nurse can think about emotional or learning needs.

If a patient has a problem meeting needs for oxygen, fluids, food, elimination, and rest, the needs should be ranked in that order, oxygen being the first priority and rest the fifth. Safety needs, if they exist, would be sixth; emotional needs follow.

Occasionally, a patient comes into the emergency room needing oxygen but experiencing such a high level of anxiety that the nurse can't put the oxygen equipment in place. In this case, dealing with the anxiety would take highest priority in order to get oxygen to the patient.

Maslow provides a guideline for planning, but in any situation other factors may alter the plan and have to be accounted for. If you need to rearrange priorities and they are inconsistent with Maslow's guidelines, you should be able to explain the rationale for your decision.

If your instructors give you other guidelines for establishing priorities of care, discuss how to use those guidelines. Compare them with the guidelines given here and understand how they are similar and different.

Goals

Outcome criteria and goals are the means by which the nurse can measure the quality, quantity, and suitability of the nursing care given.

It is first necessary to establish objective criteria. To do this, decide what needs to be measured. Use the manifestations and symptoms in the nursing diagnosis to write the desired criteria. Example:

Nursing Diagnosis	Goal	Outcome Criteria
impaired gas exchange related to pneumonia manifested by decreased breath sounds and chest x-ray, respiratory rate 20, frequent productive cough		Lung sounds clear, chest x-ray clear, respiratory rate 14, decreased coughing

Also, state the *degree* of observable change and a *time period* to observe. In the example above, quality is indicated but not quantity or frequency. We could say that the criteria would be met in 2 days. Some goals can be met in a *short* period of time, while other goals may require a *longer* time for achievement. It is important to set realistic goals for patients.

Nursing Diagnosis	**Expected Outcomes (Goals)**	**Nursing Interventions**
Alteration in nutrition: more than body requirements related to lack of information re calorie requirements and foods low in calories	Able to plan 1200-cal diet for 3 da. Eats only foods allowed on diet Loses 2 lb/wk til desired wt of 150 lb is achieved	Review 1200-cal diet 12/6 Assess recall of foods allowed and foods to be avoided 12/7 Wt every T & F Assist with menu selection × 3 da. 12/7–9
Altered comfort: chest pain related to lack of oxygen to heart muscle manifested by pt. statements, use of pain med. q4h, P 100, R 20	Pt. states no pain or states relief with pain med. P 72, R 16	Decrease O_2 need of heart Give Rx when pain occurs

Interventions

Before care is given, nursing interventions need to be selected to prevent, alter, or remove patient problems. They may include observing or collecting additional data (further assessment), nursing activities to provide assistance, regulating the environment or preventing injury, carrying out the medical therapies prescribed, and health teaching or education.

Nursing interventions should be chosen for the individual patient. There are many ways of providing comfort. Choose those that will work with this patient.

Interventions should be specific, telling what, when, and how. If you want to increase fluid intake, indicate kinds of fluids (it may be important for the fluid content to be protein as opposed to coffee), amount to be increased (total for one patient may be 1500 ml/day and for another 3000 ml/day), and when offered (could be increased with between-meal drinks at 10, 2, and hs if patient drinks freely, or if unable to tolerate much at a time, may need to be increased in lesser amounts every 2 hours).

To increase your learning and understanding of nursing intervention, include in your nursing care plan a *statement of rationale for your actions.* A rationale is the scientific reasons or the principles upon which you base your action. It is a broad, widely accepted physiologic or psychologic concept or principle that explains why a particular intervention is suitable for your patient. It may also explain what has gone wrong in illness.

Implementation

Implementation is the *activation* of the written nursing care plan. It includes written documentation of the effectiveness of the interventions. It includes further assessment, nursing activities, teaching, and carrying out prescribed medical orders. The nurse is responsible for the planning, communication, and coordination of care, but may delegate actual care to others. This is the only step of the nursing process that can be delegated to others.

Independent nursing actions include management of patient care by assessing and identifying patient problems and planning for their elimination, supervision, and teaching of others who participate in patient care, the performance of nursing procedures, observation of signs and symptoms and the response to therapy, and accurate recording, reporting, and evaluation.

Dependent nursing actions involve carrying out the doctor's orders regarding treatments and medications.

Documentation is also part of implementation. Every doctor's order must be documented as having been carried out. All assessments and responses to therapies, whether favorable or unfavorable, must be recorded. Remember—if you didn't document it, you didn't do it.

Evaluation

Using your outcome criteria, observe behavioral responses of the patient and record in the care plan and the nurse's notes. These observations might include the patient's verbal or nonverbal actions and the presence or absence of clinical symptoms. The actual outcomes of patient care are compared with the desired outcome.

If the care plan worked, the interventions may be continued. If the care was ineffective, then the plan needs to be revised. You may need to choose alternative interventions, collect and analyze more data, or establish a new nursing diagnosis.

Ask your instructor to share with you a sample of how your nursing care plan for Volume II should look. Be sure you understand how to formulate a nursing diagnosis, goals, outcome criteria, interventions, and rationale statements. Refer to the Data Base Form (DBF) and Nursing Care Plan (NCP) that follow.

DATA BASE FORM (DBF)

1. Physical Description:
2. Social Data: Initials:
   Sex:
   Marital Status:
   Age:
   Religion:
   Education:
   Occupation:
3. Physiological Data: Diagnosis: Hospital Day ______
   Surgery: Days Post-op ______
   Other Hospitalizations, Operations:
   Physical Examination and Medical History Highlights:
   Baseline Vital Signs: Ht.: Wt.:
4. Environment (Home Situation): Family Members:
   Living Accommodations:
5. Average Day (Lifestyle): Hygiene:
   Rest/Sleep:
   Meals/Diet:
   Activity:
   Elimination:
6. Chief Complaint or Concern of Patient (in patient's words):
7. Mental/Emotional Status:
8. Current Medical Orders: Expected Outcome:

9. Current Lab Exams and Results:

Nursing Care Plan (NCP)					
Nursing Diagnosis	Rank	Goal/Outcome Criterias	Nursing Interventions	Rationale for Intervention	Evaluation

Why Should I Study?

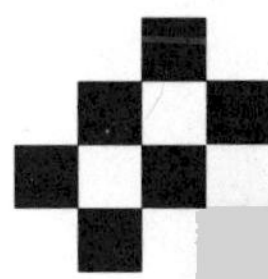

Level Six

Level Six includes one LEG in each component of care: **A. Crisis, B. Regulatory,** and **C. Body Systems.** Information included at this Level will give you some background materials for the rest of this Volume and help you utilize the theory and skills learned in Volume I as you focus on specific health problems of patients.

You will find that patients' physical and emotional problems can be studied in all settings: general medical-surgical, pediatric, psychiatric units, outpatient departments, and physicians' offices.

In your clinical experiences, you will want to perfect and improve the basic skills you learned in Volume I (for example, giving medications to a group of patients instead of one patient), improve your ability to work with patients, and increase your manual dexterity, in addition to learning new theory and skills in this Volume. To help you do this, in each Level we have identified general clinical performance expectations for you.

To meet the **Clinical Performance Expectations** at the end of Level Six, you should be able to:

1. Use time with patients for learning more about health problems.
2. Show increased skills in organizing and giving nursing care.
3. Make a written plan for your learning experiences for the day.
4. List your plan of actions, either in writing or verbally, for your instructor to check before you begin a new procedure.
5. Identify and report verbal and nonverbal communication problems of patient and family.
6. Use basic verbal and nonverbal communication skills to identify and reduce anxiety in your patient, your patient's family, and yourself.
7. Make nursing assessments that can be used as a guide for planning nursing care.
8. Identify and rank nursing diagnoses using basic needs.
9. State or write nursing interventions to be used for each nursing diagnosis.
10. Provide care based on nursing diagnoses.
11. Evaluate nursing care according to expected outcomes (goals).
12. Teach patients about self-care and preventive measures according to a teaching plan.

The clinical experiences described with each group of Objectives are not meant to limit your practice but to offer you new areas for learning. Be sure that you are building and working toward giving more complete care to patients. At the end of this Level, reread the 12 expectations above and evaluate your progress.

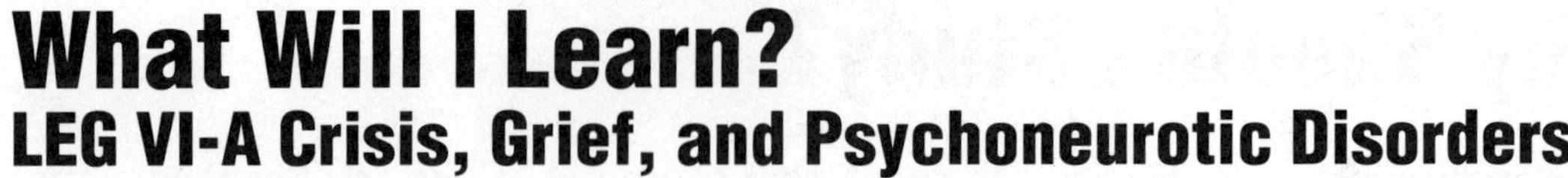

What Will I Learn?
LEG VI-A Crisis, Grief, and Psychoneurotic Disorders

Since the beginning of your nursing program, you have spent a great deal of time, effort, and possibly frustration while learning and beginning to perfect your communication skills. You have learned some basic knowledge about how personality develops and how the mind protects itself from painful experiences through the use of defense mechanisms. In this LEG you will begin your study of crisis intervention and grief reactions that include depression.

A **crisis** is considered to be occurring when a person's customary methods of problem solving do not work. The person becomes upset and loses mental and emotional equilibrium. The person searches for new methods of solving the problem and may adapt by finding a solution. A state of equilibrium then develops that may be better or worse than the one the person experienced before the crisis event occurred. Experiencing a crisis is not necessarily unhealthy. Each crisis event can be a maturing experience since it stimulates a person to learn new and better coping behaviors. When a crisis is unresolved, the person relives the event with each succeeding life crisis; this pattern continues until that person can be helped to develop successful coping behaviors for dealing with such events.

You might be the key person who can help a family member to assist the patient in developing problem-solving skills. Or you might recognize the patient's need for a professional therapist and be able to communicate your assessment so that help can be obtained during those critical times. No longer do we close our eyes to a patient's problems and say "Oh, it will go away with time. He'll get over it," or "She'll be O.K."

In addition, you will look at what happens when a person is unable to successfully adapt to stress or crisis by using normal conscious and unconscious coping and defense mechanisms. How do the growth and development of the child and environmental stressors and influences help determine the mental wellness or illness of a person?

When a patient is dying, your own coping behaviors will be stressed. You will learn how to recognize your own feelings so that you will be able to help a person who is dying. Then, you will prepare the body after death.

For review of earlier related information, see:

LEG I-B	Listening to and Observing Communication
	Beginning a Nurse-Patient Relationship
LEG II-C	Ways to Encourage Patient Decision Making
LEG III-A	Planning, Giving, and Reporting Total Patient Care
LEG III-C	Anxiety and Defense Mechanisms
LEG IV-A	Therapeutic Communication Skills
LEG V-B	Helping a Patient Clarify and Solve a Problem
	Communication Methods When Patient Has Speech or Hearing Problem
LEG V-C	Communicating with a Blind Person

What's Ahead in Later LEGs

You will be expected to apply your knowledge of crisis theory when caring for patients in the following LEGs:

LEG VII-A	Surgery
LEG VIII-A	Labor and Delivery
LEG VIII-C	Emotional Needs before a Colostomy

LEG IX-A Patients with Mental Illnesses (Psychoses) and Other Emotional Problems

You can see that this LEG is another step in your learning how to aid patients with their emotional levels of wellness. Take good notes because you will be referring to LEG VI-A frequently.

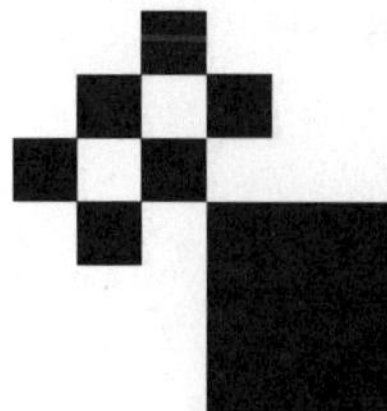

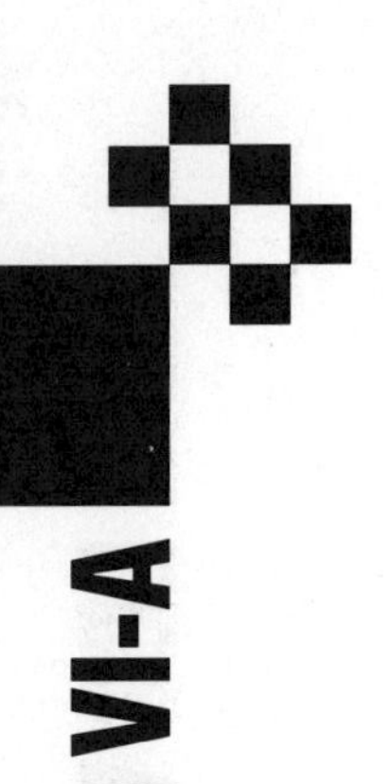

■ Overview of Learning Experiences in LEG VI-A

Objectives	Campus Lab/ Self-Practice	Group Discussions/Lectures	Clinical Lab Focuses
Therapeutic Relationship and Psychosocial Assessment			
1. Therapeutic relationship **2.** Psychosocial assessment		**B1.** Therapeutic skills necessary for making a psychosocial assessment	**B2.** Psychosocial assessment Observe self-help groups Observe interviews for psychosocial status Evaluate relationship
Crisis Intervention			
3,4. Crisis events and nursing interventions **5.** Healthy response to crisis **6.** Using nursing process in crisis intervention		**B7.** Nursing process and crisis intervention	**B2.** Care for patients at risk for crisis Record conversations and feelings Observe in crisis clinic
Assisting the Patient in Coping with Grief and Death; Providing Postmortem Care			
7. Normal grieving process **8.** Helping people express grief **9.** Helping adapt to loss **10.** Coping with a fatal illness **11.** Caring for a dying patient **12.** Postmortem care	**B1.** Care of body after death	**A6.** Hospice care (guest speaker) **B3.** Nursing process and loss **B5.** Care of the dying patient	**B6.** Care for patient with terminal illness; write a nursing care plan and a process recording Talk with nurses about caring for dying patients Attend a nursing conference on planning care Find out about postmortem procedures Visit morgue

Overview of Learning Experiences in LEG VI-A (cont.)

Objectives	Campus Lab/ Self-Practice	Group Discussions/Lectures	Clinical Lab Focuses
Depression			
13. Differences between grief and depression **14,17.** Behaviors in depression **15.** Nursing interventions for depressed patients **16.** Therapeutic communication with depressed patients **18.** Antidepressant drugs		**B1.** Nursing process in depression	**B2.** Talk with and care for depressed patients Observe medications and complete drug cards Identify your strengths and weaknesses in helping patients
Disturbed Coping Patterns: Anxiety and Psychophysiologic Disorders			
19, 20. Neurotic disorders **21.** Nursing interventions for patients with neurotic disorders **22.** Psychophysiologic disorders **23.** Antianxiety agents (minor tranquilizers)		**B3.** Anxiety disorders and nursing process	**B4.** Look for patients taking medications listed in Objective 23 Practice describing patient behavior

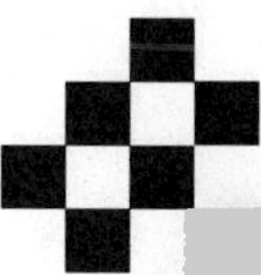

New Terms

It's your responsibility to know the meaning of these terms.

agoraphobia
alienation
amnesia
antidepressant
anxiolytic
apathy
autopsy
bereavement
body image
compulsion
crisis
depersonalize
depression
dissociative
endogenous
equilibrium
exogenous
factitious
fugue
grief
hospice
hypochondriasis
hysterectomy
malingering
neurosis
obsession
phobia
postmortem
premortem
psychiatry
psychoanalysis
psychology
psychophysiologic
resolution
restitution
self-concept
self-esteem
somatoform
sex role identity

Abbreviations

MAO
PTSD
SAD

Therapeutic Relationship and Psychosocial Assessment

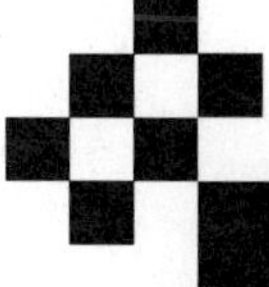

LEG VI-A

Objectives

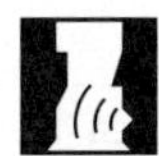

1. Describe what is meant by having a therapeutic relationship.

2. State the rationale for making a psychosocial assessment. *

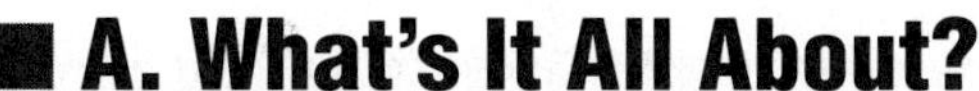

A. What's It All About?

1. Think about the number of patients you have talked with during the past few weeks. How many times did you use your therapeutic communication skills? It's hard to get in the habit of focusing most of your attention on the patient's needs when your own needs are causing you such anxiety. But you should have developed some self-confidence by now and be able to perform many of your nursing skills more routinely and efficiently. If you can, you are ready to take the next step toward helping patients with emotional problems. These problems will often accompany a physical disorder and can be found on any medical, surgical, obstetrics, or pediatrics unit. In this LEG you will learn to assess for emotional problems and see the resultant changes in behavior. So don't delay any longer in perfecting your communication skills.

2. Read in psychiatric nursing and communication textbooks about *therapeutic relationships psychosocial assessment*, *self-concept*, *role function*, and *interdependence.*

3. Write the answers to these questions.

(a) Briefly describe what is meant by a therapeutic nurse-patient relationship. List the essential ingredients and skills.

(b) List your personal strengths and weaknesses in developing nurse-patient relationships. Refer to the example below.

Strengths	*Weaknesses*
Am very aware of nonverbal communication between myself and the patient	Am ill at ease when talking with children

*Note: The ladder symbol means the objective may be omitted or reworded for VN/PN students.

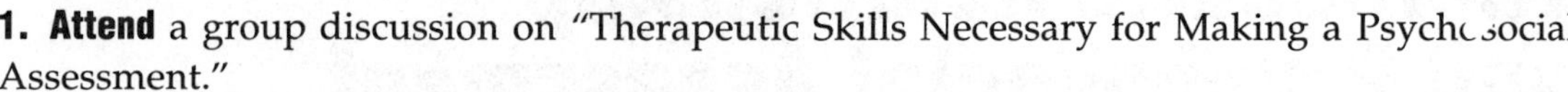

■ B. Putting It into Action!

1. Attend a group discussion on "Therapeutic Skills Necessary for Making a Psychosocial Assessment."

■ What factors or influences in the hospital make it difficult to make an accurate psychosocial assessment? List at least six reasons for making such an assessment.

■ What information should be obtained from a psychosocial assessment and why? Which categories on the data base form would give you this information? How is it listed in your agency's nursing history forms or admission forms?

■ Discuss your feelings regarding the importance of religious beliefs in a person's life. Why is it important to be aware of a patient's beliefs? What do you do if you disagree with them?

■ Role play giving a response to the following patient statements:

"Do you believe in God?"

"God is punishing me."

"Would you say a prayer for me?"

■ Discuss self-concept. Review how an individual develops a concept of self. Development begins in early infancy and is continuously revised as one grows and develops and has life experiences.

List some events that can affect an individual's self-concept. Place them in one of the following categories:

altered appearance

altered function

altered control

How can the nurse help patients recognize and adapt to threats to their self-concept?

■ Discuss the need for including significant others in case planning. How do people meet their social needs? Can we be totally independent of others?

Would it be important to find out about a patient's educational background, culture, feelings about work, and significant other people in the patient's life? Why? Could you find out about the amount of stress a person has recently experienced? How? What is the difference between defense mechanisms and coping strategies?

■ Practice interviewing each other in order to assess psychosocial needs, paying special attention to how you word your questions and how you respond to the answers. If you have a video recorder, record yourselves before class and then help each other review your tapes and suggest improvements. How are the following skills helpful in making the assessment?

active listening

accurate observations

empathetic responses

showing respect

being genuine and warm

■ Does the therapeutic relationship encourage or discourage patients from making decisions regarding their own health care? Explain how. How does this affect the traditional caregiver role of the nurse? Discuss specific examples of conflict between the caregiver and therapeutic nursing roles. How can these conflicts be resolved?

■ Review the "ANA Standards of Psychiatric and Mental Health Nursing Practice" found in psychiatric nursing textbooks. How do these standards guide the professional nurse's actions? Which standards are being met when you use therapeutic intervention and make a psychosocial assessment?

2. **Plan for** a clinical experience.

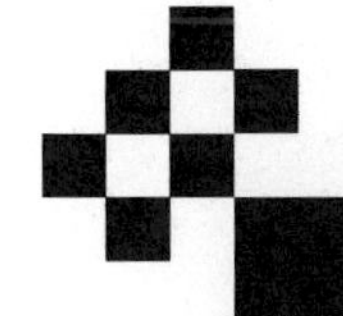

▲ Complete a psychosocial assessment on a patient. Use sections from the data base form or a form provided by your clinical agency or instructor. Analyze this assessment along with the physical assessment and complete a nursing care plan using the nursing process.

▲ Evaluate your relationship with your patient. Identify the helping skills you were able to use. Which decisions did the patient make? Which did you make? Were any made jointly (shared) by the patient and you? Share a list of these decisions in post-conference. What is the value of recognizing who is making the decisions?

▲ Observe nurses and other health care professionals interviewing patients to determine their psychosocial status.

▲ Observe some self-help groups. Find out what has been important to people as they attempt to adapt to demanding events in their lives.

Crisis Intervention

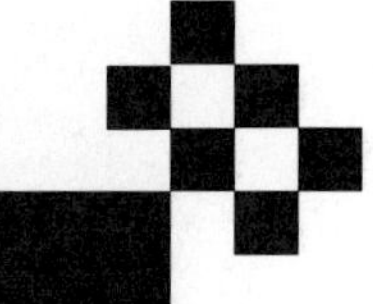

LEG VI-A

O b j e c t i v e s

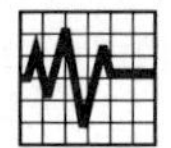

3. Given a list of events, select those that could result in crisis situations. Identify if they are situational or maturational, and state your rationale.

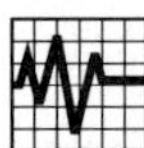 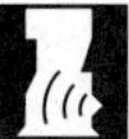

4. Given a list of statements, select the ones that best describe why a person requires therapeutic intervention in time of crisis.

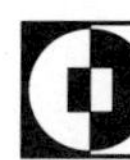  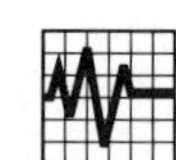 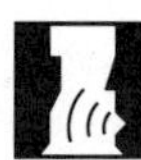

5. Given an example of a crisis event, describe healthy and unhealthy behavioral responses and the long-range consequences of each for the person or family experiencing the crisis.

 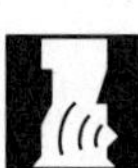 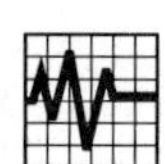 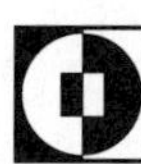 

6. Given an example of a patient anticipating or experiencing a crisis event, demonstrate using the nursing process to offer crisis intervention.

■ A. What's It All About?

1. Think about the stressors of everyday living that create tension. We have all developed methods of coping. Some of us yell or cry, some escape through sleep, and some jog. Now imagine yourself in your doctor's office for your yearly checkup. You learn you have a lump in your abdomen and further tests are needed and surgery may be necessary. Do you feel overwhelmed and speechless or do you feel angry and hostile? How well are you functioning at the moment, during the drive home, and later with your family? Are your usual methods of coping or adapting working? Do you feel in control? Do you need help from others close to you to manage even the simplest of decisions? In your imagination you have gone from experiencing a normal stressful doctor's exam to being in a *crisis* in which your normal state of health is in jeopardy. What losses or potential losses do you experience? These "crisis" Objectives will increase your understanding and teach you ways to help patients and yourself to manage crisis in healthy ways. Consequently these situations can become positive growth experiences.

2. Review:

LEG I-B Holistic Health Care and Stress

Listening to and Observing Communication

LEG II-B Fetal Development

LEG II-C Ways to Encourage Patient Decision Making

Growth and Development of the Infant

LEG III-A Growth and Development during Early Childhood

LEG III-B Middle Childhood

LEG III-C Adolescence

LEG IV-A Normal Growth and Development: Older Adult

Therapeutic Communication Skills

LEG IV-C Terminating Relationships

Caring for the Dying Patient

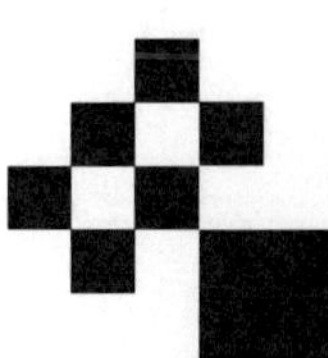

LEG VI-A

3. Read about *crisis intervention, grief, mourning, denial, change in body image, loss of body function* in medical-surgical, psychiatric, geriatrics, growth and development, and nurse-patient relationship references.

4. View audiovisuals and read articles and books from a list given you by your instructor.

5. Preview:

LEG IV-B Stress and Adaptation

LEG X-A Support for Patients with Fatal Illness and Their Families

LEG III-B Nursing Process with Terminally Ill Child and Family

6. Write your answers to the following study questions as you read, view tapes, and listen to information about crisis.

(a) Write statements that give you a clearer understanding of the meaning of the word *crisis*. Get at least one statement from each article you read. For example: "A period of disequilibrium results after coping has been ineffective," and "Coping mechanisms are used to solve problems, while defense mechanisms are attempts to avoid problems."

(b) List the phases or stages of a crisis event and describe the behaviors of people in each stage. Give examples of behavior at higher level and lower level functioning.

(c) Fill in examples of crisis. This will give you a sample list for Objective 3.

Situational Crisis Event

1. Loss of body part
2. Loss of body function
3. Premature delivery
4. Loss of home in fire
5. A past crisis of your own
6. A past crisis in your family
7. A crisis you have seen in the hospital
8. A crisis you can anticipate happening to a patient

(d) List potential developmental or maturational crises in the following age groups (review Erickson's eight stages of growth and development):

children

adolescents

young adults

middle adults

aged

LEG VI-A

(e) What is the "Life Change Scale?" If this tool is available at your school, answer these questions. How can it be used to decrease stress and possible crisis situations in our lives? Give an example.

(f) What stress is present in your life this week? When will this stress create a crisis situation and why? How do you react to stress during a crisis?

(g) Explain the time periods of a crisis.

(h) List some factors that make us prone to crisis. Select one patient who has the potential for developing a situational crisis event. List two actions you could take to help prepare to cope with the crisis.

How would you know if you had helped? Describe the behavior as if you were charting. Include a *subjective* observation such as what the patient might say and an *objective* observation that you might make while caring for the patient.

What might occur if the patient was not able to cope with the crisis event? How would you chart that behavior?

(i) How does crisis intervention for the elderly person differ from intervention for younger adults?

■ B. Putting It into Action!

1. Attend a group discussion on "Nursing Process and Crisis Intervention."

Nurses are exposed to contagious organisms and environmental hazards.

- Discuss events that can cause a crisis for the nurse. How likely are they to occur? How can the nurse cope? What changes can be made? Who can the nurse use for support?
- Describe a healthy problem-solving process that can be used by the nurse when dealing with a crisis.
- Describe assessment and nursing intervention in crisis.

  What is included in the assessment? What are the defining characteristics? What questions will you ask in interviewing the patient?

  List at least two goals.

  What could you teach this person?

  What is the focus of crisis therapy?
- In crisis, intensive interventions may be required. Your interventions depend on your skills as a nurse and a therapist. You may need to seek the assistance of someone in your community with specialized knowledge. Who is available?

■ Use the information above from your discussion to assess and intervene with the following patients.

Patricia has just lost her baby. She doesn't know if she is to blame. She is oblivious to her surroundings and stares out the window. She doesn't talk, can't eat, and refuses to get out of bed or groom herself.

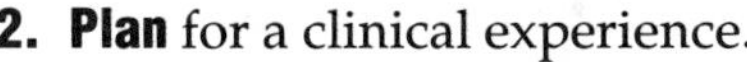

Felicia has come for help to the emergency department (ED). She is near panic, trembling, and talking rapidly. She has a hard time talking slowly enough for you to understand what she is saying. She is worried that she may have gone "too far" tonight. She went for a drive with her boyfriend and ended up parked and alone. It all started innocently, but she is now worried she may be pregnant. There is no way to reassure her that she is not. It is too soon. She is convinced that she is. She feels better after talking about how she let her father down. She thinks she can talk to her mother.

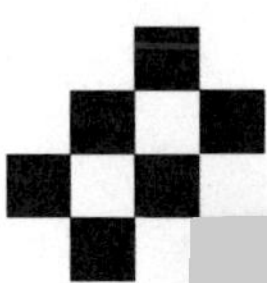

2. Plan for a clinical experience.

▲ Select patients that have experienced or are at risk for experiencing a crisis. While caring for them, determine their responses and apply the theory you have been practicing. Write a nursing care plan.

▲ Record your conversations and feelings immediately after leaving the patients' rooms. Share in postconference.

▲ Observe in a crisis clinic or listen to volunteers on a crisis hot line. Listen to their assessment of patients.

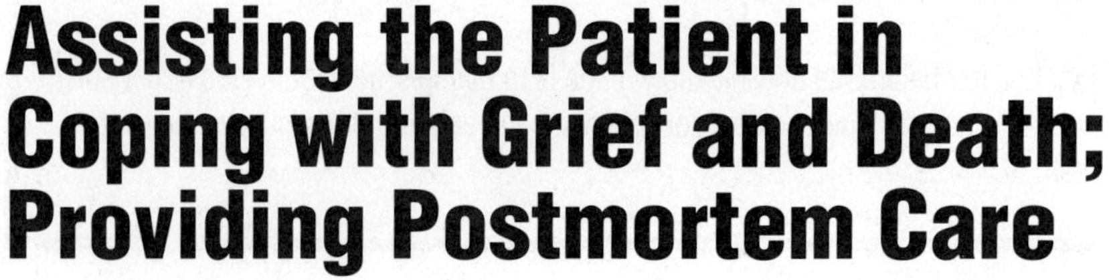

Assisting the Patient in Coping with Grief and Death; Providing Postmortem Care

Objectives

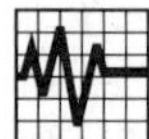

7. Given a list of behaviors, select those that could occur during a normal grieving process.

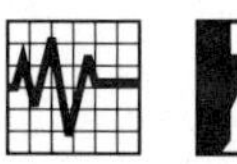

8. List three reasons nurses find it difficult to help people express grief.

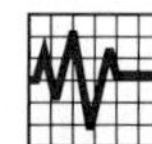 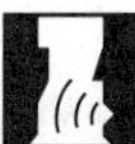

9. Given a list of statements, select the ones that could be used to help a patient begin adapting to a loss.

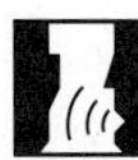 

10. Describe three coping behaviors that a nurse might recognize as adaptive responses to the diagnosis of a fatal illness; write a nursing intervention that would be appropriate and give your rationale.

11. Given a real or hypothetical patient who is dying, use the nursing process to help the patient emotionally and physically achieve a dignified death.

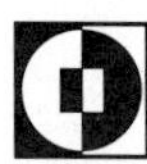

12. Describe the procedure followed in your hospital for the care of the body immediately after death: notification of family, nursing supervisor, and physician; and obtaining of permission for organ donation or autopsy.

Note: Objectives 11 and 12 were Extra Added Objectives in LEG IV-C.

■ A. What's It All About?

1. Think about what subjects you avoid in conversation. Do you ever discuss the death of members of your family or loved ones? Do you ever find out how a mother feels who has just delivered a dead fetus? How about the single mother who has given her baby up for adoption? The patient who asks, "Do I have cancer?" will resent being offered a statement of reassurance. It is easy to avoid these painful subjects and leave patients to find other sources of help.

Why are these subjects so painful to us? Are we threatened by the possibility of seeing ourselves in our patients' places? What causes us to be so uncomfortable with these subjects and to be so unhelpful to patients? There is no easy answer to these questions. But we can begin to find our own answers. We must first recognize these reactions in ourselves, then stop and look at our behavior, share it with other people who are looking for their own answers, and study what the experts in the fields of psychology and psychiatry have to offer us.

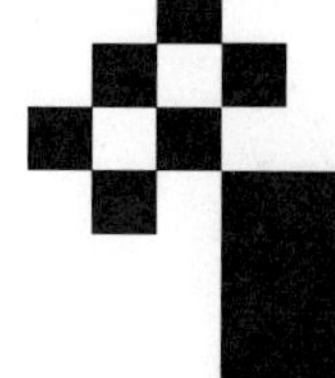

LEG VI-A

Think about your *true* feelings about the patient who is dying. Begin to do preparatory work toward the day that you will be caring for dying patients. Which of the following statements best describes your attitude?

_____ If I had a choice, I would not care for dying patients.

_____ I'm afraid I won't know what to say to a patient who is dying.

_____ I look forward to the opportunity to comfort a dying patient.

_____ I think children should freely discuss death from the age of 4 or 5 years and older.

_____ I think children should not be told about death until they are 8 or 9 years old.

2. Review LEG IV-C, Caring for the Dying Patient.

3. Read about *death, terminal illness, grief, mourning, change in body image, loss of body function, denial, hospice,* and *postmortem care* in medical-surgical, growth and development, nurse-patient relationship, and psychology references.

4. View audiovisuals and read articles and books from a list given you by your instructor or read from the following:

Grainger, R.D. "Successful Grieving." *AJN,* September 1990, p. 12

"Meeting the Challenge of a Dying Patient. An Interview with Joy Ufema." *Nursing91,* February, pp. 42–46.

5. Preview:

LEG X-A Care of Terminally Ill Patients

LEG XIII-B Care of Children with a Fatal Illness

Comments on Timetable for Grief

There are three plateaus in the timetable for grief. Many people who grieve for a loved one wonder why they haven't "recovered" from their grief after a few months and, in fact, often seem to feel worse as time passes. While the patient should know that there is no "normal" or "right" timetable for the grief process, an explanation of the phases and their potential duration can be very comforting and reassuring to grieving people and significant others in their lives.

First plateau: Numbness may last several weeks or months. An emotional distance is often kept from everyone, but much physical contact is needed. The person appears to function normally but it is usually mechanical.

Second plateau: Disorganization often occurs around 6 months after loss. The person may feel lonely, depressed, full of self-pity, and experience hallucinations. There is a need for intimacy, for a chance to express feelings, and to acknowledge the impact of the loss. There may be a need to discuss the details of the death.

Third plateau: Reorganization usually occurs between 7 and 9 months or even several years after the death. The person can talk about the loss without tears, can rejoin life and have a complete relationship with another person. There is occasional peacefulness.

LEG VI-A

6. Listen to a guest lecturer on "Hospice Care."

Come prepared with questions about the philosophy of care, the types of care and treatments used in the patient's home and hospice or hospital, the members of the hospice team, and how a hospice can be started or, if one is present, supported in your community.

■ B. Putting It into Action!

1. Practice in campus lab.

■ **Check out** materials on "Care of Body after Death." You will find the items used in your hospital and instructions for preparing the body for the mortuary. Read through the directions and become familiar with the tags, shroud, ties, and so on. Be aware of your feelings as you check out and examine the materials. How are you feeling now as you are reading this paragraph? We all view death differently and yet in many ways the same. It is frightening, puzzling, elusive, incomprehensible, and therefore easier to try to ignore and avoid than to think about. It will help you and your patients if you will take this opportunity to examine *some* of your feelings, at least the ones on the surface. You might want to use these materials in a small group and sit on the floor in a circle, hold the items jointly, and share your experiences with death. How does the body appear after death? After being prepared for burial? Why does the body look different once life has stopped than it did a few moments before when the heart was pumping and the alveoli were receiving and releasing air? What is death and when does it begin? What kind of religious or spiritual support can *any* nurse offer a patient?

■ Following this experience, record your thoughts in writing and share them with your instructor.

2. Apply the Facts about Grief to the patient situations that follow them. Write the number(s) of the statement(s) that explain or describe each of the patients' behavior. You will use this exercise in the group discussion in B.5.

Facts about Grief

1. The normal healing process of grieving cannot be accelerated.

2. The healing process can be interfered with.

3. Grieving takes certain predictable steps.

4. Familiarity with cultural patterns is necessary in evaluating the grief response.

5. A child has less capability for resolving a loss than does an adult.

6. Any impending loss revives unfinished grief work from previous losses.

7. Preparation for a loss allows some of the grief work to go on before the loss occurs.

8. Grief is a response to loss.

9. Threats to self-image and life itself arouse anxiety, and, through defenses, the individual will strive to retain equilibrium, to maintain a consistent self-concept.

10. Anticipation of own death allows patient to progress through grief process and obtain peace of mind before dying.

1. A student had a date with a boy she had secretly admired for weeks. When the night of the date came, the boy didn't show up, nor did he call. The girl said she must have misunderstood him and that she had a headache, anyway, so it was a good thing he didn't come. Later, she was crying in her room and called her girl friend to tell her she'd been stood up and how awful she felt. The following Monday, she planned what she would say to the boy when she saw him at school.

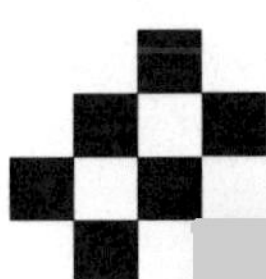

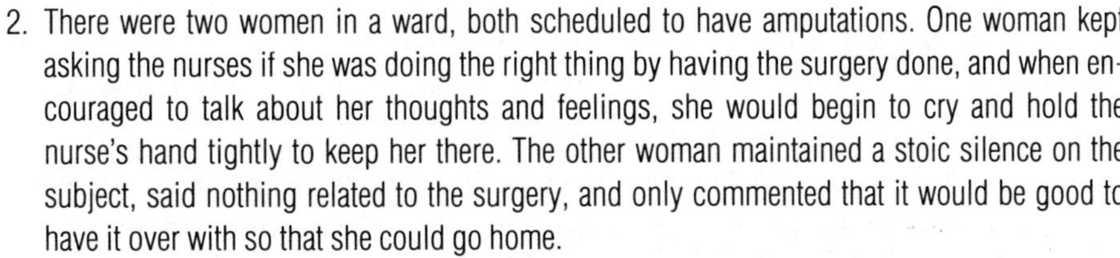

2. There were two women in a ward, both scheduled to have amputations. One woman kept asking the nurses if she was doing the right thing by having the surgery done, and when encouraged to talk about her thoughts and feelings, she would begin to cry and hold the nurse's hand tightly to keep her there. The other woman maintained a stoic silence on the subject, said nothing related to the surgery, and only commented that it would be good to have it over with so that she could go home.

After the surgery, the first woman was able to get out of bed on her second postoperative day and was able to obtain relief from her pain with medication. She continued to talk about the loss of her leg but now related it to using crutches. The second woman refused to be turned in bed and required pain medication more frequently than was ordered. She became delusional for a short period of time.

3. A middle-aged man suffered a heart attack and was confined to bed on absolute bed rest for a period of at least 1 week. He was allowed up for use of the commode once a day only. He refused to allow the nurses to wash him and said, "There is nothing wrong with me except for a little indigestion." One nurse was adamant in telling him that he had had a very severe heart injury, and unless he stayed in bed, he could die.

4. A third-grade class visited an animal reservation where a freak accident occurred. A lion dug a hole underneath his fence and pulled a little girl from their class into his cage where he mauled her severely. She was hospitalized. The next day in class no one mentioned the incident. The students did not ask about her, and the teacher had decided not to bring up the subject unless one of the students did. Many of the parents noticed an increase in bedtime problems, bad dreams, bed wetting, and fears.

3. Attend a group discussion on "Nursing Process and Loss."

Share your reactions to the films and personal experiences you have had with loss. Bring questions that have occurred to you on this subject during the past few days and learn what others think and feel.

- Review the grieving process, the behaviors seen in each phase, and the factors that influence loss. Discuss differences that occur during the life cycle.

  How can the nurse promote healthy grieving and assist the patient to work through the phases of normal grief and adapt to the loss?

- Discuss the following questions in relation to the patients described in B.2.

  Which of these methods of responding to a loss are considered healthy and which unhealthy? Why? What phases of grief are demonstrated? What loss is each person experiencing or anticipating? What would your nursing goals be for situations 2 and 3? Are these long- or short-term goals? What difficulties would you personally encounter in helping each patient? Why?

What exactly would you say to each patient in order to be helpful? Why do you think the nurse in situation 3 was so abrupt? List nursing interventions for each patient.

What will happen if a person cannot adapt to the loss? What are the symptoms of dysfunctional grieving?

■ Role play situations 2 and 3 after you have identified your nursing interventions. Don't expect to be perfect or know exactly what to say. Try some conversation and see how it sounds. Let group members make suggestions and try it again.

Role play situation 2 preoperatively as well as postoperatively. What feelings are you aware of as you role play each situation? Are some changes in body image easier to discuss than others? Why?

If the teacher in the class in situation 4 were your friend, what would you suggest the teacher say to the students? Why was there no mention of the incident? What helpful actions could the parents take?

■ How would you know if your crisis intervention had been helpful in situations 2 and 3? What criteria can be used to evaluate?

■ Is crisis intervention intended to be short- or long-term? Why?

4. Videotape, with another student, a nurse-patient conversation for one of the following situations:

Preparing a 55-year-old patient for surgery for removal of the prostate gland.

Helping a newly delivered mother with her disappointment at having her third boy when she was "so looking forward to a girl."

Caring for a 37-year-old man with a diagnosis of advanced cancer.

Critique the tape with your instructor.

5. Attend a group discussion on "Care of the Dying Patient."

■ Sign up to read at least one article on death. By signing up, you will have less chance of using the same article another student uses. If you select a book, it may be broken into chapters or sections. Take notes on your article for sharing with the group.

■ Discuss your feelings, attitudes, and experiences that have taught you about death. Use these questions to get you started if necessary.

How have your feelings changed with age? Compare your concern about and acceptance of death as a final stage of life in your teens, twenties, thirties, forties, fifties, and sixties. Do you imagine death seems as "real" when you are in your twenties as when you are in middle age?

Do you think children should be told if a grandparent is dying? Should they be allowed to visit dying people in the hospital? How would you answer the following questions:

"Is Grandpa going to die?" (a 5-year-old)

"If we put Teddy (the hamster) in the ground, how does he get to heaven?" (a 7-year-old)

"Do children die?" (a 6-year-old)

■ What will you say if a patient says, "I want to die"? What is your initial reaction or response? What need does this patient have at this time? What therapeutic communication skills could you best use at this time? How can you assess the patient's and family's needs for spiritual assistance? What goals might be set for therapeutic intervention? How can you use the nursing process to help a patient achieve a dignified death?

■ Contrast caring for a patient who has a written nursing care plan and one who has only a medical diagnosis, medical orders, and nurses' notes. Which one would receive the best care? Which patient would you prefer to care for, if you had a choice? Why?

■ What can you say and do for the family of a patient who is dying? What support do they need?

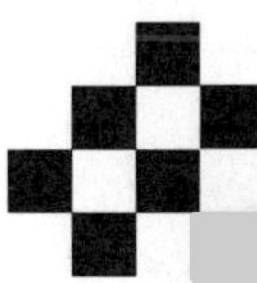

■ How might the following *views toward death* be shown in the behavior of the patient, family, and nurse? Which stage of the grief process does each illustrate?

an adventure, a welcomed new experience

a way of showing vengeance to others and forcing them to give attention

an enemy who is to be fought to the bitter end

a friend who brings release from pain

an escape from an unbearable situation to a new life

a punishment for one's sins and a way of atonement

a terrifying experience

LEG VI-A

You are caring for Ruth Jackson who is dying. Her eyes are closed and she appears to be in a stupor. She is somewhat dysponeic and is breathing through her mouth. Profuse perspiration is present over her entire body, and her feet and legs appear mottled.

■ List three nursing actions that you will take to meet this patient's needs and state your rationale.

How does a nurse or physician know that a patient is dying?

When does the reflex of swallowing cease?

How can thirst be decreased when a patient can no longer swallow?

Why does a dying patient perspire profusely? What actions should the nurse take when this occurs? What accompanying body changes might be occurring? When is the sense of hearing lost? What is the "death rattle"?

Why do you flatten the bed, close the eyes, replace the dentures, and position the jaws after death? What other actions do you take to prepare the patient's body for viewing by the family after death and before preparing the body for the mortuary?

■ What behavior will you encourage in your nursing assistants when they are assisting you in preparing a body for the mortician? How will you feel and what will you say and do when you are preparing a body for the first time and your nursing assistant has obviously done it many times? What if the roles were reversed and it was the assistant's first time—what would you say and do then?

6. Plan for a clinical lab.

▲ Care for a patient with a terminal illness. Identify in writing the behavior that is being used by the patient, family, and yourself to cope with the prognosis. Write a process recording of an interaction with the patient or the family or both and a nursing care plan.

▲ Talk with nurses about their experiences with dying patients and death. Ask them what questions the patients and family ask and how they answer them, how they feel about caring for patients who are dying, and how their staff reacts both before and after death occurs. (This conversation might best be held in a relaxed, unscheduled atmosphere such as during a coffee break.)

▲ Attend or organize a nursing conference to set up or update a nursing care plan for a patient with a terminal illness. Identify the problems that are present for both the patient and the staff and make decisions on ways to solve them. Encourage group participation in order to improve the follow-through on the plan when it has been put into action.

▲ Find out what the procedure is in your hospital for care of the body after death, what forms need filling out, who calls the family if they are not in attendance and what is said over the phone, who notifies the physician, who obtains the autopsy permission and what is said, who needs to be notified in the nursing office, and so on.

▲ Visit the morgue in your hospital and look at a body prepared for the mortician. Where are the items (valuables, dentures, and so on) kept that are to appear on the body when it is prepared for viewing?

Depression

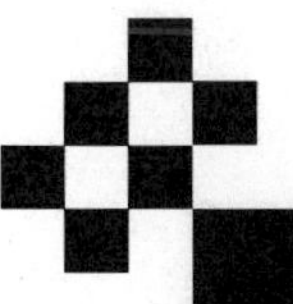

Objectives

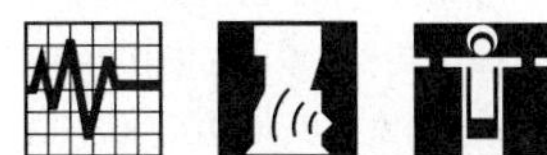

13. Differentiate between the cause and duration of grief and of depression.

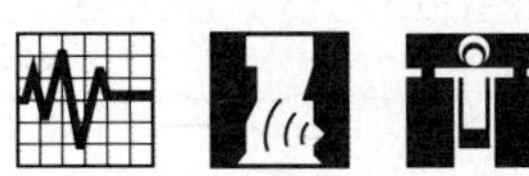

14. Given a list of behaviors, select those that could indicate a depression.

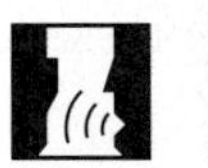

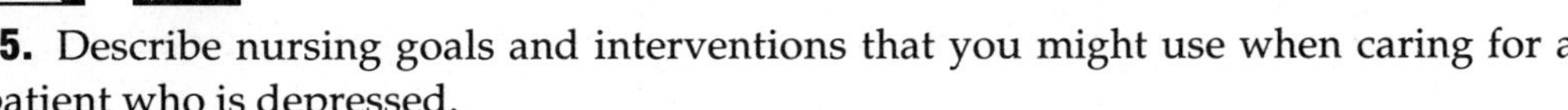

15. Describe nursing goals and interventions that you might use when caring for a patient who is depressed.

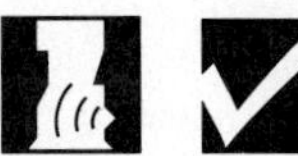

16. Given a list of statements, select those that would be helpful to the depressed patient.

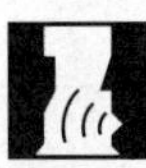 

17. Chart a description of typical behaviors of a depressed patient, including one subjective and one objective observation.

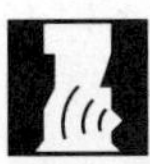 

18. Describe the action/use, side effects, and two nursing implications for the following groups of antidepressant drugs: MAO inhibitors and tricyclic compounds. (Complete drug cards on antidepressant drugs as directed by your instructor.)

■ A. What's It All About?

1. Think about the times when you feel "blue" or sad or the times when a friend says, "You seem down in the dumps today." What does that observation do for you? Do you feel relieved that someone cares enough to notice and ask? How do you feel if you then start to tell your friend how you feel and your friend interrupts with, "Yes, I know exactly how you feel. Just last week the same thing happened to me. Let me tell you about it." Do you now feel more alone and sadder than before, plus having the added burden of having to listen politely to your friend's problem?

LEG VI-A

Comments on Depression

It is hard to listen to someone tell you how bad he feels. But it is a skill that you must acquire in order to care for patients with emotional illnesses. And depression is a real illness! We're not talking about the blues that last only a day or two, but the deep-down, energy-draining bouts of gloom that drag on for several days to weeks and cripple the daily pattern of living (no energy to clean house or care for the children, unable to concentrate at work or school, unable to sleep at night). Probably each of us knows of someone who has had such a depression, whether or not it was recognized. The majority of these depressions result from a loss, from unresolved grief. And many result in suicide, divorce, or drug or alcohol addiction. Depressed people often go unnoticed or untreated until too late. Yet the symptoms of depression are unmistakable, and a helping relationship is crucial in treating it. Learn the symptoms and ways to help, then look around you.

2. View audiovisuals on loss, grief, depression. Write down your immediate impression and feelings while viewing and listening to the films.

3. Read about *depression, helplessness, hopelessness, suicide, grief, loss, antidepressants,* and *nurse-patient relationship* in psychiatric and pharmacology references.

4. List behaviors that might be seen in an assessment of a person who is depressed. Write some nursing diagnoses and develop a plan of care.

How is the care of the depressed patient different from that for an elated or overactive patient?

What precautions can you observe that might prevent a suicide? Why is prevention of suicide important?

5. Fill in this chart:

Antidepressant	Action/Use	Side Effects	When Action Begins	Nursing Implications
MAO inhibitor				
Tricyclic compounds				

■ B. Putting It into Action!

1. Attend a group discussion on "Nursing Process in Depression."

- Discuss the relationship between depression and each of the following factors:

  diet
  exercise
  age and stage of growth and development
  fatigue
  culture
  religious or spiritual beliefs
  physical environment
  previous education
  feeling of self-worth
  personal values and goals
  relationships with significant others

living environment: alone or with others

use of alcohol or drugs

employment or retirement

heredity

medical illness

chronic illness

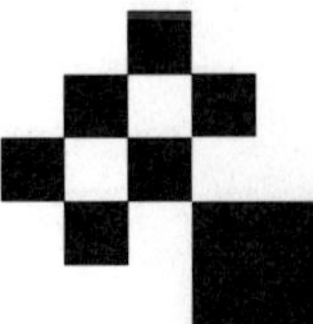

■ How would holistic health advocates treat a problem of depression?

■ There is a higher incidence of depression among women than among men. Why do you think this difference occurs? What sociocultural influences might predispose women to having less coping ability? What are women doing to change this situation?

■ How do you think a high unemployment rate affects the incidence of depression and psychophysiologic illness? Why?

■ What is the relationship between developmental or maturational crises and depression? Describe some personal examples of depressive reactions.

■ Break into groups of three to five students for 20 minutes. Create a short story or play to dramatize one of the people described below. Include at least three examples of symptoms you expect. Include physiologic, psychomotor, and psychologic differences of symptoms in each age group.

Depressed mother at home with two young children and a newborn

Woman grieving after a hysterectomy

Depressed grandfather in the hospital, a recent widower

Child 3 years old grieving loss of a pet

Depressed teenager, male or female, in school

8-year-old child grieving loss of grandmother

At the end of 20 minutes, take turns presenting your story or play to the total group. Discuss how the behaviors would make you feel if you were a family member. Would you react the same way as a nurse?

At the end of your presentation ask the group to list the symptoms of grief or depression that they recognized. Ask for a volunteer to write charting examples describing the behaviors. Decide whether each example is an objective or subjective observation.

Take turns making statements that demonstrate how to apply the following interventions to any of the situations.

1. Help person express angry feelings through talking
2. Improve persons' feeling of self-worth by recognizing own strengths
3. Help the person recognize the event that caused the feelings
4. Encourage a moderate level of activity even though it seems meaningless
5. Accept the patient's feelings as being real and attempt to understand his point of view.
6. Confirm that patient swallows medications
7. Identify suicide potential

Add additional nursing goals you can anticipate from the symptoms presented.

2. Plan for a clinical experience.

- ▲ Talk with and care for depressed patients on a medical-surgical or psychiatric unit. Record your conversation with them, including your feelings. Write down their symptoms of depression.
- ▲ Observe the medications they are receiving. Learn about them. Can you detect any side effects? Complete drug cards.
- ▲ Identify and list your strengths and weaknesses in helping your patient. Date this evaluation and insert it into your LEGs binder so you can compare it with your self-evaluation at the end of Volume II to see if you have strengthened some of your "weaknesses."

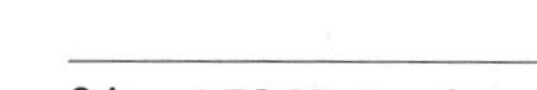

Disturbed Coping Patterns: Anxiety and Psychophysiologic Disorders

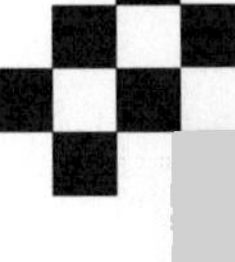

LEG VI-A

Objectives

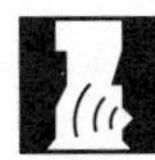

19. Given a list of statements, select those that are true about neurotic disorders.

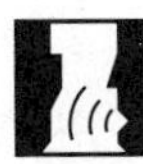

20. Describe the behaviors exhibited by people with a diagnosis of anxiety disorder, somatoform disorder, and dissociative disorder.

 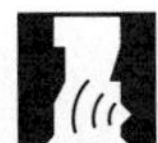

21. List nursing interventions for patients with anxiety, somatoform, and dissociative disorders.

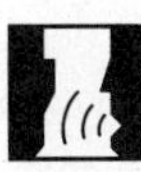

22. Given a list of statements, identify which are current definitions of the term psychophysiologic *disorders*.

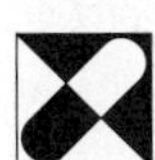

23. Describe the action/use, side effects, and nursing implications for antianxiety agents (minor tranquilizers). (Complete drug cards on minor tranquilizers as directed by your instructor.)

Note: Major tranquilizers will be studied in LEG IX-A.

A. What's It All About?

1. Think about how you cope with everyday problems. In Volume I you learned about healthy ways of coping with anxiety and stress. Did you learn something about your own patterns of behavior? Did you find out that you liked some of them more than others and, in fact, that some of your ways of coping were downright awful? We are all on a continuum of growth and are maturing and learning better ways of dealing with conflict as we age. With these Objectives you will learn about *disturbed ways of coping* with anxiety that do not bring satisfaction, but, instead, bring increased pain and distress. You will be introduced to the concept of mental illness as a behavioral pattern that causes distress and disability. For many years theorists distinguished between neuroses as minor illness and psychoses as major ones. The newer classifications no longer make that distinction. The newer Diagnostic and Statistical Manual III-Revised (DSM III-R) Classifications by the American Psychiatric Association (APA) use five categories to include all the disorders previously called neuroses.

2. Review:

LEG I-B Holistic Health Care and Stress

LEG III-C Anxiety and Defense Mechanisms

3. Read about *psychoneuroses, panic, disturbed coping pattern, psychophysiologic stress, anxiety, conflict, mental health, mental illness, reality therapy, behavioral therapy, ritualistic behavior, defense mechanisms, mental maturity, psychosomatic illness* in psychiatric, pediatrics, medical-surgical, geriatrics nursing and psychology references.

4. View audiovisuals and read articles and books from a list given you by your instructor or read from the following:

Paiva, Z. "Sundown Syndrome." *RN,* July 1990, pp. 46–51.
Strome, T., and T. Howell. "How Antipsychotics Affect the Elderly." *AJN,* May 1991, pp. 46–49.

5. Preview LEG IX-A Habitual, Inflexible Behaviors and Anxiety.

6. Review child growth and development, especially during the toddler and preschool years. Look for the emergence of defense mechanisms and how the child's level of anxiety and degree of parental influence affect the way the mechanisms are used to maintain control through later life.

Comments on Mental Illness

As you read about mental illness you will notice that earlier developmental experiences play a role and influence the mental health of the adult person. How easy it is to read and understand physical illness and describe the nursing care needed. If you compare several books, you may find that the trend in psychiatric nursing references is to group patients by the *behavior* they exhibit instead of by the names of specific diagnoses. For these reasons we caution you not to be discouraged as you read and fail to find ready answers to your questions or clear-cut definitions. This is part of the evolving body of knowledge about mental illness. The Objectives are intended to increase your awareness of illness that is widely seen both in and out of the hospital.

You will recognize many of the behaviors in yourself and might wonder if you are mentally ill. This is the beginning of your awareness of the continuum between mental health and illness. Why are you healthy when someone else with the same but more exaggerated behavior is ill?

What determines the degree of wellness? These are fascinating and at the same time threatening questions. It may be frightening to look (closely) at yourself. This is the time to use small group discussions and your instructor to help you understand yourself and others.

■ B. Putting It into Action!

1. Write the effects of anxiety that may occur to the body systems listed. The first listing is an example.

Body System	Immediate Effect of Anxiety	Chronic Effect of Anxiety
gastrointestinal	heartburn, cramps	peptic ulcer
musculoskeletal		
respiratory		
integumentary		

Write the answers to the following questions in preparation for your discussion.

(a) What is the difference between a functional illness and a psychophysiologic illness?

(b) In your own words, describe how anxiety causes disturbed coping behavior.

(c) Give six examples of emotional symptoms of excessive anxiety that can incapacitate a person. Next to each example try to write which defense mechanism is being used.

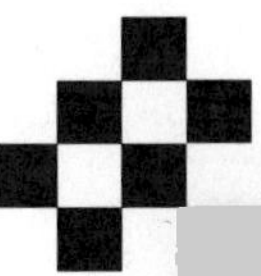

LEG VI-A

2. Write an example of a behavior and a nursing approach for each disorder below and bring to the group discussion.

Disorder	*Behavior*	*Nursing Approach*
Anxiety disorders		
Panic disorder		
with agoraphobia		
generalized anxiety disorder		
obsessive-compulsive disorder		
posttraumatic stress disorder (PTSD)		
Factitious disorders		
with physical symptoms		
with psychologic symptoms		
Somatoform disorders		
conversion disorder		
hypochondriasis		
Dissociative disorders		
multiple personality		
Sexual disorders		
paraphilias		

3. Attend a lecture or a group discussion to share your information on "Anxiety Disorders and Nursing Process."

■ Apply your information to the following patients. Which have symptoms of anxiety? How does each deal with anxiety?

Johnny, age 9, skips to school each day but is very careful to avoid stepping on a crack in the sidewalk. If he does, he repeats a poem.

Bill, age 25, is unable to get the job he wants because it would involve crossing a high bridge, and he is "deathly" afraid of heights.

Jean, age 45, is invited to attend a bridge club, but when the first day to meet comes around, she is incapacitated with a severe headache and is unable to attend.

LEG VI-A

> Jacob, age 75, a recent widower, is physically well, yet is not interested in doing anything but sitting at home. He talks about a variety of illnesses that he could be getting and has very little interest in food. He has stopped reading the newspaper and talking with his neighbors.

- How do defense mechanisms help a person handle anxiety?
- What is the difference between

  normal fear and a phobia?

  obsession and compulsion?

  factitious and somatoform?

- When does anxiety become a problem for patients?
- What guidelines should the nurse follow when planning nursing care for patients with ritualistic behavior or patients with physical symptoms that have no organic cause?
- Name some major anxiety disorders that affect the elderly.
- What is Sundown Syndrome?
- Complete a nursing care plan using the nursing process for a patient with a specific disorder from the list in B.2.
- What are the dangers of using minor tranquilizers over a long period of time? What alternatives are there to drug therapy?
- What are the adverse effects of antipsychotic drugs on the elderly patient?
- Discuss the case of the following patient. What would you expect the doctor to do when this problem is discovered? How can you help?

> Mercedes, age 69, has had musculoskeletal pain for some time. She constantly feels depressed and in pain. She is taking a narcotic analgesic, a NSAID, an antidepressant, an antianxiety agent, a sedative, and an antipsychotic.

4. Plan for a clinical experience.

▲ Look for patients taking medications listed in Objective 23. Visit and observe them. Study their charts for evidence of side effects. What precautions would you take when caring for these patients to prevent injury to them? What dietary restrictions would you recommend? Whose responsibility is it to teach them about their drugs?

▲ Practice describing the behavior of the patients you care for, using both objective and subjective assessments.

Have I Learned?

The following questions are for you to answer in order to find out if you have met the Objectives. All of the Objectives in LEG VI-A are covered in this series of questions. Pick a quiet time and answer them. Answers follow this selftest.

No space has been left for answering the questions related to the "doing" Objectives. Use a separate sheet of paper for your answers and then use the answers in clinical or campus lab for your own evaluation.

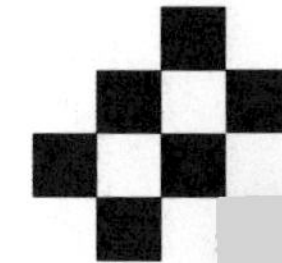
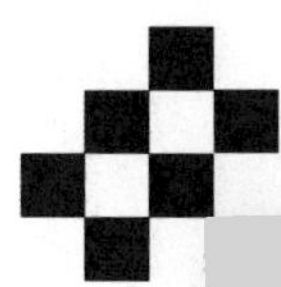

LEG VI-A

Objective **Question**

1 **1.** A student spent about 20 minutes with Mrs. Jensen giving her morning care. Which of the following descriptions would show that the student was attempting to have a therapeutic relationship with Mrs. Jensen?

(a) The student asked Mrs. Jensen how she slept, what she ate for breakfast, if she had any visitors, and if she had gotten out of bed the evening before.

(b) Mrs. Jensen told the student a joke and then they discussed the Phil Donahue show that was on the TV at the time. The subject was food and they shared some favorite recipes.

(c) Mrs. Jensen commented that she had had trouble sleeping last night. The student replied, "You feel tired this morning because you didn't sleep much." The patient then described her problem of insomnia at home, which had been especially pronounced since her husband had passed away. Using active listening skills and some probing, the student discovered that this was a source of great concern for the patient at home. Together they discussed conditions related to the problem.

(d) Mrs. Jensen was very irritable when the student came in to give her a bath. She complained of the "lousy" food, noise at night that kept her awake, and the length of time she had to wait for someone to answer her light. The student listened politely, explained that she should have asked for another sleeping pill before 3:00 A.M., and that the floor was temporarily short-staffed due to vacations.

2 **2.** When the nurse admitted a 72-year-old woman to the hospital for cataract surgery, a psychosocial assessment was done for which of the following reasons:

(a) To recognize the presence and effect of stress in the patient's present life.

(b) To identify significant others or a social network in the patient's life.

(c) To evaluate her mental status.

(d) To obtain a medical history.

(e) To recognize the patient's stage of maturity.

(f) To learn about religious, racial, cultural, and ethnic identification and beliefs.

3 **3.** From the following list of events, select those that could be crisis events and state why. State whether they are situational or maturational.

(a) marriage

(b) pregnancy

(c) children starting school

(d) children leaving home for college or to be married

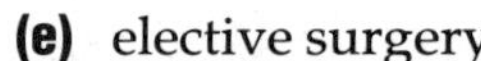

(e) elective surgery

(f) surgery that changes your body such as prostatectomy, hysterectomy, amputation, or radical mastectomy

(g) illness that changes your body image such as heart attack, stroke, arthritis, or any chronic disease

(h) admission to the hospital as a patient

(i) retirement

(j) terminal illness of yourself

(k) terminal illness of a loved one

(l) failing a test

(m) loss of a loved one by death

(n) loss of a job

4 **4.** Mr. Graves, age 76, had been living with his married daughter since his wife died 4 years ago. He was hospitalized because of a stroke last month and needs considerable assistance in his daily activities. The family decided to place him in a nursing home nearby where he could receive the care he needed and they could visit frequently. Which of the following statements best describe *why* Mr. Graves and his family require crisis intervention at this time.

(a) The incidence of later mental disorders may be reduced by providing therapeutic intervention to people while they are in crisis.

(b) The adjustment process cannot be completed satisfactorily without outside help.

(c) The person undergoing the crisis event needs to be allowed to express his feelings during each phase of the process.

(d) The person needs to be given outside interests until the crisis event has passed.

(e) This period presents an individual with an opportunity for personality growth but also with the danger of increased vulnerability to mental disorder.

5 **5.** Describe how Mr. Graves could respond to this crisis event in his life in (a) a healthy manner and then (b) in an unhealthy manner, and state the long-range consequences of each.

6 **6.** Mrs. Phillips had radical surgery for cancer of the right breast. After the surgery, she avoided looking at the dressing or wound during dressing changes. She never discussed her surgery with the nurses or appeared upset. She spent her days reading and watching TV.

(a) List at least three observations you would make of Mrs. Phillips that would be relevant for a crisis assessment.

(b) Describe at least three items of information you would need in order to begin a nursing care plan.

(c) Which of the following characteristics might be valid for Mrs. Phillips?

1. Failure to express sorrow at the loss of her breast and change in body image.

2. Inability to talk with new people about personal matters.

3. Loneliness for her family, friends, and familiar belongings.

4. Poor adjustment to the hospital routine.

(d) Which of the following nursing goals would be of prime importance for Mrs. Phillips?

1. To include the family in much of her care.

2. To increase her physical activity.

3. To help her become aware of her emotional needs.

4. To teach her self-care of her incision and dressing.

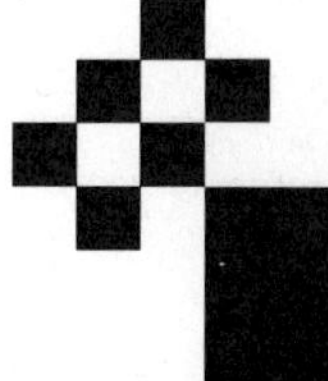

(e) List one or two other goals that would be appropriate at this time.

(f) Which of the following nursing interventions would be most helpful in implementing your goals?

1. Confronting her with the need to face her problem more directly in order to prevent future depression.

2. Saying, "It must be hard to realize that you've had surgery or that your breast has been removed."

3. Providing privacy.

4. Asking her if she has any questions about taking care of herself at home.

(g) List several other nursing interventions that would help you implement the goals.

(h) Which of the following criteria would be most important in evaluating your goal in question?

1. The patient's amount of daily physical activity.

2. The husband's interest in helping care for the patient after discharge.

3. The amount of crying observed.

4. The ability to express both positive and negative feelings about the surgery.

(i) List other criteria you could use for evaluating the patient's progress.

7 **7.** Which of the following behaviors can normally occur during grieving?

(a) crying

(b) indifference

(c) anger

(d) feelings of guilt

(e) joy

(f) wish to commit suicide

8 **8.** List three reasons nurses might find it difficult to help the following patient to express his feeling of grief over the loss of his leg: Mr. Stone, age 46, is a diabetic and developed gangrene in one of his toes several months ago. Now an infection has developed and amputation of the lower leg was advised in order to stop the process and promote healing. It is now 3 days after surgery, and Mr. Stone is asking for pain medication frequently before he is allowed to receive it, and very often he wets the bed because he cannot reach his urinal or spills it. The nursing staff has not talked with Mr. Stone about his feelings, about how he sees this amputation as changing his image of himself as a man, husband, and father.

9 **9.** Which of the following statements could a nurse make in order to help the patient, Mr. Stone (Question 8), begin to adjust to his loss?

(a) "Do you have hospitalization insurance, or will you have to pay the cost of this surgery, Mr. Stone?"

(b) "It must be hard to realize that this surgery, which removed your leg, has really happened to you."

(c) "Having this happen to you must make you want to strike out at the world."

(d) "I wonder if you feel bad inside and maybe even wish you had never consented to the operation."

(e) "You will probably feel better if you would start getting out of bed more often."

(f) "Tomorrow the physical therapist is going to measure you for crutches so you can start getting around again. Then you can start making plans to go home."

10 **10.** Describe three behaviors that show that a person is coping with a diagnosis of a fatal illness, a nursing intervention, and a rationale for the action.

11 **11.** Write a nursing care plan for a patient who is dying. Use the nursing process to help meet the patient's emotional and physical needs.

12 **12.** Imagine that you are the night nurse and one of your patients dies at 5 A.M. The death is expected by the physician and family. No family member is present. Describe the procedure that you will follow to accomplish each of the following:

Care of the body immediately after death

Notification of the family, the nursing supervisor, and the physician

Obtaining permission for organ donation

Obtaining permission for an autopsy

13 **13.** What are the differences in the cause and duration of grief and of depression?

14 **14.** Which of the following behaviors that describe patients could make you suspect that that person is depressed?

(a) Did not want to eat for several days.

(b) Skipped one meal.

(c) Had difficulty sleeping for two nights in a row.

(d) Complained of insomnia for the past 2 weeks.

(e) Sits in room and never talks unless spoken to directly.

(f) Greets each person who enters the room with a cheery hello but is found crying late at night by a nurse.

(g) Is depressing to be around, saying things are hopeless.

(h) Won't even make his own bed; says he's not up to it and can't do it right away.

(i) Takes a long time to answer any question.

(j) Takes no interest in fixing hair or putting on makeup.

(k) Complains and acts cranky. Used to be so nice.

15 **15.** You are having your clinical experience in a nursing home one week and see that your previous patient Mr. Graves (see Question 4) is a resident. The nurse tells you that he is not doing well. He is eating poorly, sleeps most of the day in his chair, and has numerous complaints about his bowels not moving. He refuses to bathe or dress himself without a great deal of assistance or to walk to the bathroom. He prefers to remain alone in his room. At night he urinates in his bed instead of putting on his call light. He cries when the night aide comes in to change him. The physician diagnoses his condition as a depressive disorder associated with his stroke.

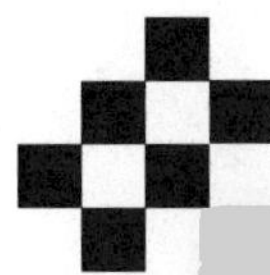

List at least three nursing goals and nursing interventions for depression that you would include in your care plan for Mr. Graves.

16 **16.** Which of the following statements would be helpful for a nurse to use with a patient in an acute depression?

(a) "You feel that there is nothing to look forward to, and you don't know how to change that feeling. Having to think about living without your wife is such a terrible thought, you can't even let yourself think about it."

(b) "Your dinner will be ready in a few minutes. It will be necessary for you to get out of bed and sit in the chair to eat. I know you don't want to get up, but I will help you."

(c) "It will do you good to get out of bed more. There is no reason for you to stay in your bed all day. The more you get up, the sooner you can go home."

(d) "You must feel very unhappy. You want someone here in the room with you, yet we never seem to find out what is really bothering you. Maybe you feel caught in a problem and don't know how to change it."

17 **17.** Write a charting example that describes the behavior of a person who is depressed. Include one subjective observation and one objective observation.

18 **18.** List the action/use, side effects, and the nursing implications for each of the following types of antidepressants.

Antidepressant	Action/Use	Side Effects	Nursing Implications
MAO inhibitors			
Tricyclic compounds			

19 **19.** Which of the following are true statements about neuroses?

(a) A neurosis involves complete disorganization of the personality.

(b) People with neuroses usually have insight.

(c) People with neuroses usually have hallucinations.

(d) People with neuroses use suppression and repression to deal with conflicts.

(e) Neurosis does not inhibit normal developmental and peer relationships.

(f) In neurosis there is no thought disorder.

20 **20.** Describe one behavior that would be seen on assessing a patient with each of the following diagnoses:

- **(a)** Anxiety disorder
- **(b)** Somatoform disorder
- **(c)** Dissociative disorder

21 **21.** List four nursing interventions you would take while caring for the following patient with an anxiety disorder.

> Mrs. Slaker, age 46, was admitted for diagnostic tests for complaints of chronic fatigue and backache. She was treated with bed rest and mild analgesics. When the tests revealed nothing physically wrong with her, she was discharged. Two months later she was readmitted with functional paralysis of her lower extremities. The tests again revealed no physical cause for the paralysis, and the diagnosis of conversion disorder (somatoform disorder) was made.

22 **22.** Select from the following descriptions the one that best explains the current medical opinion of the relationship between an organic disease and the psychologic status of a person.

- **(a)** Psychologic factors can cause physiologic changes in the body that are either temporary or permanent.
- **(b)** Psychologic factors can cause temporary physiologic changes in the body that are always reversible.
- **(c)** Psychologic factors can cause irreversible structural changes in the body.
- **(d)** There is no relationship between structural changes in the body and the psychologic status of a person.

23 **23.** Write nursing implications and two side effects of the minor tranquilizing agents.

■ Answers to Have I Learned?

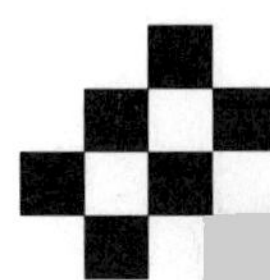

LEG VI-A

1. **(c)** The student focuses on the patient's story and encourages a better understanding of her problem by exploring it together, moving toward possible solutions. Decision making is centered on the patient.

2. All but **(d)** are correct. All this information is useful to the nurse when assisting a patient to identify threats to coping and adaptation.

3. All of these could be correct. Crises vary in severity. A crisis occurs when a person is unable to deal effectively with an emerging problem. The familiar problem-solving mechanisms do not work, and the usual patterns of life are affected.

(e), **(f)**, **(g)**, **(h)**, **(j)**, **(k)**, **(l)**, **(m)**, **(n)** are situational.
(a), **(b)**, **(c)**, **(d)**, **(i)** are maturational.

4. **(a)** and **(e)** are best, **(c)** is correct but does not answer the question why. **(b)** and **(d)** are incorrect statements.

5. **(a)** A healthy response to the events occurring might be to talk about the decision not being "definite" or about staying in the nursing home only "a short time." He may become uncooperative, dependent, angry toward his daughter or the staff. This reaction will be followed by expressing wishes that he will like the home, how he will miss the staff, making plans for belongings. The long-range consequence is one of acceptance and normal mental health.

(b) An unhealthy response might show immediate approval of the idea and eagerness to tell everybody about what a fine home it is at the same time that he avoids talking about his true feelings, or he might become quite passive about the whole idea and avoid talking about the subject at all. If the staff allows this silence to continue without an attempt to help the patient resolve his feelings, he will probably suffer an acute depression when moved to the nursing home.

6. **(a)** *Objective observations:*

1. Not looking at her incision.
2. Not talking about her surgery.
3. Not expressing any feelings of sadness or loss.
4. Not weeping.

(b) You would need information about:

1. Previous crises she has experienced, how she coped, and what happened.
2. The available support persons in her life.
3. Her understanding and feeling about her current situation and how she will deal with it.
4. Her current ability to complete the activities of daily living.

(c) **1.** Avoidance of looking at the surgery and talking about the subject makes one think this patient is in a period of disequilibrium which is characterized by discomfort, anxiety, or depression.

(d) **3.** The patient needs an opportunity to explore and experience her feelings in a nonjudgmental setting with an empathetic nurse and needs to be able to rally her own resources and to set goals for herself.

(e) Other goals might include: to improve communication between patient, family, and staff; to support and strengthen normal coping behaviors or normal problem-solving skills.

LEG VI-A

(f) 2. This acknowledges the difficulty in facing the truth but confronts the patient with the fact. The patient has the choice to either change the subject or continue the conversation with the nurse, who obviously cares enough to want to listen. The nurse knows that if the patient does not progress beyond the stage of denial while in the hospital, she will receive little professional help at home and is a good candidate for a later depression.

(g) Other interventions may include:

1. Provide an unhurried atmosphere for talking and listening for clues.
2. Promote crying, expression of feelings, and offer feedback.
3. Keep interaction goal-oriented: talk about the present and avoid superficial subjects.
4. Explore available resources.
5. Encourage sharing common problems with others, such as members of a mastectomy support group.
6. Avoid criticizing.
7. Approve of normal use of coping mechanisms.
8. Assess to see if family needs help.

(h) 4.

(i) Other criteria for evaluation might include observing for:

1. Verbal acknowledgment of a need for assistance to adapt.
2. Expression of feelings both verbally and nonverbally.
3. Acceptance of suggested referrals.
4. Decision making and realistic plans for the immediate future.

7. All but **(e)**.

8. Possible answers are: Afraid he will cry, and they are uncomfortable seeing a man cry. Afraid he will say something they won't know how to answer and make them feel ill at ease. Irritated at his behavior of demanding medication and wetting the bed. Threatened by the thought that this could also happen to them. Easier to attend to the physical needs than the emotional.

9. (b), **(c)**, **(d)** are correct. The nurse is accepting his behavior and feelings, encouraging him to have feelings and show them, and confronting him with the fact of the surgery.

(a) is incorrect and avoids the subject.

(e) and **(f)** are incorrect and are false attempts at cheer. Instead of feeling better, the patient, when faced with the prospect of being out of bed where everyone can see he is missing a leg, may withdraw.

10. There are numerous behaviors, most of which are action-oriented. One example is the *asking of questions about what the next weeks or months will bring in terms of symptoms or problems.* The nursing response to this question can have two purposes: *to find out what preconceived ideas the person has* that might need correcting and *to give information.* The nurse could say, "Tell me what you imagine some of the problems will be or that your doctor has told you will occur and then I will tell you what I can." After determining what the patient knows, the nurse can give information, such as: "We can keep you from suffering by giving you medications to relieve pain," or, "You are wondering if you can cope with the future weeks as the disease worsens. It seems overwhelming to look ahead to it." This last response helps the person to ask an answerable question, to identify concerns about self, and to handle them using a problem-solving method. Remember, people have the ability to handle their own problems if given support and guidance along the way. That is what this nurse is giving.

Additional coping behaviors:

Expresses feelings openly

Plans realistically for the future

Expresses feelings, such as sorrow, depression, and anger and realizes reason for these emotional reactions

Problem solving

11,12. Attend a GES. Share your answers with your instructor and discuss your rationales.

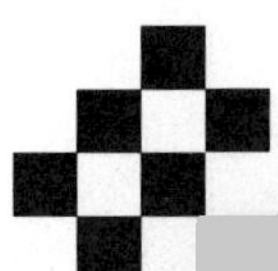

13. *Grief* is caused by a loss or a threat of loss of anything that is highly valued, such as self-esteem, a loved one, or body image. Duration of grief may be short or may take up to a year or more to resolve, but restitution begins in a few weeks. *Depression* is also caused by a loss. Patient may be unaware of the meaning of the loss. Depression is prolonged, severe, and incapacitating and continues on beyond the period of normal grief. Patient may need professional help.

14. (a), (d), (e), (f), (g), (h), (i), (j), (k).

15. Goals and nursing interventions might include:

(a) Establish a therapeutic relationship by sitting and talking with him so he can express his anger and talk about what happened before he became depressed.

(b) *Increase his self-esteem* by recognizing his strengths and accomplishments, but avoid praise, as that may overwhelm him and he will have to prove his worthlessness.

(c) *Prevent further vegetation* by providing a schedule that includes ambulation to meals and bathroom at regular intervals.

(d) *Increase social interaction and stimulation* by making sure Mr. Graves is included in group activities and programs.

(e) *Prevent alienation from his family* by explaining to them what is happening to Mr. Graves and why, and encouraging them to share their own feelings of loss with both you and their father. You may have more.

16. (a), (b), and **(d)** are correct. The nurse is trying to help the patient recognize that his feelings of worthlessness and demanding behavior are indicators that he is bothered by something else and that it is important for him to move around even though he doesn't feel like it. You care for him by helping him out of bed and talking with him.

17. *Subjective:* When his supper was served, he said, "Why should I eat? The future is hopeless."
Objective: Weighed 174 lb, refused entire meal except for glass of milk.

18.

Antidepressant	Action/Use	Side Effects	Nursing Implications
MAO inhibitors	Depression	Dry mouth, blurred vision, urinary retention; hypertensive crisis	Observe for BP, urine retention; omit cheese and wine from diet
Tricyclic compounds	Depression	Drowsiness, dizziness, dry mouth, constipation	Assess for urine retention; assess closely if suicidal

19. (b), (d), and **(f)** are true.

20. **(a)** *Anxiety disorder:* Feeling forced to carry out some act partly against conscious wishes.

(b) *Somatoform disorder:* Hypochondriasis. A severe preoccupation with the state of one's own body; many physical complaints with no organic findings; lack of interest in environment.

(c) *Dissociative disorder:* Total loss of memory of events that occurred during a specific period of time. Ideas, feelings, memories are repressed into unconsciousness, but can return spontaneously.

21. **(a)** Recognize that the paralysis is not consciously motivated by the patient, and the need for treatment and cure is real. The paralysis is a symptom of a problem that needs attention. Share feelings and opinions about patients with functional problems.

(b) Give physical care, encouraging the patient to be only as involved as she desires.

(c) Make observations of patient's conversation and behavior and record these in the nurse's notes. Avoid reinforcement of symptoms.

(d) Talk with other members of the health care team about your feelings toward the patient and how they affect the patient.

22. **(a)**.

23. *Side effects:* Initial diminishing of motor coordination, alertness. Drowsiness.
Nursing implications: Monitor BP; assess for ataxia, slurred speech, vertigo.

What Will I Learn?
LEG VI-B Stress, Adaptation, and Diabetes

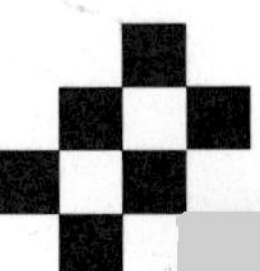

LEG VI-B

In your first **Regulatory** LEG (VI-B) you will review stress and how stressors affect the human body. In discussion groups you will consider many types of stressors, how they affect you as an individual, how you react to stressors, and how physiologic and psychologic stressors can make a well person ill. Think about the stress of beginning Volume II! How will this affect you? Fight or flight? A constant state of readiness to work, work, work, or just put it off until tomorrow? You may learn some very interesting things about yourself as you continue to study stress.

Hospitalization is a multiple stressor with all its rules, diagnostic tests, and medical and surgical treatments. One nursing goal is to help individuals cope with the stressors before they become crises, to maintain a patient in a regulated (homeodynamic) level.

Diabetes mellitus is a chronic disease that can affect any age group. It is a regulatory dysfunction of the pancreas involving the hormone insulin. Symptoms of diabetes mellitus can be classic or disguised, sudden or insidious. It won't take long before you are alert to even the most covert signs and symptoms.

Diabetes affects people of different ages in different ways. Patients with juvenile diabetes require different care and teaching than do older people who have the disease. Most people with diabetes manage their disease without hospitalization. Time in the hospital is for diagnosis, adjusting medication, and teaching self-care.

Many diabetic patients are hospitalized for other reasons such as surgery or heart disease. Diabetes can be mildly or severely complicating to other medical or surgical conditions. You must learn what diabetes is, why it does what it does, how to recognize and prevent complications, and how to help patients help themselves.

This is your first LEG to study and apply the nursing process to patients experiencing alterations in metabolism. Patients need to be involved in their own care and able to make their own decisions because this is a chronic illness. Take the initiative and teach your patients how to help themselves lead healthy lives.

What's Ahead in Later LEGs

There will be more on helping people cope with stress and on diabetes:

LEG VI-C	Respiratory Problems
LEG VII-C	Cardiac and Hypertensive Problems
LEG VII-B and VIII-C	Gastrointestinal Problems
LEG IX-A	Nursing Intervention for Patients with Long-Term Emotional and Physical Illness
	Working toward Restoring Persons to Highest Level of Wellness
LEG XI-A	Complications of Pregnancy
LEG XIII-C	Hyperglycemia

Overview of Learning Experiences in LEG VI-B

LEG VI-B

Objectives	Campus Lab/ Self-Practice	Group Discussions/Lectures	Clinical Lab Focuses
Stress and Charting **1,2.** Adaptation to stress **3.** Charting		**B1.** Stress, stressors, you and your patients	**B5.** Look for signs of stress Evaluate charting Obtain nursing audit checklist
Living with Diabetes **4.** Actions of insulin and glucagon **5.** Comparing types of diabetes **6,7.** Signs, symptoms, and lifestyles **8,9.** Diet history, planning, and teaching		**A8.** Interview a dietitian **B2.** Teaching diabetics **B3.** Assessing the diabetic patient GES Objective 9	**B4.** Give morning care to diabetic patients Help patients with diets Care for patient who has had diabetes a long time
Testing Blood and Urine **10,11.** Testing blood and urine **12.** Diagnostic testing		**B1.** Preparing diabetic patients for diagnostic tests GES Objectives 10,11	**B2.** Collect urine specimens and test for sugar and ketones Assist with diagnostic tests Teach or observe patients testing blood
Pharmacology **13–15.** Antidiabetic drugs **16.** Teaching insulin administration	**B4.** Insulin measurement **B5.** Teaching people to give insulin or oral hypoglycemic agent	**B1.** Caring for patients receiving insulin GES Objectives 15,16	**B9.** Give insulin Give insulin according to a sliding scale Find out hospital insulin policy Go with home health nurse on visits to diabetic patients
Preventing Acute and Long-Term Complications **17.** Hypo- and hyperglycemia **18,19.** Preventing long-term complications of diabetes **20.** Altered sexual function		**B2.** Nursing process for diabetic patients with complications	**B6.** Look for insulin reaction and symptoms of diabetic acidosis Plan for teaching self-care to a diabetic patient Care for diabetic. Write a nursing care plan
Community Resources **21.** Community resources for diabetics			**B1.** Visit local ADA **B2.** Attend special classes for diabetic patients

New Terms

adaptation
adult onset or maturity
anabolic
cachectic
distorted
equilibrium
GAS
gastroparesis
glycosuria
homeostasis
hyperglycemia
hyperinsulinism
hyperosmolality
hypoglycemia
insidious
juvenile
ketoacidosis
ketonuria
ketosis
Kussmaul respirations
neuropathy
osmotic diuresis
perception
polydipsia
polyphagia
polyuria
postprandial
realistic
regulation
retinopathy
stressor

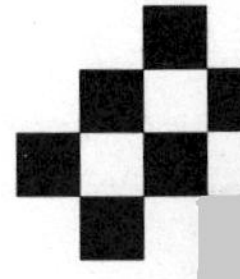

LEG VI-B

Abbreviations

ADA
DKA
DM
HHNC
IDDM
NIDDM

Stress and Charting

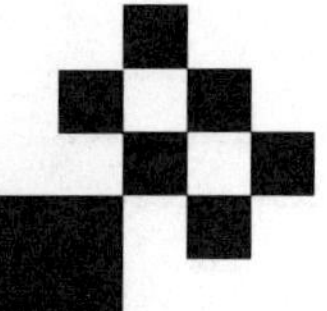

LEG VI-B

O b j e c t i v e s

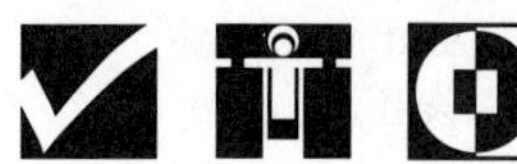

1. List assessments that might indicate that a person is adapting (maintaining homeostasis) to stress and some possible assessments of deficient coping.

2. Given descriptions of patients experiencing stress, identify at which stage of adaptation each person is: alarm reaction, stage of resistance, stage of exhaustion.

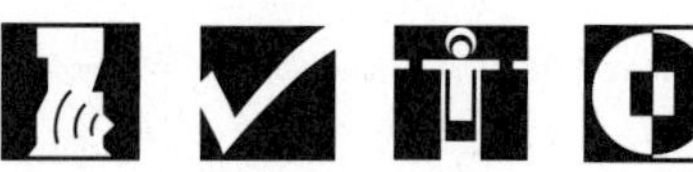

3. Given an example of charting, identify which of the following steps of the nursing process are missing: nursing assessments; nursing interventions given; patient responses or behaviors.

■ A. What's It All About?

1. Think about what stress means to you. How do you cope with the wear and tear of living? Stressors are the factors in life that require us to make adjustments, to adapt sometimes even to survive. List some stressors that you know cause you to adjust. For example, cold is a stressor. How do you react to too many stressors or pressures of living? Anxiety is the most common psychologic reaction to a stressor. Your body's ability to cope physically and mentally with stressors makes the difference in your feeling well or ill.

2. Write the definition of homeostasis as you find it in the dictionary. Write your own thoughts about the meaning of homeostasis as you maintain health. After you have read and have met the Objectives above, write a comparison of your understanding of homeostasis and the dictionary definition.

How do they compare?

What are the most important factors in successful adaptation?

3. Review:

LEG I-B Holistic Health Care and Stress

LEG II-A Charting Assessments

Assessing and Charting TPRs

4. Read fundamentals, medical-surgical, psychiatric, pediatrics nursing references on *stressors, stress, need deprivation, homeostasis, adaptation, psychologic stress, anxiety, nursing process, charting,* and *general adaptation syndrome.*

5. Identify the *alarm reaction, stage of resistance,* and *stage of exhaustion* for the following patients:

Marian Faul fractured her humerus when she fell down the stairs. She also bumped her head and was unconscious for a few minutes. When she came to, she realized that her left arm hurt and was beginning to swell. She dismissed this as a bruise and rested at home until late evening, when she realized she was unable to sleep and aspirin was not helping the pain. At this point she called her physician. She told him she felt "too faint" to drive to the emergency room.

Mike Nelson had a speech to give to his class. He had not volunteered but finally did agree to write and give the paper. As he worked on it, he became very unsure of its merits and of his own ability to deliver the paper. As he began to memorize the words, he realized that he was unable to remember whole sections. Panic set in; he couldn't eat or sleep.

Mr. Asman woke up with a cold after a weekend fishing trip. By the end of that day it was worse, and he complained of wheezing and sat up most of the night. He took home remedies for the cold, and by morning he was extremely weak and realized he needed more than "cold pills."

Mrs. Sucar has had diabetes mellitus for many years. She has learned to live with the disease and with very minimal complications. She tests her urine daily and watches her diet. Her daughter is getting married and she is very busy with wedding plans and showers. She notices that her urine has become more orange than blue when tested. She tries to compensate by taking a little more insulin and watching her diet.

Note: If you are unfamiliar with some of the terms in these situations, look them up. Mrs. Sucar leaves you in doubt as to the outcome. Finish the story any way you wish but identify the stages.

Bring your answers to the group discussion (B.1).

Facts about Stressors and Illness

Stressors are factors that tax an individual's adaptive capacities. How one individual reacts to a particular stressor compared with how another person is affected by the same stressor is determined by:

- How suddenly the stressor happens
- How long the stressor lasts
- How forceful the stressor is
- The individual's own limitations and capabilities

These factors show us how important the history (both nursing and medical) is for a patient. For example, heredity, experiences, and successes and failures all influence an individual's adaptive mechanism.

Illness is characterized by:

- Lack of energy in both mind and body
- Inaccurate perceptions of routines
- Feelings of uncertainty
- Loss of private or unique abilities
- Loss of routine way of life and personal involvement

Independent nursing actions can help a person conserve energy, help with feelings of security, and create situations that keep people private and uniquely involved in the business of getting well.

You won't always "read" your patients right, but now is the time to begin. You are the one who can help each patient help herself.

LEG VI-B

Facts about Charting

Charting is the method used to pass information from person to person and shift to shift. The information charted must be clear, concise, meaningful, comparative, and accurate.

There are excellent tools to chart a patient's progress from illness to wellness—the highest level that can be attained. Whatever type of charting forms are used in your hospital, information can be recorded in such a way as to be a valuable tool in improving nursing care.

For each problem that is identified, your charting should include all the steps of the nursing process, your assessment, diagnosis of problems, what you did about them, and whether it worked.

- Assessments and interventions must be recorded as they happen without waiting to summarize so that details and sequence will not be forgotten later.
- Additional information should be added as needed, dated and signed. Information already recorded should not be repeated.

Look at your own chart forms and think how you can use them in the most efficient manner.

■ B. Putting It into Action!

1. Attend a small group discussion on "Stress, Stressors, You and Your Patients."

- Prepare for this discussion by reading one chapter from a book and one article, preferably on stress and children, and viewing one audiovisual.

  One purpose of this discussion should be to find out more about stressors and your own responses so that you can recognize stages of adaptations for your patients of all ages and be better able to help them cope.
- Discuss the nursing actions below as they did or might apply to your patients this week. Describe an event that would indicate the need for each intervention. Give your rationale for the action, including how that person must feel.

Nursing Actions That Help Patients Cope with Stress

(a) Acknowledging pain

(b) Appearing to know what to do

(c) Able to assess a situation quickly and initiate action

(d) Taking over when the patient is overwhelmed and knowing how to do the right thing

(e) Being there when needed (patients feel loss when staff is rotated and a "favorite" nurse is no longer there)

(f) Identifying and providing needed information

(g) Finding out what the patient expects and helping to correct misunderstandings

(h) Encouraging patient to be self-sufficient

(i) Helping patient become aware of even small gains

(j) Demonstrating sensitivity to and concern about feelings

(k) Taking care of patient's personal belongings and environment

(l) Paying attention to what is important to patient, such as right to privacy

(m) Keeping informed about changes in therapy—keeping up the nursing care plan

(n) Reviewing with patient those events that caused anxiety

(o) Anticipating and rehearsing in preparation for threatening event

(p) Listening for lack of hope and providing hope that things can change

2. Practice charting for the following situation. Use the forms for your clinical agency. Compare your charting with that of another student. Include all the steps of the nursing process.

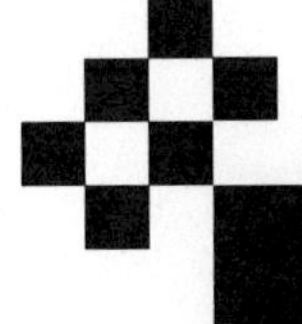

LEG VI-B

Notes on 8–11 A.M. Clinical Experience

Miss Brown, freshman nursing student, arrived for nursing lab at 8:00 A.M. She was introduced to Mrs. Smith, the team leader, who gave her information about Mr. Coles, the patient she was to care for during lab. The information Miss Brown received about her patient was as follows:

1. Mr. Coles had been in the hospital 3 days because of a back injury.
2. He could be up to the bathroom with crutches.
3. He continued to have pain in his low back and right leg.
4. He was to have a heating pad on his back when he was in bed.
5. He needed some assistance with his bath. The amount needed had varied from day to day, depending on his discomfort.
6. He was not to sit in the padded chair; he could use only a straight chair.

The nurse's notes from the 11–7 shift stated the following:

"12 sleeping, 4 A.M. awake—severe right leg pain. Medication given. 6 A.M. dozing."
— *A. Smith, R.N.*

When Miss Brown entered Mr. Coles's room, he said, "I'm not sure I want a bath this morning. All I want to do is sleep. I had a bad night." After talking with Mr. Coles, Miss Brown identified that the patient had experienced much leg pain during the night and that this pain had been more severe than ever before. He asked Miss Brown for medication for pain relief and described his present situation as "not bad now, but I don't want it to get as bad as last night." Miss Brown also noticed that Mr. Coles's breakfast tray was almost complete, with only the coffee and a half a piece of toast gone.

After giving Mr. Coles a medication for pain, Miss Brown helped him with his bath, gave him a back rub, and made his bed. She noticed transitory redness in his low back; this disappeared during the back rub. She gave Mr. Coles fresh ice water and helped him into a clean pair of pajamas. He asked her to clip his toenails, so she obtained a nail clipper from central supply and helped him trim his nails. Mr. Coles said, "Thank you for your care. My leg feels better than it has for a long time. There is still a dull ache running down my calf, but the throbbing pain is gone."

Mr. Coles walked (with crutches) to the bathroom while Miss Brown made the bed. When he returned to the room, he sat in the big chair by the window. Miss Brown said, "Oh, has the doctor given you the O.K. to sit in that chair?" Mr. Coles replied sharply, "Well, I never heard that he didn't want me to sit in this chair." Miss Brown explained what the team leader had told her and explained that the soft slant-back chair did not help to keep his body in good alignment. Mr. Coles stated, "Well, I suppose I can go along with that, but I wish they'd let you know about these things before you go ahead and do them."

After Mr. Coles got back into bed, Miss Brown sat and talked with him. "You know," he said, "this having a back injury really bugs me. I have a brother-in-law who hurt his back lifting a sack of grain the wrong way. He's had surgery on his back three times, and he still has to wear

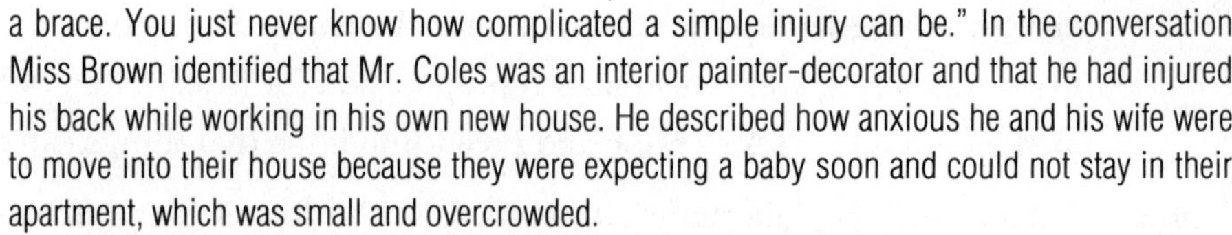

a brace. You just never know how complicated a simple injury can be." In the conversation Miss Brown identified that Mr. Coles was an interior painter-decorator and that he had injured his back while working in his own new house. He described how anxious he and his wife were to move into their house because they were expecting a baby soon and could not stay in their apartment, which was small and overcrowded.

Before leaving Mr. Coles's room, Miss Brown changed the heating pad cover and checked the water level.

During the morning Miss Brown gave Mr. Coles the following medications:

Valium 10 mg p.o. at 9 A.M.—given to him daily to help relax him

Tylenol 650 mg p.o. at 9 A.M.—for pain in back and leg

Mr. Coles was to receive one Stress Cap, a multivitamin, at 9 A.M. but he refused this. He stated, "I don't think I want that capsule this morning. Yesterday I felt nauseated about a half hour after I took this. The morning before I experienced the same thing."

3. List at least three examples of adaptations to stressors in the following chart:

Stressor	**Psychologic Adaptations**	**Physiologic Adaptations**
Amputation		
Traffic ticket		
Hospitalization		

Add signs and symptoms of *not* coping with stressors to your list above.

What differences would you expect in the response and reactions of children or teenagers compared with those of an adult? List these differences.

List the differences you would expect in the reactions and responses of aged adults compared with those of children, teenagers, and middle-aged adults. Refer to your geriatrics nursing references if necessary.

List possible environmental stressors for patients who are in the hospital.

How do rules affect patients? Are they a help or a hindrance to the patient? Are they made to be broken? Are they for staff or patient comfort and safety?

4. Match the signs of adaptation in the right column that might be used for each of the stressors listed in the left column.

Stressor

_____ 1. Infection

_____ 2. Smog

_____ 3. Fear of failure

_____ 4. Anger

_____ 5. Nutritional deprivation

Sign of Adaptation

(a) Increased attention paid to finding food and less attention to learning, social behavior, appearance.

(b) Denial of fact at the conscious level of the mind.

(c) Develops backache and is unable to meet obligation.

_____ 6. Loss of loved one

(d) Increased adrenalin supply, increased cholesterol deposits on blood vessel linings, increased blood pressure, increased viscosity of blood.

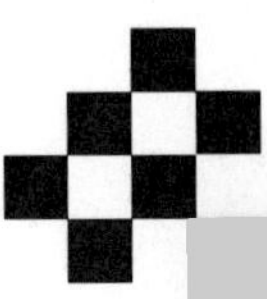

(e) Increased temperature, malaise that increases desire for rest.

(f) Increased mucous production, cilia action, and cough.

LEG VI-B

Answers:

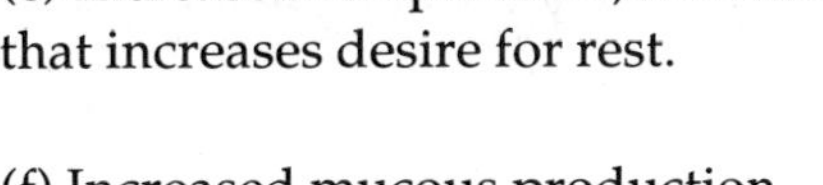

1(e), 2(f), 3(c), 4(d), 5(a), 6(b).

Label the defenses above as either psychologic or physiologic.

Comments on Stressors

Homeostasis is a word that explains the mechanisms that make our life not only possible but downright exciting! It is a regulatory function (a balancing system) to keep the body in equilibrium. The disease condition of diabetes mellitus is a stressor that requires constant regulation, both external and internal, so that the patient can maintain an optimum state of health.

Stressors abound as conflicts, grief, shock, loss, and fear. Hospitalized patients can be in a stage of exhaustion. Having expended human, physical effort to overcome stressors, these people need your help to restore them to a state of physical and psychologic stability. For example, surgery for a patient, whether lifesaving or elective, inflicts multiple stressors. The patient experiences a period of confusion immediately after surgery. Later, a slow recognition of what has happened begins, followed by a lag while the patient assesses the damage or change before progressing to recovery.

Recovery may not be a return to the original condition (the tonsils or gallbladder is gone; the prediabetic state cannot be reached), but rather the patient must achieve a new balanced state.

You must learn to recognize the descending stages of alarm, resistance, and exhaustion and the ascending return to physiologic and psychologic stability. Your patient requires a different kind of care and support during the different phases of recovery (for example, your patient needs to receive care and support passively during the early phase of confusion and slow recognition, which continues during the lag of assessment, then needs encouragement for self-help, patient participation, and involvement from that stage up to the new balanced state.

5. Plan for a clinical experience in combination with others in this LEG.

▲ Look for signs of stress. Identify the stressor(s) if you can. Note the stage of reaction and state how you would help these patients ascend to their new state of balance. How much stress can be tolerated before illness results? Can you tell by looking and listening when a person is sick even though he may say, "I feel fine"? You must learn to recognize the signs of disease. Watch closely for signs that your patients may feel worse than they say, or better. What behaviors of children make you think stress and anxiety are becoming too great?

▲ Attend postconference. As you listen and discuss your experiences of the day, write on the chalkboard the stressors mentioned. Note the nursing actions taken and discuss the rationale.

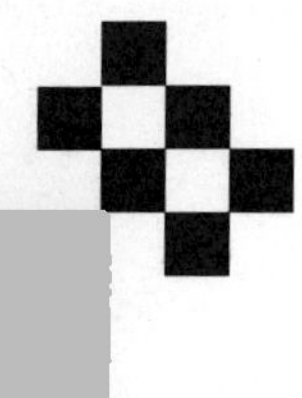

LEG VI-B

▲ Bring a copy of your charting on one patient to postconference. Evaluate each other's charting. Are the steps of the nursing process covered? What more would you want to know? What more could you have done for your patient if you had seen the "picture" as charted?

▲ Obtain your clinical agency's requirements for charting or a nursing audit checklist. Evaluate your examples of charting and decide if they meet your clinical agency's standards for being accurate, adequate, and meaningful.

Living with Diabetes

O b j e c t i v e s

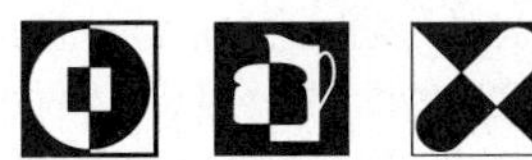

4. Compare the actions of insulin and glucagon in the body.

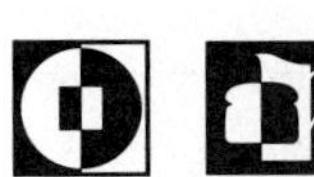

5. Compare the age of onset, predisposing factors, severity, and treatment for insulin-dependent diabetes (IDDM or juvenile-onset) (Type I) with non-insulin-dependent diabetes (NIDDM or maturity-onset) (Type II).

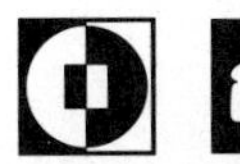

6. Given a list of statements of cause and a list of signs and symptoms of diabetes mellitus, match the ones that best explain the cause of the symptom.

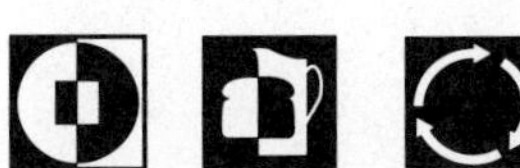

7. Describe how diet, exercise, stress, weight, and illness affect the insulin-dependent and the non-insulin-dependent diabetic.

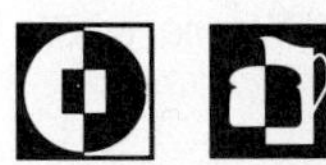

8. Given a prescription for a diabetic diet, demonstrate planning meals for 2 days using the ADA exchange lists.

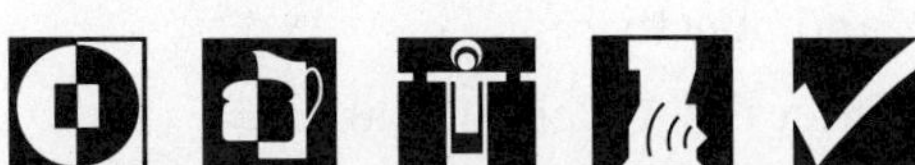

9. Demonstrate or role play taking a diet history and teaching an insulin-dependent patient or a family member to use a diet exchange list.

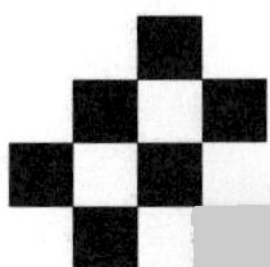

LEG VI-B

A. What's It All About?

1. Think about diabetes as a regulatory dysfunction and as a chronic disease. The implications are numerous. All the patient's activities, whether planned or unplanned, will be influenced by the lack of regulation and loss of equilibrium. Instead of depending on an autonomic (automatic) system, the patient must become the controller. You must be able to tell the patient not only how but also why!

2. Review LEG IV-C, Making Assessments Related to Fluid and Electrolyte Balance.

3. Read in medical-surgical, pediatrics, nutrition and pharmacology references about *diabetes, insulin, diet, teaching, exercise, stress, autoimmune disease, hypoglycemia, hyperglycemia.*

4. View audiovisuals and read articles and books from a list given you by your instructor.

5. Preview:

LEG VII-B Dehydration in All Ages
Causes of Respiratory and Metabolic Acid-Base Imbalances
LEG XIII-C Diabetic Emergencies

Note: If you are taking a separate course in nutrition, this is the time to apply your basic information to special diets that are ordered for patients with specific disease conditions, such as diabetes. If you do not have a separate course (and most students do not), you must use the information learned in Volume I. Refer to the index under nutrition and diet for the nutrition content in the four LEGs volumes. Review the basic nutrients and diet principles each time you come across new special diets.

---

6. Explain to another person why these symptoms of diabetes occur:

polyuria
polydipsia
hypoglycemia
hyperglycemia
polyphagia
glycosuria
dehydration
weight loss
fatigue

7. Answer the following questions.

(a) Why is the incidence of diabetes increasing in the United States?

(b) List the actions of insulin and the actions of glycogen. Where is each produced?

(c) Describe what occurs to the blood sugar level of a normal healthy person after eating and during a period of hunger. Include what hormones are secreted and what effect they have on carbohydrate, fat, and protein metabolism. What is the relationship between diabetes and obesity?

(d) Explain why dehydration would occur in a diabetic patient.

(e) Explain the chain reaction of symptoms that results after a meal when there is a deficiency of insulin in the body. What metabolic changes occur with severe insulin deficiency (DKA)?

(f) List the triad of symptoms in diabetes and explain why they occur.

(g) What is the effect of exercise on blood sugar? What are some exercise guidelines for a person with diabetes mellitus?

(h) Explain the relationship between hyper- and hypoglycemia and hyper- and hypoinsulinism.

(i) Compare diabetes mellitus with other carbohydrate metabolic disorders such as galactosemia and glycogen storage diseases, including their onset, pathophysiology, nursing assessment, and care.

(j) Compare the early signs of diabetes in a child with those typically found in a young adult and in the elderly.

(k) What medical conditions might cause diabetes?

8. Interview a dietitian to gain insight into how to work with patients to educate them about their dietary needs and how to learn about their personal food preferences and patterns. Discuss with the dietitian the complementary roles of the dietitian and the nurse. With your classmates and the dietitian, consider ways in which dietitians and nurses can enhance their mutual effectiveness in patient education regarding dietary management of diabetes by the patient.

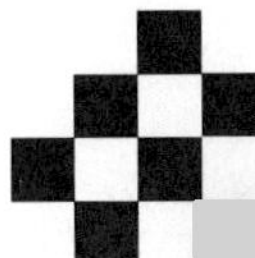

9. Visit a local supermarket. List all the special dietetic foods you find. Be sure to look in the frozen food section for egg substitutes and in the soft drinks, jams and jellies, and other sections where sugar substitutes may be found. Compare the cost of these special items. Be sure to note the price of fructose. After surveying this information and considering the choices available to a diabetic, discuss with another classmate or several classmates whether diabetics need to buy these special products and, if not, what are some alternatives?

10. Write a diet plan for one day for the following patient using either the diet exchange lists or the point system. Find out which method is used in your area.

> Mr. Gower, age 65, has non-insulin-dependent (NIDDM) (Type II) diabetes.
> He is on Orinase (tolbutamide) 250 mg b.i.d. His diet prescription is 2000 calories a day, which should be divided into 260 gm of carbohydrate, 125 gm of protein, and 60 gm of fat.

Using the following guidelines, figure out how many calories each of the patients described in B.2, below, should be eating each day and write a sample meal plan for at least two of them.

Decide which people are insulin-dependent and include at least one of them when writing your meal plans. Bring your plans to the group discussion to share and discuss any problems you encountered.

Meal-Planning Guidelines

To maintain weight, eat 30–35 calories a day per kg of ideal body weight.

If there is a tendency to gain weight, eat 30 calories a day per kg of weight.

If you are physically active most of the day eat 35 calories per kg of weight.

If you are trying to reduce your weight eat 15–20 calories per kg of weight.

Children through late teens should not eat less than 1200 calories per day.

Elderly people should reduce fat and increase protein to reduce the risk of atherosclerosis.

Midafternoon or evening snacks must be included if the person takes insulin.

Alcohol should be deducted from the fat exchange (45 calories equal 1 fat exchange). Omit sweet wines and liqueurs; artificial sweeteners are allowed. (Alcohol proof × 0.08 × fluid ounces equals calories.) Physician approval regarding recommendations on alcohol in the diet should be obtained before working with the patient.

Carbohydrates should make up 50% of the calories.

Proteins should make up 20% of the calories.

Fats should make up 30% of the calories (may be reduced but should never exceed 30%).

Be consistent in dividing calories between CHO, P, and F.

Eat at regularly scheduled times each day!

LEG VI-B

Fill in these blanks to use as a reference:

A kilogram equals ______________________ pounds.

I weigh ______________________ kilograms.

One gram of carbohydrate equals ______________________ calories.

One gram of protein equals ______________________ calories.

One gram of fat equals ______________________ calories.

■ B. Putting It into Action!

1. Plan and eat your own ideal meals for one day using the guidelines in A.10. Calculate your ideal caloric intake and use the diet exchange lists to select your foods. Complete this experience before the group discussion so you can share your reactions. Why is it said that diabetics often live healthier lives than the average person? Do you feel any different after eating your planned meals? Can you think of ways you might benefit from changing your own dietary habits?

2. Attend a small group discussion on "Teaching Diabetics."

■ Be sure there are several diet prescriptions and exchange lists available for your role playing.

■ Role play with two of your classmates. One person should assume the role of the insulin-dependent diabetic, one the role of the non-insulin-dependent diabetic, and the third person the role of the dietitian. The dietitian can review with the patients the importance of following the dietary strategies for the specific type of diabetes each patient has. This can be done by asking each patient to outline the usual diet plan to be followed and then to identify changes that may be necessary for each of the following: exercise, stress, weight control, and illness. Be sure the dietitian summarizes the significant differences between the dietary strategies for the two different types of diabetic patients. Here are some possible patients to use:

Peggy Posy, age 6, has diabetes and weighs 40 pounds.
Her mother is a teacher and seems very anxious to learn everything to help the child.

Joe Jones, age 16, weighs 150 pounds. He is withdrawn and uncommunicative. He states that he does not want to talk about diabetes and shows little interest in discussing diet exchanges. He likes soda and chips and is on the school baseball team.

Mrs. Middling, age 50, weighs 180 pounds. Her diabetes was recently diagnosed and she seems agreeable to most of your suggestions. She loves to eat and cook.

Mr. Elderly, age 72, is also recently diagnosed. He seems confused by this disease and can't seem to understand the diet exchange lists. He says, "My wife always took care of the meals. Since she's been gone, I haven't paid much attention." His daughter visits him daily and is concerned about his living alone. He weighs 185 pounds.

■ Review the developmental tasks of each of the patients above. How will they affect their learning?

■ Relate stress and crisis to the regulatory aspect of caring for diabetic patients. How are they interrelated?

■ Explain the theory that diabetes may be the result of an autoimmune process.

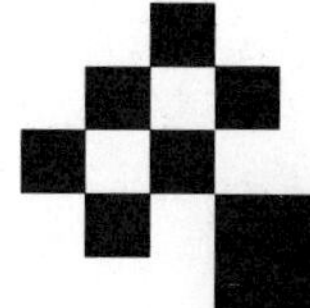

■ Assume that you are working with Mrs. Middling, who is interested in modifying her living pattern to reduce the possible complications of diabetes. What suggestions would you make to help her? Why are these ideas likely to help? What cautions would you need to include when working out a plan with her?

Assume you are working with Mr. Elderly who likes to have a little alcohol in his diet. How would you approach your discussion about the consumption of alcohol, or would you feel it wise to ignore the subject? Discuss this issue with your classmates. Would this matter need to be discussed with a patient who makes no mention of alcohol consumption? How does alcohol consumption fit into the 2-day diet plan you are developing?

■ Explore the changes that would occur in a diabetic woman during pregnancy.

LEG VI-B

3. Attend a group discussion on "Assessing the Diabetic Patient."

■ Compare the assessment data for a patient with IDDM with that of a patient with NIDDM.

■ What nursing diagnoses might be assumed by the assessment data?

■ Name three nursing goals for the care of a diabetic patient.

■ Discuss the case of the following patient:

> Jim Daniels, a 34-year-old white male, is admitted to the ED with nausea and vomiting and states he has not eaten in 2 days, has not checked blood sugar regularly, and has had no doctor's care for some time. He is currently taking Insulin NPH 35 units and Reg 25 units at 8 A.M. and 4 P.M. but did not take it today. VS are stable. Lab studies include:
>
> pH 7.3 — Na 131 — Blood sugar 560
>
> CO_2 32 — K 4.7 — Blood ketones 160
>
> UA: 2+ ketones
> 2+ proteins
> 4+ glucose
>
> Doctor's admit orders were:
>
> Hydrate with NS 300 cc/hr.
> Insulin 5u/hr til BS 240 then decrease 1u/hr.
> Give D-5 if needed for BS <100
> ADA diet
> Compazine 5 mg for nausea prn
>
> You are caring for him 3 days later. His current orders are:
>
> IV NS 300 cc/hr with 5 units/hr Insulin
> Blood glucose every hr till BS <240 then ↓ insulin infusion to 1u/hr and ↓ BG to q2h × 2 then q4h
> Tylenol 650 mg q4h prn
> Valium 5 mg qhs

DSS 250 mg p.o. daily

Mylanta 30 cc q2h abd. pain prn

While you are caring for the patient, the FBS was 160. The doctor orders:

In A.M. stop insulin infusion.

Start Reg Insulin 25 units and NPH Insulin 35 units q A.M. and q 4 P.M.

While talking with the patient, you learned that he was first diagnosed as diabetic when he was 30 years old. He is single and does not pay much attention to his diet. He also mentioned that he has been having some problem with his vision. His feet are in good condition. He has no insurance.

■ Using your data base format, identify what data you have and what assessments need to be made. Explain the metabolic changes that are occurring. Identify any teaching needs that may be present.

Note: Save this care plan and your notes to use as you proceed through this LEG. Look back at the patient data and discuss as you study diet, drugs, complications, and teaching.

---

4. Plan for a clinical experience.

▲ Give morning care to diabetic patients with or without complications and of different age groups. Look for symptoms of diabetes. Ask patients to tell you about past symptoms. Chart your care and observations. Make notes on your speculations or care you would want to give. Bring them to postconference.

▲ Help patients with diets. Use diet exchange lists. Is soluble fiber a part of the diet? Feed as necessary. Help with special preferences. Find out how the patient's food intake is reported and by whom—dietitian, aide, RN? What is not eaten? How will religious beliefs affect the diet?

▲ Care for a patient who has had diabetes for many years. Give general morning care. Do not look at the patient's chart, but listen to the patient. Find out how she copes with the disease—which routines work, which don't work; how illness, such as a cold, affects the balance; how did she learn to take insulin, measure diet amounts, and so on. Chart and work up a nursing care plan so that others can benefit by what you have learned.

■ C. Extra Added Attraction!

1. Create a teaching pamphlet or poster for children or older adults on a diet that has food exchange lists, types of foods that can be exchanged, and so on. Plan this project either in a group or individually and then try using it with some well-planned objectives, such as: Using a 1000-calorie menu, accurately select one food exchange from lists 4, 5, and 7 for breakfast, lunch, and dinner one day.

■ Role play teaching these patients (or others) how to use exchange lists.

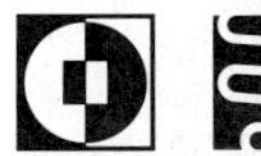

Testing Blood and Urine

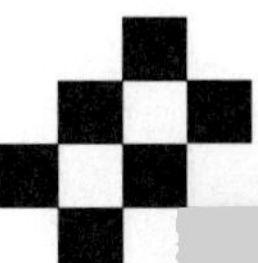

LEG VI-B

O b j e c t i v e s

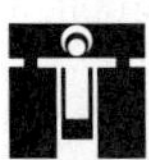 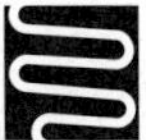

10. Demonstrate and describe in writing testing a blood and urine specimen for sugar and/or ketones, including the reasons for the test.

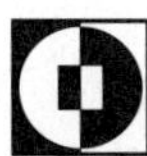 

11. Demonstrate and/or describe in writing teaching a patient how to test urine and/or blood for sugar and/or ketones and state the normal results.

12. Describe the purpose and patient preparation for each of the following: fasting blood sugar, glucose tolerance test, and postprandial blood sugar.

■ A. What's It All About?

1. Think about urine specimens and testing. Is this an appealing subject to you? It is probably no more appealing to your patient. The patient may have to collect and test urine specimens for the rest of her life or she may need frequent needle sticks to obtain blood samples. Your attitude is vitally important as you teach the patient *how* and *why* so that a positive, rather than depressed or denying, attitude can be developed.

2. Read medical-surgical, pediatrics, laboratory test, and pharmacology references on *collecting* and *testing specimens, blood sugar tests, glucose tolerance tests.*

■ B. Putting It into Action!

1. Attend a small group discussion on "Preparing Diabetic Patients for Diagnostic Tests."

■ Explain what you would tell each patient. How will you know whether your patient understands?

■ Role play the activities with which a nurse will need to be concerned for each of these patients, on each of the next three shifts. Include giving a shift report about what is to be done and what was done. (Don't forget to include the patient, the lab, the diet kitchen, and the physician.) Are fluids restricted? What results would be expected and desirable for an IDDM patient? For an NIDDM patient? What is the purpose of the glycosylated hemoglobin (GHb) test? How is it helpful?

Mrs. Manson has an order for a fasting blood sugar and a 2-hour postprandial in the A.M.

A glucose tolerance test is ordered for Mr. Morgan in the A.M.

Mary Sixtine has an order for a glycosylated hemoglobin.

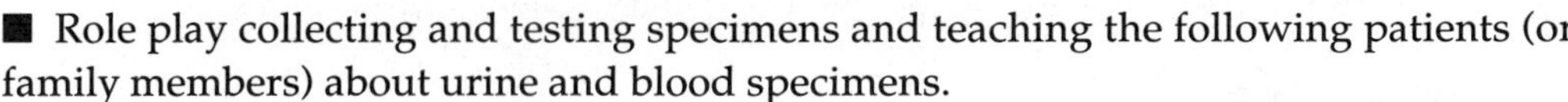

■ Role play collecting and testing specimens and teaching the following patients (or family members) about urine and blood specimens.

A 35-year-old postoperative patient with an indwelling catheter. (An insulin-dependent diabetic hospitalized for surgery unrelated to diabetes.)

An 18-month-old boy whose mother is ready for teaching.

A 66-year-old man who has newly diagnosed diabetes and is up and about with bathroom privileges.

A 17-year-old girl who is used to testing her own blood at home and is going away to college next month.

■ After you have evaluated your role playing of the situations, change them: What if one patient is color-blind? How would you know? What if one patient is incontinent? Has cataracts? Has had a stroke and has little or no use of her right hand?

2. Plan for a clinical experience.

▲ Collect urine specimens from patients. Test the specimens for sugar and ketones. Report or record the results, either routine or sliding scale. Why is urine that has been collected from a drainage bag likely to give an error in testing? How would you collect a specimen from a child?

▲ Assist with diagnostic tests for diabetes mellitus.

▲ Teach or observe at least two patients testing blood for sugar and ketones. Follow up to be sure your teaching is successful. See clinical experience for Objectives 17–20 for more on teaching and the value of the time spent on teaching.

■ C. Extra Added Attraction!

1. Create a teaching poster or pamphlet that teaches how and why to collect and test blood or urine and also depicts attitudes. Make it as positive and motivational as you can. What differences would you want to include for the different age groups? How can the patient keep daily records to take to the doctor's office? You may want to practice this yourself at home. Go through the whole procedure and take notes on how you feel and what you do before making the teaching tool. What questions do you have? Would you feel or do anything differently if you had to collect and test blood or urine every day?

Pharmacology

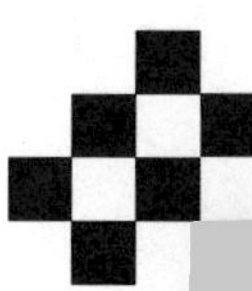

Objectives

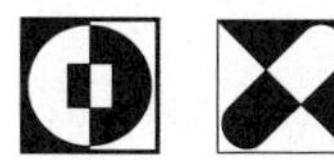

13. Differentiate between the action/use, route of administration, and untoward effects of insulin, oral hypoglycemic agents, and glucagon.

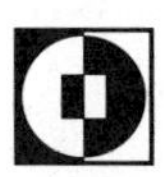 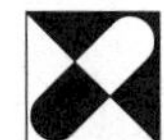

14. Differentiate between short (rapid), intermediate, and long (slow) acting insulin in relation to the onset, peak, and duration of effect, and give an example of each.

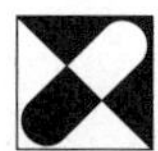 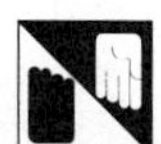

15. Demonstrate and/or describe in writing preparation and administration of a prescribed dose of insulin to a patient, including mixing two types of insulin in one syringe.

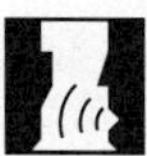  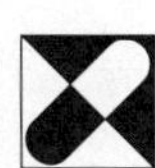 

16. Write a plan for teaching a patient (teenager, middle adult, and aged adult) how to give insulin to herself stating your rationale for each step in your teaching plan, and then role play or demonstrate teaching a patient according to your plan.

■ A. What's It All About?

1. Think about what insulin means to the diabetic patient. It is lifesaving, and it will need to be taken by most patients for the rest of their lives. Patients must be responsible for taking their own insulin at home. To be informed they must learn about the drug—when to expect the peak effect and when the least. Most of your patients will have ambivalent feelings about insulin and their need for it.

2. Review:

LEG II-B	Nutritional Assessment and Teaching
	Preventing Problems during Pregnancy through Teaching
LEG II-C	Ways to Encourage Patient Decision Making
LEG III-A	Patient Discharge
LEG III-C	Anxiety and Defense Mechanisms
LEG IV-B	Preparing Parenteral Medications
	Selecting Sites and Giving Injections
LEG V-B	Helping a Patient Prepare for Discharge
LEG V-C	Teaching Patients after Eye Surgery
	Teaching Breast and Testicular Self-Examination

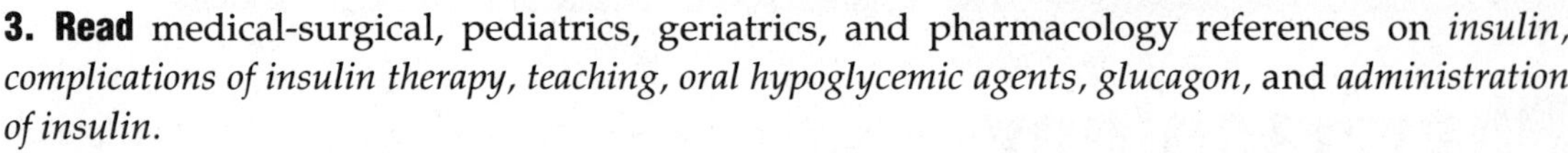

3. Read medical-surgical, pediatrics, geriatrics, and pharmacology references on *insulin*, *complications of insulin therapy*, *teaching*, *oral hypoglycemic agents*, *glucagon*, and *administration of insulin*.

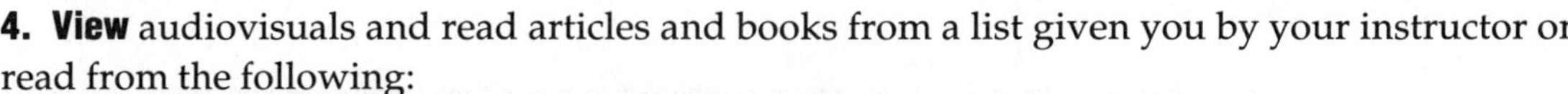

4. View audiovisuals and read articles and books from a list given you by your instructor or read from the following:

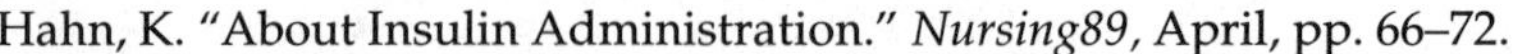

Hahn, K. "About Insulin Administration." *Nursing89*, April, pp. 66–72.

Mackowiak, L., and R. McCarthy. "Managing Diabetes on Sick Days." *AJN*, July 1989, pp. 950–951.

Steil, C. F., and D. A. Deakins. "Today's Insulins. What You and Your Patient Need to Know." *Nursing90*, August, pp. 34–39.

LEG VI-B

■ B. Putting It into Action!

1. Attend a small group discussion on "Caring for Patients Receiving Insulin."

■ Consider the following patients. When would you look for the beginning effect from insulin? How will you know? What would alert you to a problem? Why? Which of the following patients would be a candidate for an insulin pump?

> Mrs. Nelsen, age 54, is hospitalized because of pneumonia. Her long-standing insulin-dependent diabetes is out of control. She is receiving NPH insulin qd and regular insulin on a sliding scale.

> Mary Deaton was admitted in diabetic coma. She is 15 years old and has had insulin-dependent diabetes for 2 years. She is now being regulated on a sliding scale. Her appetite is poor, and she has many food idiosyncrasies. She must be urged to eat her evening meal. She frequently uses antacids at home.

> Mr. Barrotti has severe vascular disturbances and several ulcerous lesions on his right leg. A "brittle" insulin-dependent diabetic of long standing, he takes NPH insulin on a regular basis. He is scheduled for a fasting blood sugar this morning, so has a "hold" breakfast and "hold" insulin. He is 39.

■ Which patients are likely to need an early breakfast or a little orange juice? Why? Discuss alternate types of insulin for those patients.

What particular precautions or observations would you make or take if you were the evening nurse? Night nurse? Why?

What symptoms of fluid and electrolyte imbalance might occur? Why?

■ You are caring for a diabetic patient at night. You know that visual observation is not enough. When you go into the room and feel her bed clothes, you notice that they are damp from perspiration. What is your next move? Why?

■ If your patient is scheduled for x-ray or surgery and is NPO, should you give the morning insulin?

■ An adolescent patient wants to sleep until 11 A.M. on Saturday morning. Is that all right?

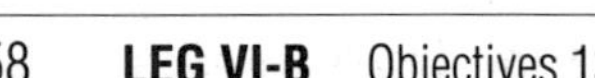

- What is the largest amount of insulin you would give subcutaneously without questioning the doctor's orders?
- A patient likes to drink alcohol socially and also smokes cigarettes. What is the effect of these on insulin requirements?
- What is the Somogyi phenomenon?
- What is the effect of surgery on the control of diabetes? How is control maintained before, during, and after surgery?
- How do purified and human insulin differ? When would they be preferred over beef or pork insulin? Do they have the same effect on your patient as beef and pork insulin?

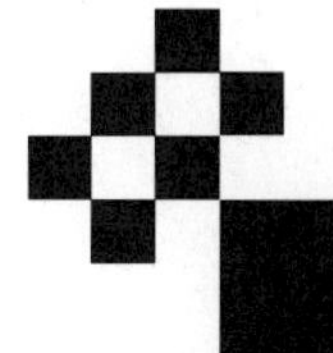

LEG VI-B

2. Create a teaching tool to explain the amounts of self-administration of insulin.

Example: Large syringe with movable plunger; markings clearly readable for U 100 insulin.

3. Write teaching objectives for your patients. Include what you want to do for them and what they must learn from you. For example, demonstrate to a patient the sites for self-administration of insulin. Demonstrate to a patient how to give insulin sq. Have patient return the demonstration to the nurse. List ways for them to learn and how you will find out if they did learn. (You may find that you are writing a tiny LEG for self-administration of insulin.)

4. Check out self-practice materials for "Insulin Measurement." Practice drawing up solutions in unit amounts on both an insulin syringe and a tuberculin syringe. (Label them according to "pretend units" for practice.) Check your measurement with other students.

- Is insulin given sq, IM, or IV? When? Why? Which types? How do you mix insulin in the vial? Shake? Rattle? Roll? Why?
- When mixing two insulins in a syringe, Regular and NPH, which would you draw up first and why?

5. Practice in campus lab (with another student playing the part) teaching the following people to give insulin or an oral hypoglycemic agent; consider each of these patients to be a newly diagnosed diabetic.

Mother of a 4-year-old diabetic girl
14-year-old boy
30-year-old primipara
56-year-old obese man
86-year-old woman

How would you adapt your teaching methods if these patients had had diabetes for a year or more? How will you find out how much they already know and how much they need to learn? How would you adapt your teaching if one of these patients were blind? Had hand tremors? Spoke no English?

What would you do if the 4-year-old's mother was unable to prepare herself psychologically to give her injections? There are no other close members in the family.

What if one patient takes aspirin for arthritis and is now taking glyburide?

How do you communicate with the other nurses on each shift about the progress of the patient's learning? How many nurses will be involved in teaching the patient and why?

LEG VI-B

6. Draw in the areas on the two figures below where it is safe to give insulin. Circle the areas that are usable by the patient for self-administration of insulin. You may need to do some practicing on yourself (using a syringe without the needle) to find out which are possible.

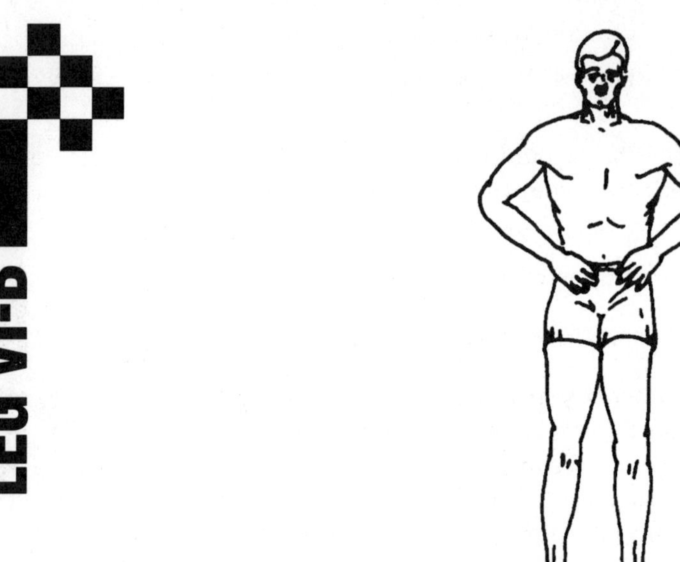

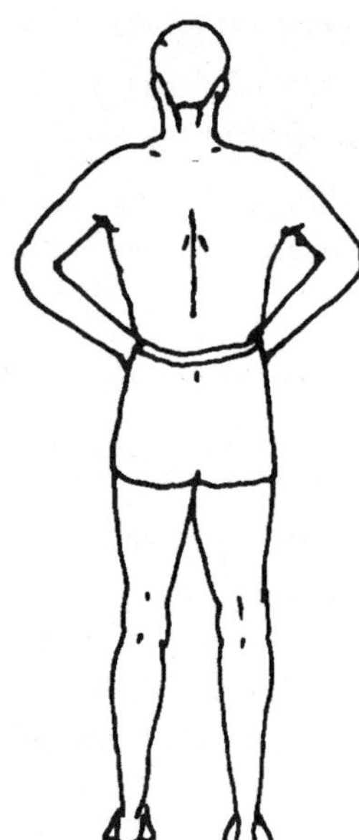

How would you teach the patient to rotate sites? How often can the same site be used? What can happen if the same site is used too often?

7. Write or discuss your reaction to the following order for a patient who is being admitted to the ED and whom you have not yet seen.

> Glucagon 0.5 mg IM stat

- What would the patient look like? Why do you think this drug has been ordered?
- In what form is the drug available? How do you mix it? Is it an emergency drug?

8. Write what you would do to carry out the following orders on your patient:

> bG q6h
> Sliding scale
> 4 + 15 U Regular Insulin
> 3 + 10 U Regular Insulin
> 2 + 5 U Regular Insulin
> 1 + None

9. Plan for a clinical experience.

▲ Find out what your hospital's procedure is before giving insulin. It may be necessary to verify that you have drawn up the correct dosage with an additional person before giving it. What can you do to ensure accuracy when no one else is available?

▲ Give insulin to a variety of patients: child between 3 and 8 years, teenager, middle or older adult.

▲ Give insulin according to sliding scale or before breakfast as ordered. Teach the parent or patient about giving insulin.

▲ Go to a pharmacy. Look at drug labels. How many drugs have sugar as one of their ingredients?

▲ Go with a home health nurse on visits to diabetic patients. Notice how the patients keep records of their medications and tests. Who needs help with preparation of injections, and what help do they receive? Which insulins are stable in a syringe without refrigeration? Which must be given soon after they are mixed?

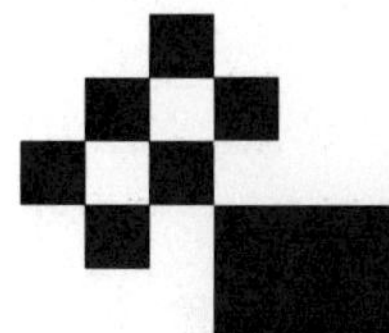

Preventing Acute and Long-Term Complications

LEG VI-B

O b j e c t i v e s

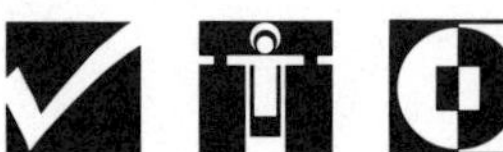

17. Given either a patient situation or an assessment of hyperglycemia and hypoglycemia, identify which condition exists, and given a list of nursing actions, select which action would be best for each situation (or symptom) and state your rationale.

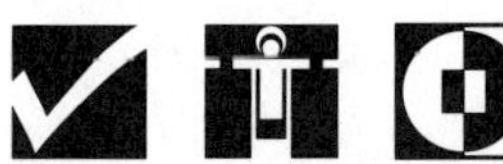

18. State why long-term complications of diabetes mellitus (e.g., infections, visual disturbances, neuropathies, vascular problems) are likely to occur and how they may be prevented or eased, including teaching about infection, trauma, healing, and foot care.

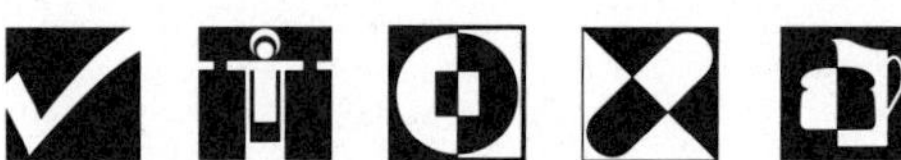

19. Demonstrate caring for a patient who is diabetic, taking measures to ensure that the patient is receiving diet and medication as prescribed and planning nursing interventions to prevent complications of the disease. Write a nursing care plan.

20. Describe why the sexual pleasure of a person with diabetes might be altered.

A. What's It All About?

1. Think about complications. They are always dreaded and often can be avoided by an astute patient or nursing assessment and excellent care. Learn how to recognize signs and symptoms of complications when they are still in an early treatable stage. Teach patients how to watch for them and to prevent them. What would you do if your patient had long, ragged toenails and cracked, dry skin between the toes?

2. Review LEG V-A, Circulatory Problems in the Extremities.

3. Read medical-surgical references on *acidosis, diabetic coma, complications of diabetes, retinopathy, nephropathy, neuropathy, gastroparesis, moniliasis, HHNC,* and *collaborative problems.*

4. View audiovisuals and read articles and books from a list given you by your instructor or read from the following:

Christensen, M. H., M. M. Funnell, M. R. Ehrlich, E. P. Fellows, and J. C. Floyd. "How to Care for the Diabetic Foot." *AJN,* March 1991, pp. 50–57.

Huzar, J. G. "Diabetes Now. Preventing Acute Complications." *RN,* August 1989, pp. 34–40.

Lumley, W. A. "Recognizing and Reversing Insulin Shock." *Nursing89*, September, pp. 34–41.
Robertson, C. "Coping with Chronic Complications." *RN*, September 1989, pp. 34–43.
Sabo, C. and S. R. Michael. "Managing DKA and Preventing a Recurrence." *Nursing89*, February, pp. 50–56.

5. Preview:

LEG VII-B Regulation of Fluid and Electrolyte Balance
Causes of Respiratory and Metabolic Acid-Base Imbalances

LEG XIII-C Diabetic Emergencies

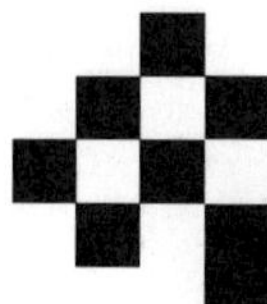

LEG VI-B

6. Underline the signs and symptoms in each patient situation and then write out the problem(s) (e.g., complication, varicose ulcer) on the blank lines.

- Identify the condition that exists.
- List as many nursing actions as you can think of or find that would assist a patient who has hyper- or hypoglycemia. From this list write which ones you would use for each of the situations below and state your rationale.

Martha Baker, 19 years old, studying for exams. She has had diabetes for 5 years and has difficulty keeping it under control. She is slightly obese and loves to nibble at food while she is studying. She finds it increasingly difficult to study because of blurred vision and difficulty with lines of print. ____________________

____

Robert Worldson has just returned from a trip to South America. He is 52, a successful businessman who has had mild diabetes for 4 years. He knows about the importance of diet and has been maintained on an oral hypoglycemic agent. He contracted an intestinal parasite while traveling and has had violent bouts of diarrhea, nausea, and vomiting even though he is on antibiotics. He "can't eat," and after 2 weeks he was admitted to the hospital with a rapid, weak pulse, flushed, dry, hot skin, and was semiconscious. ____________________

____

Madge Sommer, age 66, has had diabetes since she was 38 and has maintained fairly good control with diet. She has arthritis and finds it difficult to "get around as much as I used to." She has noticed that her legs "tingle" and that she has very dry skin, itching, and an open sore on her right shin where she "bumped it over a month ago," while going to the bathroom at night. She notices some swelling in her ankle in the evening, and her lower legs are bluish and mottled. Her toes are becoming stiff and the joints deformed, making wearing shoes difficult. She notices that she has many more "corns" than ever before. ____________________

____

Marilyn Popula is 25, newly married, newly pregnant, and has been a diabetic for 8 years. She has had her ups and downs with diabetes. She gives herself insulin, and when she remembers and cares enough, she regulates her diet very well. She is finding meal preparation more difficult now because she is frequently nauseated and has little interest in food. She complains of frequent sudden attacks of nervousness and tremors; her skin becomes pale and moist. ____

____

Roger Robust, age 37, has had insulin-dependent diabetes for 10 years. He takes daily insulin and is in good control. He has just been admitted to the emergency room because of injuries in an auto accident. He has multiple bruises and bleeding from a compound fracture of the left femur. He is scheduled for emergency surgery in 1 hour. He was alone in the car, and next of kin cannot be found. He has Kussmaul respirations. ______________________

____

Because of excellent nursing care and teaching, Mrs. Popula found relief from her negative gastrointestinal symptoms (nausea and anorexia) in her second trimester. She went to many parties and coffees with her friends. She took a cooking course and created many delicious "out-of-bounds" dishes. But she was faithful about taking her insulin. She had gained 5 pounds by her next prenatal checkup, her blood pressure was low, and the nurse cautioned her to "watch her diet." Poor Marilyn Popula had gotten into a pattern of wanting the extra food and socialization that went with it; for 2 weeks she continued to eat and gain weight; her skin became dry and hot. Her urine tests were alarmingly orange, and then she became too drowsy to bother to cook. She was not hungry, and her husband called the doctor because he could not arouse her one morning. He told the doctor: "Her breath smells sweetish, and she is gulping for air." ______________________

____

■ Using the steps of the nursing process, determine nurse-patient goals and identify the nursing interventions that you could employ or observe related to these patient situations. Practice charting.

■ B. Putting It into Action!

1. List the signs and symptoms, causes and treatment for ketoacidosis and hyperosmolar hyperglycemic nonketotic coma (HHNC).

2. Attend a small group discussion on "Nursing Process for Diabetic Patients with Complications."

■ Using your answers to A.6 and B.1, discuss the signs and symptoms, causes, and actions you would take because of the symptoms you observe. Discuss your rationale. What symptoms would you look for next time that might precede those observed in the situations?

■ What physiologic adaptation occurs in response to hyperglycemia? To hypoglycemia? What are the symptoms of decompensation?

■ Review the data on Jim Daniels with diabetes on p. 53. Which condition do his symptoms fit? How was it treated?

■ When would it be important for the patient at home to check urine for ketones?

- Write a description of a patient with hypoglycemia. Include a cause for it to occur. Compare your descriptions.
- Identify at least six snacks you could give a patient who can take oral food. What would you use if the patient is unconscious?
- List some other terms for hypoglycemia.
- Discuss four nursing diagnoses that would probably be on the NCP of any patient with DKA.
- In order to become self-disciplined about special daily care of the feet, a patient will need to know what can happen without special care and why. What can happen? List several possibilities. Make a teaching plan.
- Review the long-term complications of diabetes. How can infections and neurological and vascular changes affect the sexual function of men and women? Be specific. What factors lead to these changes? What is the nurse's role?
- Review what is meant by independent nursing actions by a nurse. How are they different from dependent or interdependent actions?
- Some of the complications of diabetes require both medical and nursing interventions. The nurse's primary role may be to continuously assess to prevent or detect symptoms early so that medical care can be given. For instance, hypoglycemia is a complication that the nurse monitors but requires medical intervention for treatment. Review collaborative problems with your instructor and use them in writing your NCPs.
- Discuss the process of psychologic adaptation to diabetes. What styles of coping are used? Which would be healthy? Which unhealthy? What could happen to relationships with the family? In the community?

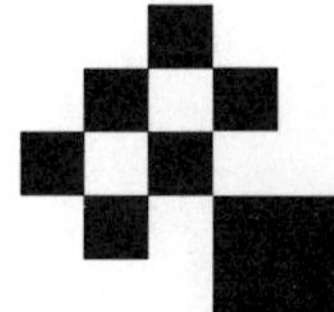

3. Write a paragraph on the difference between causes of fluid loss (e.g., polyuria because of glycosuria in diabetes mellitus and diaphoresis due to fever or anxiety). State how these different causes of dehydration influence nursing action.

4. Create a card to carry with you that gives you reminders of the signs and symptoms of insulin reaction and diabetic acidosis. Use whatever terms will help you remember. Under the symptoms write one or two nursing actions you would take.

5. Examine the following:

> Jenny Day, 6 years old, was admitted to the pediatric unit at 9 A.M. Her father and mother came with her. Her diagnosis: probable diabetes.

Use the doctor's order sheet and the notes made by the nurse to compare the course of the illness, the characteristic symptoms, and lab work with what you have read about diabetes. Try to determine from each assessment what is happening and why the doctor wrote those orders. What nursing actions were taken and why?

It might be easier to see what is going on if you first organize and summarize the notes and chart the pertinent information on the chart form used in your facility.

Doctor's Orders

4/15 9 A.M.

VS q4h

1200 cal diet, no extra sugar or sweets.

bG now. Repeat 3h after insulin given and at 2200.

D-5-1/2NS to run at 25 cc/h

Give Regular Insulin 5u. sq after IV is started.

Parents may visit anytime.

4/15 3 P.M.

Reg. insulin 5u. sq now.

Sliding Scale Insulin to start at 0200 4/16.

4+, sm-lg 3+, lg	5 units, Reg. insulin sq
4+, neg 3+, sm-mod	4 units
3+, neg 2+, sm-lg	3 units
2+, neg 1+, sm-lg	2 units
1+, neg neg, neg	none

Notes on Patient Care

4/15

0900	Routine admit procedure. States inc. thirst and inc. urine. Looks well nourished. Grandmother diabetic. Skin warm, dry; mouth dry. Oriented. States had O.J. for breakfast.
1000	Urine, blood spec. to lab; Voided 200 cc. S & A 2% mod. TPR 99.5-112-20; BP 108/80; Ht. 44 ½" Wt. 42¼ lb. IV started, #22 angio, left hand, TKO D-5-0.45% NS-500 cc. Up and about room. Diet soda, 80 cc.
1100	Admit lab: Blood glucose 450 (65–110 mg/dl); Ketones 250 (↓ 5 mg/dl); Na 137; K 51; Bicarb 18; Cl 97.
1130	Reg Ins. 5u sq
1200	Lunch 75%; 240 cc milk.
1400	Voided 200 cc, Blood glucose 435, ketones 100. Patient Education Coordinator here. Diet Coke 70 cc.
1500	Total IV 100 cc; watching TV; parents here. Reg. Ins. 5u sq; Diet Coke 100 cc. Lung sounds clear, upset about having injections every day.
1600	TPR 99.6–80–20. Dietitian here.
1800	Feeling shaky and hungry Voided 250 cc; blood glucose 65, ketones 10. Dinner 90%; O.J. 240 cc.
2100	Diet Coke 200 cc; Jell-O 120 cc. Voided 250 cc; blood glucose 115, ketones neg.
2200	Diet Coke 180 cc, then sleeping. Total IV 200 cc.

LEG VI-B

4/16	
2300-0700	Slept, afebrile, no oral fluids, 215 cc IV
0400	TPR 97.8–120–18.
0645	Voided 300 cc.
0800	Voided 150 cc; Reg. Ins. 3u sq
	TPR 98.6–100–20; lung sounds clear, states not very hungry.
	No c/o abd. pain, nausea.
	Breakfast: applesauce, 2 bites egg, 240 cc milk.
0900	Tub bath, oral care. Still upset about idea of daily injections.
1030	Voided 200 cc; Reg. Ins. 5u sq.
1200	Lunch 50%, 150 cc juice.
1430	IV dc'd; voided 200 cc; Reg. Ins. 5u sq.
1500	Total IV 160 cc.
1600	TPR 99–100–24; juice 90 cc.
1700	Dinner 95%, Diet Coke 100 cc.
1800	Voided 300 cc.
2000	TPR 98.8–100–24.
2200	Juice 55 cc.
	Voided 300 cc, Reg. Ins. 4u sq.
2300	To bed, feet cold.

6. **Plan** for a clinical experience.

▲ Look for examples of situations in which nursing interventions could be employed. Make notes, and bring them with you to postconference. Compare your observations and discuss your feelings about taking independent action.

▲ Look for signs and symptoms of insulin reaction and diabetic acidosis, either as the primary or secondary cause for admission to the hospital.

▲ Plan for teaching self-care to a patient with either insulin-dependent or non-insulin-dependent diabetes. Determine how long it would take you to teach the patient. Limit the teaching to one aspect of self-care, such as blood testing or self-administration of insulin.

Find out what audiovisual materials are available. How long would it take a patient to learn to use the audiovisual equipment? Figure this into your overall time.

▲ Find out what *nursing time* is worth (financially) per hour or minute. What do patients pay as an hourly rate for nursing care in your hospital?

When you have the answers to all these questions, then you will know approximately what a patient would have to pay if the teaching of self-care by a staff nurse were a separate charge. How would the cost of teaching compare with the cost of medications, lab tests, and physical therapy if it were a separate item on the patient's bill? Compare its value in relation to its cost. Discuss your findings in postconference.

▲ Care for a diabetic patient. Check the diet and medication orders. Find out what the patient eats from each tray and whether the diet is satisfying. Review the complications that are likely and take special measures to prevent complications. What drugs do you find being used to treat complications? Write a nursing care plan and present a summary of your care in postconference.

▲ Look for some patients who have collaborative problems identified on their NCPs. What is the nurse's role? What is the medical care?

C. Extra Added Attractions!

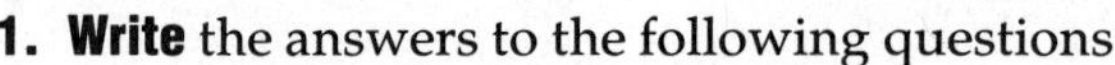

1. **Write** the answers to the following questions:
    - **(a)** Define metabolic acidosis.
    - **(b)** What conditions cause the body to accumulate excess acid?
    - **(c)** How does acidosis occur in diabetes?
2. **Look** ahead to LEG VII-B for more on acidosis.

LEG VI-B

Community Resources

O b j e c t i v e

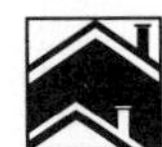 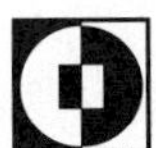 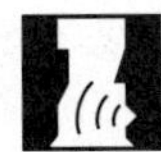

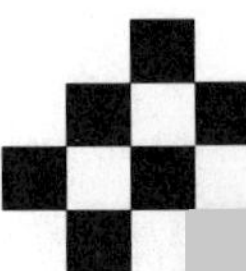

21. Given a list of patient problems, select those that could benefit from or be helped by the American Diabetes Association (ADA).

A. What's It All About?

1. Think about national, state, and local official agencies. What do they do for people? The general public? Patients? Students? Medical professionals? Which agency are you most familiar with? Why?

2. Contact your local branch of the American Diabetes Association. Ask them for their objectives or purpose for being; how they remain solvent; what percentages of moneys go to direct patient services. What services do they provide and at what cost to the patient?

3. Read pamphlets from the ADA and *The ADA Forecast* (bimonthly magazine for diabetics and their families).

B. Putting It into Action!

1. Visit your local ADA office (after making an appointment).

2. Attend special classes for diabetic patients, if any.

3. Match the following (use more than one answer if necessary):

_____ 1. Give daily insulin	(a) ADA (National)
_____ 2. Speaker for civic club meeting	(b) VNA
_____ 3. Treatment of diabetic coma	(c) Local ADA
_____ 4. Provide caloric diabetic menus	(d) Local hospital
_____ 5. Sponsor annual case-finding clinic	(e) Drug companies
_____ 6. Provide educational materials	(f) Pharmacist
_____ 7. Teach patients about foot care	(g) Other
_____ 8. Provide sample blood-testing equipment	
_____ 9. Provide diabetic meals at home	

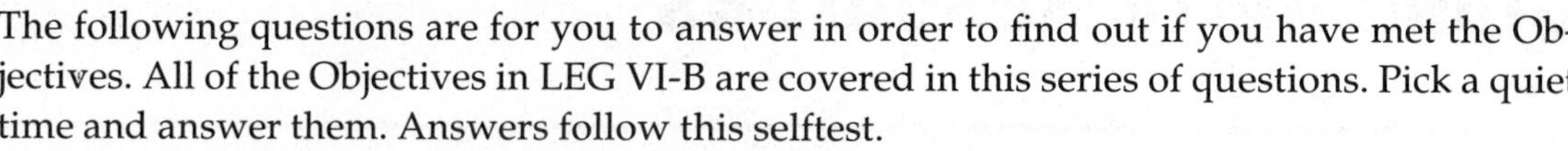

Have I Learned?

LEG VI-B

The following questions are for you to answer in order to find out if you have met the Objectives. All of the Objectives in LEG VI-B are covered in this series of questions. Pick a quiet time and answer them. Answers follow this selftest.

No space has been left for answering the questions related to the "doing" Objectives. Use a separate sheet of paper for your answers and then use the answers in clinical or campus lab for your own evaluation.

Objective **Question**

1 **1.** List three assessments that might indicate that a person is adapting to stress and three that might indicate deficient coping in the presence of any stressor.

2 **2.** Identify at which stage—the alarm reaction, stage of resistance, or stage of exhaustion—the person is in for the following. (You will have to make up some of it if the specific reaction is not stated):

a) Child playing, stubs toe; hurts, bleeds, comes in crying for comfort and first aid.

b) Husband prepares for a particular venture for many weeks; deal falls through; wife notices that her husband is irritable and very tired.

c) Mother has been harassed by a cross, whining child and cries when husband criticizes her burned vegetables.

3 **3.** Which steps of the nursing process are *not* covered in the charting below?

Bath; special skin care; rubbed area over coccyx. Positioned on left side. Very quiet today. Said she did not sleep well. Awake, wondering how she can manage at home. Suggested social worker visit to help arrange for some care during first week at home.

4 **4.** Which of the following statements are true about insulin and which true about glucagon? Mark each with an *I* or a *G*.

(a) It is produced in the pancreas by the alpha cells in the islets of Langerhans.

(b) It is released when the blood sugar level falls, such as after several hours without eating.

(c) It helps convert glucose to glycogen for storage.

(d) It is produced in the pancreas by the beta cells in the islets of Langerhans.

(e) It stimulates moving glucose out of the bloodstream and into the cells.

(f) It helps convert glycogen to glucose in the liver in order to raise the blood sugar level.

(g) It promotes all processes that lower the blood sugar level.

(h) It is released by the islets when the blood sugar level is high, such as after eating.

(i) It promotes a rise in the blood sugar level when the glucose level in the blood drops too low, such as after skipping a meal.

5 **5.** Imagine hearing the following statements by a patient or friend. Write true or false in front of each statement.

(a) Insulin-dependent diabetes usually appears after the age of 30.

(b) The non-insulin-dependent diabetic often has a family history of diabetes.

(c) Obesity will often cause symptoms of non-insulin-dependent diabetes.

(d) The symptoms of non-insulin-dependent diabetes are less severe than those of insulin-dependent diabetes.

(e) An infection, stress, or pregnancy can create excessive demands for insulin and cause symptoms of non-insulin-dependent diabetes to appear.

(f) People with non-insulin-dependent diabetes must take insulin regularly.

(g) Insulin-dependent diabetics can stop taking insulin when they increase their exercise and reduce their weight.

(h) Insulin-dependent diabetics must follow a prescribed diet carefully and must usually have more than three feedings a day.

(i) Non-insulin-dependent diabetics must take insulin the rest of their lives.

(j) Hyperglycemia is a problem for both insulin-dependent and non-insulin-dependent diabetics.

(k) Vascular problems can affect the coronary and peripheral arteries, the kidneys, and the eyes in both insulin-dependent and non-insulin-dependent diabetes.

6 **6.** Match the following lists (one answer only):

_____ 1. Carbohydrate metabolism inefficient	(a) Polyuria
	(b) Polydipsia
_____ 2. Kidneys attempt to dilute urine	(c) Polyphagia
_____ 3. Ingested food cannot be utilized	(d) Hyperglycemia
	(e) Glycosuria
_____ 4. Hormone lacking that changes glucose to glycogen for liver storage	(f) Hypoinsulinism
_____ 5. High blood sugar "spills" into urine	
_____ 6. Dilution of urine may cause dehydration	

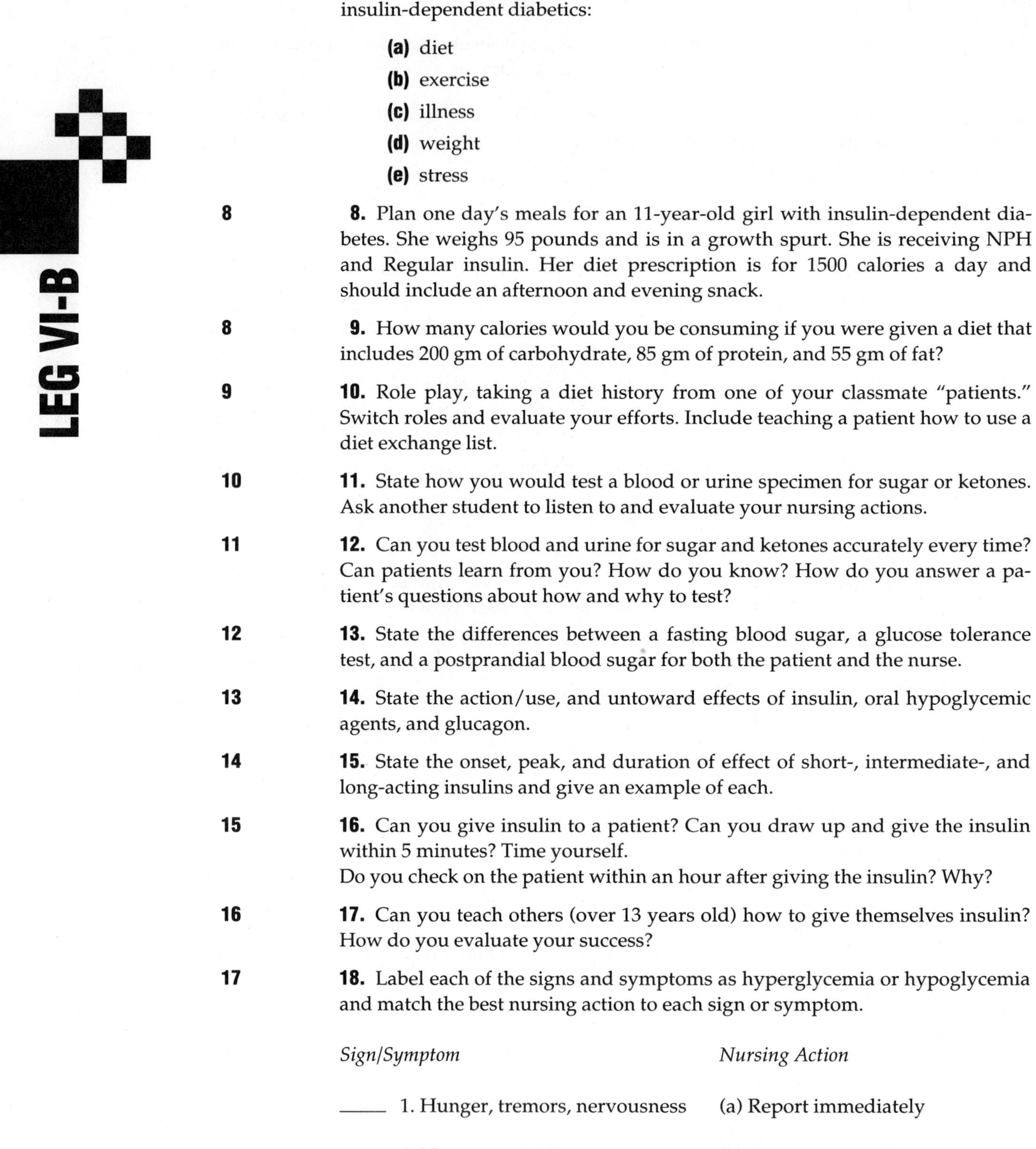

7 **7.** Describe the effect the following have on insulin-dependent and non-insulin-dependent diabetics:

- **(a)** diet
- **(b)** exercise
- **(c)** illness
- **(d)** weight
- **(e)** stress

8 **8.** Plan one day's meals for an 11-year-old girl with insulin-dependent diabetes. She weighs 95 pounds and is in a growth spurt. She is receiving NPH and Regular insulin. Her diet prescription is for 1500 calories a day and should include an afternoon and evening snack.

8 **9.** How many calories would you be consuming if you were given a diet that includes 200 gm of carbohydrate, 85 gm of protein, and 55 gm of fat?

9 **10.** Role play, taking a diet history from one of your classmate "patients." Switch roles and evaluate your efforts. Include teaching a patient how to use a diet exchange list.

10 **11.** State how you would test a blood or urine specimen for sugar or ketones. Ask another student to listen to and evaluate your nursing actions.

11 **12.** Can you test blood and urine for sugar and ketones accurately every time? Can patients learn from you? How do you know? How do you answer a patient's questions about how and why to test?

12 **13.** State the differences between a fasting blood sugar, a glucose tolerance test, and a postprandial blood sugar for both the patient and the nurse.

13 **14.** State the action/use, and untoward effects of insulin, oral hypoglycemic agents, and glucagon.

14 **15.** State the onset, peak, and duration of effect of short-, intermediate-, and long-acting insulins and give an example of each.

15 **16.** Can you give insulin to a patient? Can you draw up and give the insulin within 5 minutes? Time yourself.
Do you check on the patient within an hour after giving the insulin? Why?

16 **17.** Can you teach others (over 13 years old) how to give themselves insulin? How do you evaluate your success?

17 **18.** Label each of the signs and symptoms as hyperglycemia or hypoglycemia and match the best nursing action to each sign or symptom.

Sign/Symptom	*Nursing Action*
_____ 1. Hunger, tremors, nervousness	(a) Report immediately
_____ 2. Nausea, vomiting, abdominal pain	(b) Give 3 sugar cubes or 4 oz juice
_____ 3. Fruity breath odor	(c) Prepare for emergency IV, fluids, insulin, glucose
_____ 4. Dizziness, headache, blurred vision	(d) Prepare for emergency IV glucose

_____ 5. Thirst, parched tongue

_____ 6. Kussmaul breathing

_____ 7. Soft eyeballs, coma

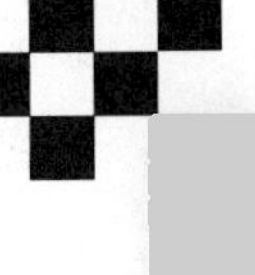

17 **19.** Look at the patient descriptions in A.6, Objectives 17–20 (pp. 63–64). Which of the patients might develop ketoacidosis? State why.

17 **20.** Which of the above patients already shows signs and symptoms of ketoacidosis and what are they?

17 **21.** What treatment will you anticipate these patients needing immediately?

18 **22.** Why are complications (for example, infections, visual disturbances, vascular problems) likely to occur in patients with diabetes mellitus? How can they be prevented or eased? (Include teaching the patient and specific nursing care.)

19 **23.** Write a nursing care plan for a patient with diabetes. Include a teaching plan.

20 **24.** List two physiologic effects of diabetes that can affect the sexual pleasure of men and women and state how the nurse can be helpful.

21 **25.** Indicate which of the following functions apply to the American Diabetes Association:

a. Publishes a magazine
b. Administers insulin
c. Provides foot care
d. Provides diabetic food exchange lists
e. Gives emergency care for diabetic coma or insulin reaction
f. Provides teaching materials for patients about care of feet
g. Provides educational materials to patients
h. Carries out research on diabetes mellitus
i. Provides educational materials for professional educators
j. Provides antidiabetic drugs for patient use

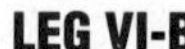

Answers to Have I Learned?

LEG VI-B

1. *Physiologic behaviors:* changes in respiratory, circulatory, or nervous system. Occur automatically (autonomically) to compensate for the problem; slow down body needs until correction can be affected; produce faintness and thus avoidance of danger; reduced movement for healing.

Psychologic behaviors: previous experiences, childhood training, personality, cultural values, all affect the psychologic or emotional reactions to stress. Some reactions may be very exaggerated (e.g., stoic or highly emotional response).

Assessment of *adaptive coping* would show that the patient is able to keep distress at a manageable level, will maintain self-esteem, and will be able to maintain a cooperative relationship.

Deficient coping behaviors include smoking, drinking alcohol, taking actions that push people away, depression, suicide.

2. **(a)** *Child's* first reaction is the alarm reaction; recognizing the hurt and injury then going for help and comfort is the resistance phase. As she responds to comforting and first aid, she can again go out to play while her physiologic forces take over. She will not reach the exhaustion phase.

(b) *Husband's* disappointment, perhaps anger, is his alarm reaction. His wife notices it as irritability and fatigue; whether his own inner forces are strong enough to combat these destructive feelings, combined with his wife's ability to take supportive action in response to his irritability, will decide whether the resistance phase will be adequate or whether this man will need to have more intensive intervention because of the stage of exhaustion (e.g., gastrointestinal symptoms or mental illness).

(c) *Mother* probably recognizes that some small alarms probably did go off during the day and that was the time of resistance; the response to the criticism indicates the stage of exhaustion.

3. Nursing assessment was missing. Assessment of skin and evaluation of interventions are missing. There was also no assessment of or intervention for lack of sleep.

4. *Insulin:* **(c)**, **(d)**, **(e)**,**(g)**,**(h)**.
Glucagon: **(a)**, **(b)**, **(f)**, **(i)**.

5. **(a)**, **(f)**, **(g)**, **(i)** are false. All the rest are true.

6. 1 **(d)**, 2 **(a)**, 3 **(c)**, 4 **(f)**, 5 **(e)**, 6 **(b)**.

7. **(a)** *Diet:* Anorexia, infrequent eating, or not eating all the food prescribed can cause an insulin reaction for patients who are taking insulin or oral hypoglycemic agents. Overeating can cause the reverse problem and create symptoms of hyperglycemia.

(b) *Exercise:* More exercise than usual (tennis for a non-tennis player) burns up carbohydrate, and thus leaves an excess of insulin in the insulin-dependent diabetic unless extra food is given. Less exercise than usual does the reverse.

(c) *Illness:* Causes more stress on the body, burning more glucose and requiring more insulin. The likelihood of ketoacidosis is great in insulin-dependent diabetics.

(d) *Weight:* Obesity increases the demand for insulin and can cause symptoms to occur in the non-insulin-dependent diabetic. These symptoms will disappear when the weight returns to normal.

(e) *Stress:* Stress increases the demand for insulin in the same fashion as illness and weight. It can cause symptoms to appear in the non-insulin-dependent diabetic also and create problems of hyperglycemia.

8. Compare your diet with another student's. Add up the calories and see if they equal 1500 and are distributed so that 50 percent are from carbohydrates, 20 percent from protein, and 30 percent from fat.

9. 1635 calories.

10. Evaluate your success with at least one other student.

11. Evaluate your success with at least one other student.

12. Evaluate your success with at least one other student.

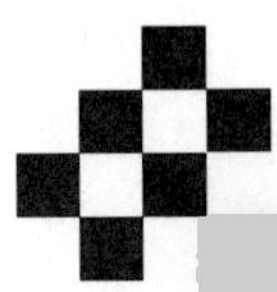

13. *FBS:* tell patient no food after midnight the morning of test; short hold on breakfast until blood drawn. Be sure that patient receives breakfast right after sample of blood is taken. Do not restrict fluids. Nurse must request lab test and be sure that diet is given after test.

GTT: no food after midnight before test; tell patient; blood sample drawn (nurse must have sent request to lab); urine sample taken (tell patient). Administer a drink of glucose proportionate to body weight. Samples of blood and urine taken at 1/2-hour intervals, 1 hour, and 2 hours after ingestion of glucose mixture. Nurse must be sure lab samples are taken. Time schedule must be written down and checked off.

Postprandial: to test blood sugar after meals usually 1–2 hours. Note time patient finishes meal. Notify lab.

LEG VI-B

14.

	Action	Use	Untoward Effect
Insulin	catalyst in metabolism	coma, severe to moderate diabetes	hypoglycemia, nervousness, local skin reactions
Oral hypoglycemic agents	increase secretion of insulin	mild, uncomplicated diabetes	GI upset, weakness
Glucagon	increases glucose concentration in blood	hypoglycemia	nausea and vomiting

15.

		Onset	Peak Effect	Duration
Short-acting	Regular	1/2–1 hr	2–4 hr	6–8 hr
Long-acting	PZI	4–8 hr	12–24 hr	over 30 hr
Intermediate-acting	NPH	1–2 hr	8–12 hr	18–24 hr

16. Evaluate yourself with at least one other student.

17. Evaluate yourself with at least one other student.

18. *Hyperglycemia:* 2, 3, 5, 6, 7.
Hypoglycemia: 1, 4.
(a) for all of them. 1 **(b)**, 2 **(d)**, 3 **(c)**, 4 **(b)**, 5 **(c)**, 6 **(d)**, 7 **(c)**.

19. Martha Baker, Marilyn Popula, and Roger Robust are all candidates for ketoacidosis if they become hyperglycemic because they are insulin-dependent diabetics.

Robert Worldson and Madge Sommer are non-insulin-dependent diabetics and can also develop hyperglycemia, but probably not ketosis because their bodies do produce small amounts of insulin.

20. Marilyn Popula has hot, dry skin, her urine tests orange, or positive for sugar, she is drowsy, her breath has an acetone odor, and she has Kussmaul respirations.

Roger Robust has Kussmaul respirations.

Robert Worldson has flushed dry, hot skin and rapid, weak pulse, and is semiconscious.

21. All need insulin to reduce the high blood sugar level.

All need fluid and electrolyte replacement to reduce the severe dehydration.

All need close observation for cardiac irregularities due to potassium imbalance.

22. *Infections:* Tissues heal slowly (circulatory problems). Prevent skin breakdown. Care for toenails, avoid cutting, use professional foot care. Avoid injury. Evaluate extremities for adequate circulation.

Visual disturbances: Circulatory problems cause retinopathy. Careful control of the disease prevents or slows this. Use care to prevent accidents from falling, stumbling into objects, and so on.

Vascular problems: Atherosclerosis of coronary arteries and other arterial changes. Changes may be reduced by careful control of the disease. The vascular problems contribute to all other complications. Meticulous cleanliness, proper-fitting shoes, rest, and exercise all play a part in keeping complications to a minimum. Plan your teaching with these facts in mind. Remember that patients are most willing to comply with instructions when they understand why!

23. Share your nursing care plan in postconference or turn in to your instructor.

24. *Effects on men:* Decreased libido, impotence.

Effects on women: Decreased ability to experience orgasm, dyspareunia if frequent vaginal infections (yeast).

Nurse's role: Assess whether problem exists, refer to community resource for help, teach patients how to keep diabetes under better control to prevent neurologic and vascular complications.

25. a, d, f, g, h, i.

What Will I Learn?

LEG VI-C Respiratory Problems

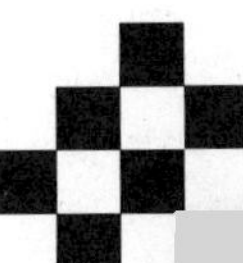

LEG VI-C

It is difficult to pick up a magazine or look at television without seeing something about air pollution, smoking, or cough remedies. We are surrounded with and very much aware of **respiratory problems** almost every day of our lives. Who in your immediate vicinity, this very minute, is coughing or sneezing or breathing noisily? When did you last cough or blow your nose?

Diseases involving the respiratory system have been known and treated for centuries. However, it is only recently that improved equipment has made it possible to measure accurately the blood components and test the air exchanged by our lungs with such precision that many patients who formerly might have died with respiratory problems have been rehabilitated and are alive today. In addition, advances in the field of inhalation therapy have made equipment available to deliver carefully measured quantities of gases, humidity, and medications that literally reach into the respiratory tract to search out and treat the problem.

In this LEG you will learn to recognize a need for oxygen and how a variety of respiratory problems can make the simple act of breathing a chore. The ability of the lung tissue to expand and contract and the presence of liquid secretions can be both a help and a hindrance to patients. Tightly contracted or swollen respiratory passages, thick, sticky secretions, and fluid or dead air filling the air sacs, where the oxygen and carbon dioxide exchange takes place, can put a life in jeopardy. How can you alleviate these problems and the resultant respiratory distress by your nursing care? How do you know which medications and treatments will help the patients in time of emergency? Only a knowledgeable nurse can make effective *decisions.* This LEG will lead you to the knowledge and give you some trial situations in which you can apply that knowledge to patients in respiratory distress as you study your first **Body System.**

This is a long LEG with many "write" experiences. As you progress through the LEG, you will find that you can complete some without having to research the answers because you will have studied the material for an earlier Objective. The repetition is intentional so that by the end of the LEG you have a good basic understanding of the principles of respiratory care and what your nursing assessments and goals should be. Answer what questions you can; then attend a group discussion for sharing. This approach will make the best use of your time.

What's Ahead in Later LEGs

LEG VII-B Fluid and Electrolyte Balance during Illness

LEG X-A Lung Cancer

LEG XII-C Acute Surgical Respiratory Problems and Tracheostomy Care

LEG XIII-C Teaching Parents of Cystic Fibrosis Child

Overview of Learning Experiences in LEG VI-C

LEG VI-C

Objectives	Campus Lab/ Self-Practice	Group Discussions/Lectures	Clinical Lab Focuses
Assessing and Preventing Respiratory Problems			
1. Factors predisposing to respiratory problems **2.** Recognizing hypoxemia and hypercapnea **3.** Respiratory assessment **4.** Analyzing data and making a nursing diagnosis **5.** Respiratory infection control	**B3.** Physical assessment of the lungs	**B2.** Physical assessment of patients with alterations in respiratory function	**B4.** Observe and assist R.T. doing chest and lung assessment Do a chest and lung assessment; check with instructor Observe patients with low O_2, high CO_2 levels Identify measures used to decrease spread of respiratory infection Institute some measures to decrease spread
Diagnostic Tests and Nursing Responsibilities			
6–8. Diagnostic tests and nursing responsibilities **9.** Arterial blood gases related to respiratory acidosis and alkalosis		**B1.** Respiratory diagnostic tests	**B2.** Care for patients with respiratory problems Care for patients before or after diagnostic tests Observe in pulmonary function lab Look for patients who are collecting sputum specimens Use oximeter to measure O_2 sats
Relieving Respiratory Distress			
10. Rationales for medical treatment of respiratory problems **11.** Aerosol medication and nose drops **12.** Drugs used for respiratory problems	**B1.** Postural drainage, clapping, vibrating Teaching breathing exercises Respiratory medications, inhalers Effective cough technique		**B2.** Patient with a metered dose inhaler Give medications to patients with respiratory distress Observe respiratory therapist Teach abdominal breathing exercises
Respiratory Alterations			
13. Nursing process with respiratory problems **14.** Understanding and intervening in respiratory alterations **15.** Effects of aging **16.** Taking action in respiratory distress		**B1.** Nursing process for patients with respiratory problems GES Objective 14	**B2.** Care for patients with alterations in respiratory function Care for child with cystic fibrosis Care for a patient with COPD. Write a NCP that includes teaching and discharge planning

Overview of Learning Experiences in LEG VI-C (cont.)

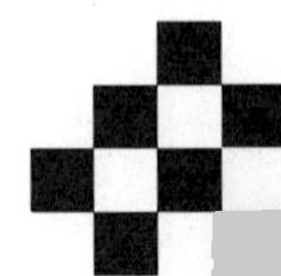

Objectives	Campus Lab/ Self-Practice	Group Discussions/Lectures	Clinical Lab Focuses
Using the Nursing Process for Common Problems Occurring with Respiratory Alterations **17.** Emotions involved in respiratory distress **18.** Cough and control **19.** Abnormal sputum **20.** Hostility related to respiratory distress **21.** Causes of fatigue and nursing interventions **22.** Dealing with anorexia		**B1.** Caring for and teaching chronically ill respiratory patients GES Objectives 17, 21	**B2.** Care for patients with respiratory problems; write a NCP and a process recording Visit community agencies Interview patients regarding cough problems and solutions. Teach relaxation techniques and effective coughing techniques Observe home health nurses caring for patients with chronic respiratory problems
Patients Receiving Oxygen and Humidity **23.** Oxygen and humidity **24.** Child in a croupette	**B1.** Oxygen equipment	**B2.** Caring for a child requiring oxygen therapy	**B3.** Observe or give care to patients receiving oxygen or humidity Care for children in croupettes Check oxygen concentration in an isolette with an O_2 analyzer Observe use of ultrasonic nebulizers or micromists
Observations for Obstructed Airway **25.** Observations for an obstructed airway **26.** Report on a child with croup		**B1.** Children with laryngotracheobronchitis	**B2.** Care for patient with upper or lower respiratory infection Review Clinical Performance Expectations
Tracheostomy Care (EAO) **27, 28.** Tracheostomy care	**B1.** Tracheostomy care and cleaning		**B3.** Observe or care for patient with tracheostomy
Intradermal Injections (EAO) **29.** Intradermal injection	**B1.** Giving intradermal injections	GES Objective 29	**B2.** Observe in allergy or immunization clinic Give intradermal injections

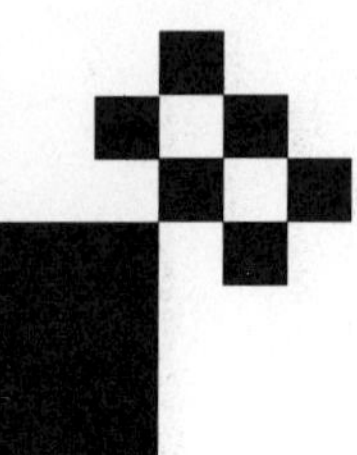

LEG VI-C

New Terms

- adventitious
- anaphylactic
- anoxia
- apnea
  - central
  - obstructive
  - pathologic
  - prematurity
- asphyxia
- atelectasis
- biopsy
- bronchospasm
- circumoral
- compliance
- cyanosis
  - central
  - peripheral
- effusion
- emboli
- epistaxis
- expectorate
- fremitus
- hemoptysis
- hypoxemia
- hypoxia
- infarction
- kyphosis
- narcosis
- oropharyngeal
- perfusion
- phlegm
- pleural rub
- predispose
- rhinorrhea
- stridor
- ventilation

Abbreviations

- ABGs
- CO_2
- COLD
- COPD
- H_2CO_3
- HCO_3
- Ig
- IgE
- PaO_2
- pH
- PND
- SaO_2
- $\dot{V}/\dot{Q}$

Assessing and Preventing Respiratory Problems

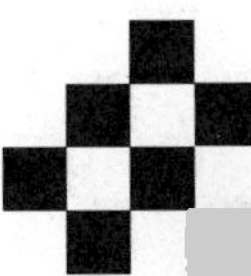

Objectives

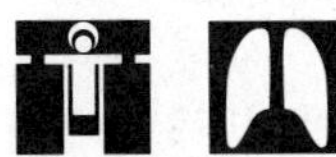

1. Given patient situations, identify those factors that predispose patients to respiratory problems (for example, receiving morphine, aspiration, air pollution).

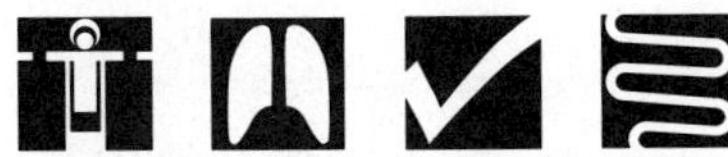

2. Given a patient situation, select those signs and symptoms that indicate the patient is experiencing hypoxemia and/or carbon dioxide retention (hypercapnea.)

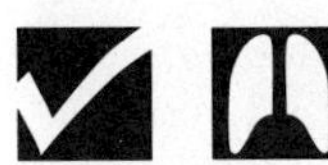

3. Demonstrate doing a physical assessment that includes lung sounds of a patient with alteration in respiratory function.

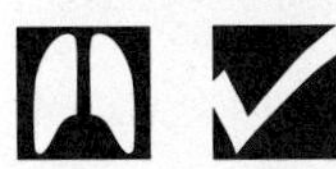

4. Given a patient situation, choose from a list of nursing diagnosis statements the one that fits the description of the patient.

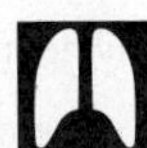

5. List three nursing measures designed to decrease the spread of respiratory infections in the hospital.

A. What's It All About?

1. Think about being able to "see inside" the lungs. When you learn to recognize the sounds that indicate the presence of secretions or fluid, you will have gained a very important assessment skill. You will need many practice sessions with a variety of patients in order to understand what you are hearing, so don't become discouraged on your first few tries. However, it is essential that you first understand the anatomy and physiology of the respiratory system in order to do an accurate assessment. If you don't understand, it will be difficult for you to recognize the signs, symptoms, and abnormal lab tests of respiratory problems.

LEG VI-C

2. Review:

LEG I-A Medical Asepsis

LEG II-A Nursing Process—Assessment: Observation and Physical Assessment
Assessing and Charting TPRs
Assessing and Charting Blood Pressure

LEG III-C Infection Control

3. Read about the *anatomy and physiology of the respiratory system, normal respiration and ventilation, hypoxia, hypoxemia, hypercapnea, physical assessment of breath sounds, oxygen, carbon dioxide excess, respiratory problems, isolation techniques,* and *nursing diagnoses related to respiratory problems* in medical-surgical, fluid and electrolyte, pediatrics, and fundamentals references. As you read, fill in the answers to the questions in A6–A12.

4. View audiovisuals and read articles and books from a list given you by your instructor or read the following:

Marchionda, K. "Flu Vaccine. Give It, Get It." *RN*, October 1991, pp. 58–64.

5. Preview:

LEG XII-C Acute Respiratory Problems

LEG XIII-C Acute Respiratory Problems of Children

6. Answer the following questions:

(a) List the major risk factors associated with pulmonary disease.

(b) How is a smoking habit documented?
Mr. Hack has been smoking three packs of cigarettes daily for 20 years. How is his smoking history described?

(c) List those people for whom flu vaccine is recommended.

7. Answer these questions.

(a) List and define words you find in your reading that can be used when charting to describe the signs and symptoms that may be seen when performing a physical assessment of the respiratory system.

(b) Fill in the blanks in the following chart to compare obstructive problems:

Assessment	Emphysema	Bronchitis	Asthma
allergy			
smoking			
loss of weight			
barrel chest			
cough			
short of breath			
lung sounds			
sputum			
cor pulmonale			
cyanosis			

8. Answer the following questions.

(a) Describe gas pressures that allow air to flow in and out of the lungs.

At rest:

On inspiration:

On exhalation:

(b) What is the pressure of gas (in mm Hg) at sea level? ______

(c) Gas moves on a gradient from ______ to ______ pressure.

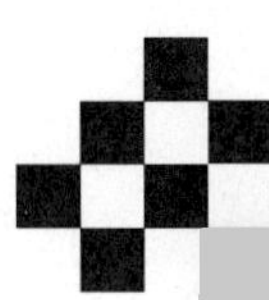

LEG VI-C

9. Fill out the chart below:

	Hypoventilation	Hyperventilation
Definition		
Resp. rate, depth		
CO_2 levels		
Causes		

What normally stimulates respirations?

What stimulates respiration in the COPD patient?

How do you breathe? What does breathing look like?

At what age would the following be normal?

Predominantly abdominal breathing

Both abdominal and costal breathing

Predominantly thoracic breathing

What type of breathing would Baby Barbara in B.3 (p. 88) normally use?

What change occurs in her breathing pattern with respiratory distress?

10. Write out the nursing measures that help to prevent each of the following respiratory problems:

	Predisposing Factors	Preventive Interventions
Atelectasis	1. Mucous plug can develop after anesthesia 2. Immobilization	1. *Example:* encourage a. deep inspirations q2h b. coughing q2h c. increase fluid intake d. turn at least q1h
Pulmonary embolism and infarction	1. Clot can develop in deep veins of legs and travel to lungs while person is immobilized. 2. Postoperative patient may develop phlebitis after discharge	1. *Example:* a. active and passive foot and leg exercises b. support hose c. no pressure on popliteal area
Aspiration pneumonia	1. Newborn taking formula with poor sucking reflex can aspirate 2. Patient with tracheostomy may aspirate 3. Unconscious patient can vomit and aspirate oral secretions 4. Patient with NG tube could aspirate	1. *Example:* cautious feeding of infant—check size of nipple hole and readiness of infant

LEG VI-C

11. Answer the following questions.

(a) List signs of hypoxemia and hypercapnea (carbon dioxide retention). List a variety of causes according to mechanism; for example: respiratory depression, airway obstruction.

	Signs	Causes
hypoxemia		
hypercapnea		

(b) In assessing the oxygenation status of your patient, you could use the following tests:

PaO_2
(partial pressure of dissolved O_2 in blood)

SaO_2
(percentage of O_2 bound to hemoglobin)

Describe each test and write the normal values. How will these normal values change with patient's age?

(c) Hypoxemia can occur in several ways. Identify when each of the following occurs:

	Description	Occurrence
↓ ventilation ↑ perfusion (thickened or destroyed alveolocapillary membranes)		
↓ ventilation ↑ perfusion (impaired blood flow to lung segment)		

(d) How do the following change the ability of hemoglobin to give up or receive O_2?

↓ pH
↑ $PaCO_2$ (partial pressure of CO_2 dissolved in blood)
↑ temperature

When a patient has a PaO_2 of 60, how helpful would it be to increase the oxygen flow rate?

Why is cyanosis a late sign of hypoxemia? What is the PaO_2 likely to be when cyanosis is present?

At what PaO_2 should treatment begin?

What are the causes of hypoxemia with a normal $PaCO_2$ or a low $PaCO_2$?

12. Answer these questions.

(a) List three measures you would take to *prevent the spread* of microorganisms from Mr. Daingero, who is coughing and expectorating a large amount of sputum, to the next patient in the room or to his visitors or nursing personnel.

1.

2.

3.

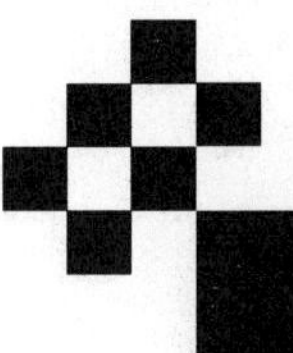

(b) List one additional measure that would be taken if Mr. Daingero were placed on infection-control precautions for a respiratory infection.

1.

(c) List three measures you could take to *protect* Mrs. Suscept, an elderly surgical patient, from being exposed to microorganisms that might cause a respiratory infection.

1.

2.

3.

(d) Which of the above measures are examples of barrier technique (preventing spread of infection)?
Which of the above demonstrate reverse protection techniques (protecting patient from additional microorganisms in the environment)?
Which of the above measures would be examples of independent nursing actions?
Which would require a physician's order?

■ B. Putting It into Action!

1. Underline possible signs of hypoxemia and hypercapnea in the following situations.

Mr. Stober was admitted with a possible myocardial infarction (heart attack). During the afternoon his BP changed from 102/68 to 120/82 and his pulse from 102 to 87. He fell asleep after receiving Demerol for pain. Two hours later he awoke, and when the nurse came in, he was quite restless, asking to get out of bed to void, and complained of a headache. His pulse was 98.

Mrs. Childer was admitted in labor. After several hours of good labor with a BP of 118/76, her blood pressure changed to 96/68. The fetal heart rate had been around 136 and was noted to decrease to 100, and the fetal activity increased. In a short while the fetal activity stopped.

Johnny, age 7, has a congenital heart defect. He was underweight, his color was slightly cyanotic, and he became short of breath when he ran more than three or four steps. His fingers and toes are clubbed. He is often seen squatting when playing with other children.

LEG VI-C

Diane, age 3, comes into the pediatric unit at midnight with acute laryngotracheobronchitis (croup). Her temperature is 102.8 R, her pulse 130, and respirations 32 and shallow. She is using her accessory neck muscles, the larynx is "tugged" down, the sternum is retracting, and her nostrils are flared with each breath. You can hear the stridor, which has a harsh, high-pitched sound with each inspiration.

Mr. Confuder, age 65, had radical neck surgery. During the surgery he lost quite a bit of blood, and several pints were replaced. Following surgery there was sanguinous drainage. He remained lethargic and often appeared confused and unwilling or unable to follow directions. He was reluctant to get out of bed and complained of being tired. His hemoglobin was checked and found to be 10 gm. He was given respiratory therapy and a blood transfusion, and a noticeable change was seen. A delightful personality emerged, and a rapid return to ambulation and recovery was expected.

Mrs. Scolder has chronic lung disease and has had repeated hospital admissions. Her respiratory rate is 28, P 110, and BP 160/90 at rest. Her lips and nails are dusky, and her skin is pale. Her speech is interrupted by labored breaths every few words. She refuses to remain with her feet in bed and insists on dangling them over the side even though her feet and ankles are swollen. She rings her bell constantly, and when the nurse appears, she asks for some item that is within her reach. She speaks crossly to everyone and never smiles. Upon waking from her frequent naps, she complains of a headache.

Lack of oxygen can be due to respiratory or circulatory difficulties, which we will discuss further in this LEG and in LEG VII-C. The signs of oxygen insufficiency are the same, however, regardless of the cause. Learn them! Remember them! When you see a patient exhibiting such behavior, showing the signs, question the cause. Notice the degree of change. Describe it well so that others can also benefit from your observations.

Which of the above patients need *protection from* respiratory infections?

Which might *spread* an infection?

2. Attend a small group discussion on "Physical Assessment of Patients with Alterations in Respiratory Function."

- Come prepared with information about each of the following:

  interview (what questions will you ask?)

  assessment (what physical clues are related to respiratory dysfunction?) Describe the assessment of dyspnea, cough, sputum, chest pain, nails, and breathing patterns.

  auscultation (identify the landmarks for assessing breath sounds; what are the classifications of the four normal breath sounds, and what are the abnormal or adventitious sounds?)

inspection (how should a normal chest appear during inspiration and expiration?)

percussion (how does normal lung tissue sound during inspiration and expiration?)

palpation (what type of information can you obtain from palpation?)

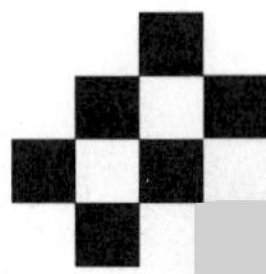

LEG VI-C

■ Which is more serious, absent or diminished breath sounds or loud crackles and gurgles?
When do you hear wheezes or a friction rub?

■ Anticipate the type of breath sounds you might hear in the patients described in B.1.

■ How do the following factors affect your assessment of skin color?

lighting
positioning
temperature of the room
emotional state of the patient

■ Where would you look for the most noticeable changes in color? Describe pallor as it appears in black skin. In brown skin.

■ Discuss some factors that would interfere with assessment. Why is chest assessment important?

■ Compare the three nursing diagnoses used for alterations in respiratory function.

ineffective airway clearance
ineffective breathing patterns
impaired gas exchange

What differences would you see in the assessment data collected? What are the independent nursing measures that you can use?

Name some complications of respiratory illness that require more than nursing assessment and independent action. Would you have to call the doctor to participate in the patient's care? How would you write these potential complications in the NCP?

Could you use any of these nursing diagnoses for the patients in B.1? What information is missing? Which nursing diagnoses are not described?

■ Discuss the effects of hyperventilation and hypoventilation on the body. Begin with the physiology of ventilation and exchange of gases, causes of hyper- and hypoventilation, the resultant symptoms and arterial blood gas analysis results, and what nursing interventions are indicated when each occurs.

■ Invite a respiratory specialist to come to your class as a resource person. Be sure to make an audio or videotape of the presentation and discussion for your reference library. After you have practiced doing an assessment, you will probably want to review the tape as new questions occur to you.

3. Practice in campus lab.

■ Review "Physical Assessment of the Lungs." Go through all the steps so you develop a pattern that you can use with patients. Try to find a student with coryza. Listen to the upper breath sounds. Are there any wheezes or crackles? What other abnormal sounds are present? Write them down and compare your assessment with another student's. Practice charting.

■ Review the following example:

> Baby Barbara, 6 weeks old, was admitted from the ED. She was having continuous coughing episodes and turned cyanotic. Her mother had been using a bulb syringe to suction out large amounts of thick secretions.
> *Diagnosis:* pneumonia.

The nurses caring for her kept the following notes. Chart this information using your own facility forms. Then, using the assessments, review the baby's response to treatment. What more do you want to know? How, in a real situation, could you have gotten this needed information?

0700 PR-149-42 Color pink. On apnea monitor. Mother here.

0730 Coughing spasm. Face cyanotic, suctioned sm amt clear white mucus. Pink. Lung sounds clear. Dr. here. Bld for CBC, ABGs, chest x-ray done.

0800 Ampicillin 200 mg IM and Gentamycin 10 mg IM

0900 TPR 100-171-51. Diaper wet. Isomil 120 cc.

1000 TPR 99^4-164-50. Coughing, suctioned sm amt cl wh mucus. Sm yellow stool.

1100 Coughing, dusky, suctioned, cried lustily.

1130 Coughing, suctioned, color pink. Diaper wet.

1200 TPR 99^3-127-35. Sleeping.

1300 Coughing, cyanotic, circumoral pallor and crowing noises, suctioned, flushed, cried, HR 100, sweat test to lab, throat culture to R/O whooping cough. Postural drainage c̄ suctioning, sm amt cl wh mucus, pink, diaper wet.

1400 TPR 99^3-166-39. Fussy, nursed by mother, color good.

1600 Purple, gagging. Turned upside down, patted between scapula, suctioned c̄ relief. Placed in mist tent c̄ 30% 0_2. Antibiotic order changed. Erythromycin 100 mg p.o. q.i.d. started.

1630 TPR 98^8-94-20. Isomil 45 cc, diaper wet.

1645 PR 146-44. Sleeping.

1700 Choking in sleep. Percussed back, relief.

1800 PR 144-25. Diaper wet.

1900 TPR 99^4-188-36. Coughing, color improved c̄ suctioning. Dr. here. Mother breast-feeding.

2000 P.T. here. Metaproterenol 0.05 in 2.0 cc saline by nebulizer. Coughing s̄ color change. PR 140-46. Lung sounds not cleared. No fever.

2030 Sleeping in tent.

■ Do you know all the abbreviations used? If not, find out what they mean.

■ What is the classification of the drug Metaproterenol? What is the percentage of the solution being administered? Is this a safe dose for Baby Barbara?

■ Describe an apnea monitor.

■ What is Isomil?

■ What would you expect the blood results to be?

■ Describe a mist tent. How does this differ from a croupette?

4. Plan for a clinical experience.

▲ Observe and assist a respiratory therapist doing chest assessments.

▲ Observe for hypoxemia and hypercapnea. Do a physical assessment of the lungs. Identify normal and abnormal lung sounds. Compare your assessment with one done by a staff nurse. Compare your observations with the patient's lab results. Are your observations consistent with the lab findings?

▲ Identify measures being used to decrease the spread of respiratory infection.

▲ Initiate some measures to decrease spread of infection.

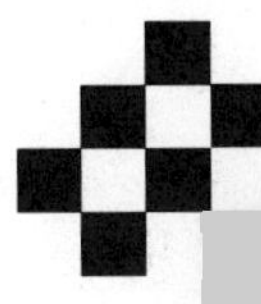

Diagnostic Tests and Nursing Responsibilities

Objectives

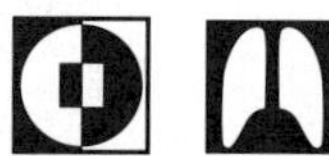

6. Given a list of statements, select one that best describes the purposes for each of the following tests: bronchoscopy, arterial blood gas analysis, thoracentesis, pulmonary function tests, lung scan, oximetry, and tuberculin skin test.

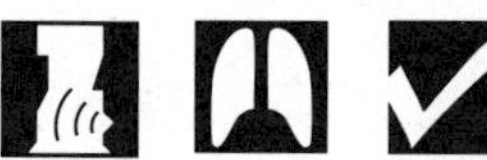

7. State the nurse's primary responsibilities to the patient and family before and after each of the following procedures is performed and the rationale: thoracentesis, bronchoscopy.

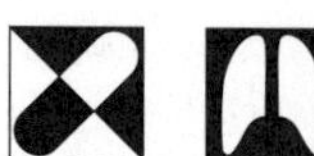

8. In correct sequence, list the actions you would take to collect an early morning sputum specimen prior to beginning a patient on an antibiotic.

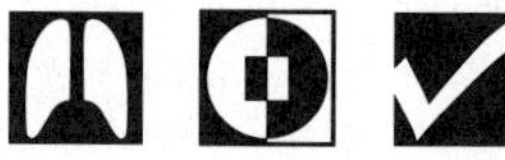

9. Given the results of an arterial blood gas analysis for a patient with alteration in acid-base balance related to impaired gas exchange; state whether the values indicate respiratory acidosis or alkalosis, what accompanying signs and symptoms should be assessed, and what nursing interventions are indicated.

A. What's It All About?

1. Think about what diagnostic tests mean to people with difficult or painful breathing. How can you make these procedures less of an ordeal for your patients? Learn the purpose of each; find out what you are responsible for doing before and after the test; do it and then spend the rest of the time observing and supporting your patient. Also, don't forget that your patient may fear the results.

Think about sputum! What feelings does it raise? Does it remind you of someone always spitting or clearing his throat and sinuses? Is it a pleasant thought? What if someone asked you to save some of your sputum so it could be looked at? Rather personal, eh? Do you recall the embarrassment of walking down a hallway in a doctor's office holding your bottle of urine for the world to see? Well, what if your sputum were in a clear glass jar and you had to take it everywhere with you—to class, out to lunch? Would you have feelings about it? Why? Why are our body secretions and excretions hidden? Yes, it is a learned cultural characteristic. Are patients immune to these feelings about their specimens? No! Think about their privacy. Help them avoid embarrassing situations. *You* take action to make sputum collection less unpleasant.

2. Review LEG III-C, Anxiety and Defense Mechanisms.

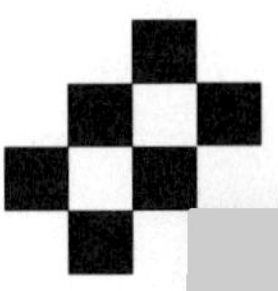

3. Read about *respiratory acidosis and alkalosis, diagnostic tests,* and *preparation of patients for procedures* in laboratory tests, medical-surgical, and fundamentals references.

4. View audiovisuals and read articles and books from a list given you by your instructor or read the following:

Ehrhardt, B. S., and M. Graham. "Pulse Oximetry." *Nursing90,* March, pp. 50–54.

5. Preview:

LEG VII-B Causes of Respiratory and Metabolic Acid-Base Imbalances

LEG XII-C Arterial Blood Gases

6. Apply the Facts about Respiratory Diagnostic Tests to the questions that follow it.

LEG VI-C

Facts about Respiratory Diagnostic Tests

1. Normally, the respiratory center is stimulated by a low oxygen concentration and a high carbon dioxide level in the blood.

2. The body then breathes faster and deeper and exhales the excess CO_2.

3. When the carbon dioxide levels in the blood remain high for long periods of time, the respiratory center becomes insensitive to this stimulus (carbon dioxide narcosis).

4. The kidneys attempt to help by sending out bicarbonate (HCO_3), which neutralizes the CO_2 for a while. The excess CO_2 then combines with H_2O in the blood and becomes carbonic acid (H_2CO_3). The normal blood pH (measurement of acidity) is between 7.35 and 7.45. Higher numbers mean alkalosis, lower numbers indicate acidosis.

5. When the carbon dioxide levels in the blood remain high, the pH of the blood falls below 7.35, and respiratory acidosis results.

6. Analysis of arterial blood gases shows the levels of CO_2, O_2, pH, and HCO_3.

7. Excessive amounts of CO_2 in the blood can cause death and coma.

8. When administering oxygen to a patient, the arterial oxygen level tells whether the oxygen reached the blood.

9. Patients with a high carbon dioxide level should receive only low-flow oxygen. A patient with chronic CO_2 retention must never get a high O_2 concentration (unless on a ventilator continuously).

10. Spirometry measures the amount of air that moves in and out—it measures the volume and capacity of the lungs.

11. Smoking reduces the function and capacity of the lungs.

12. Reduced respiratory function predisposes patients to postoperative respiratory problems.

13. A bronchoscopy allows the physician to look at the bronchus, to remove a small portion of tissue (biopsy) to study, and/or remove secretions or foreign materials.

(a) What two stimuli make us breathe faster and deeper? ____________________

(b) What happens to the excess CO_2 in our bodies? ____________________

(c) What occurs if the lung function is so poor that CO_2 cannot be exhaled, as with emphysema? ____________________

LEG VI-C

(d) How does the doctor know the amount of bicarbonate the kidneys are returning to the bloodstream? ____________

(e) The arterial blood gas measurement lab report returned with the following results. (Write in your hospital laboratory's normal values.)

pO_2	44 mmHg	(normal is______)
pCO_2	66 mmHg	(normal is______)
HCO_3	34 mEq	(normal is______)
pH	7.39	(normal is______)
oxygen saturation	80%	(normal is______)

Is the oxygen level higher or lower than normal? ____________

Is the CO_2 high or low? ____________

What symptoms would you look for if you saw this lab report? ____________

What does pH tell us? Is the patient in respiratory acidosis or alkalosis? ____________

____

What effects do hypo- and hyperventilation have on the acid-base balance? What would cause respiratory acidosis in a patient with poor gas exchange? Which imbalance occurs most frequently? ____________

(f) Complete the chart below.

	Arterial Blood Gas Results	**Signs, Symptoms**	**Goals or Evaluation Criteria**	**Nursing Interventions**
Respiratory acidosis	pH $PaCO_2$ HCO_3			
Respiratory alkalosis	pH $PaCO_2$ HCO_3			

In LEG VII-B you will learn more about the pH and acidosis. These exercises are included to get you started thinking about the subject.

(g) Why are the following tests ordered?

Mr. Dinge, admitted to the hospital for surgery, has a *spirometry* test ordered. He smokes a pack of cigarettes a day. ____________

____

Mrs. Clave, admitted for treatment of emphysema, has become lethargic. Her respirations are slow and shallow. The doctor ordered an *arterial blood gas analysis* to be done. ____________

____

Mr. Webb has complained of coughing for 2 weeks without relief from antitussives. The doctor plans to do a *bronchoscopy* this morning. ____________

____

7. **Write** answers to these questions:

(a) What will you do if the patient is unable to produce a sputum specimen and he has had the specimen cup for 2 days?

(b) How do you know if your patient needs a sputum specimen? Where are the lab slips kept in your hospital? How are they attached to the specimen, and what record is kept of the specimens being sent to the lab? What precautions are used to prevent the spread of infection?

(c) What is the youngest age that a child could be taught to raise sputum for a specimen?

(d) What if there is food or tobacco in the specimen? Do you send it? How are specimens collected when the patient is in isolation?

(e) What do you expect the sputum from a patient with chronic lung disease or with pulmonary edema to look like after a bronchoscopy?

(f) What organisms do you expect to find in the respiratory tract normally? With infection?

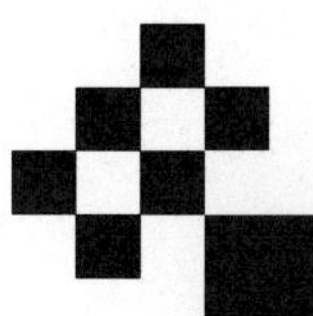

LEG VI-C

■ B. Putting It into Action!

1. **Attend** a small group discussion on "Respiratory Diagnostic Tests."

■ Assume you are the nurse caring for Mr. Webb. His medical orders are:

NPO
Bronchoscopy at 9:30

The postprocedure orders are:

NPO til gag reflex returns
Resume previous orders

Discuss how you would prepare him and his family for this procedure.

■ What specific fears might Mr. Webb have about the procedure or about the results? How can you find out what he already knows and what concerns he has? What specific information do *you* know to give him?

■ How is the patient positioned for this procedure? What medications are used? How does anxiety affect the patient's comfort during the procedure? Try lying flat and clenching your fists. Then relax and breathe through your nose with your mouth open. Could a patient practice this? When should you teach this technique?

■ While Mr. Webb was having his bronchoscopy, the nurse used pulse oximetry to measure O_2 saturation. Why did she do this? What is the acceptable range?

■ How do you observe, describe, and report bleeding? Respiratory distress? How do you know when the gag reflex has returned?

■ How would you feel if you were told you were to have this procedure done tomorrow? What specifically would help you?

■ What is the rationale for each of the pre- and postoperative orders? How will you answer each of Mr. Webb's questions:

Will I be awake?
Will it hurt?
How long will it take?
When will the biopsy report be back?

Am I supposed to be spitting up bloody mucus?

When will I be able to eat?

■ Mr. Ludmilla, age 50, is scheduled for a pulmonary function test (PFT). List two reasons why it could be ordered.
Will the test results be dependent on his size, age, sex?
Write a brief description that you could use to explain the test to Mr. Ludmilla.

The results of the test showed the following: What do they mean?

Tidal volume	700 cc
FEV_1/FVC	80%

If Mr. Ludmilla had COPD, how would these results change?

2. Plan for a clinical experience.

▲ Observe a bronchoscopy. Read the medical orders and patient's history to obtain a complete picture of the reasons for the procedure and nursing care required before and afterward. Compare bronchoscopes with fiberoptic scopes.

▲ Care for patients before or after diagnostic procedures. Learn their reactions and needs. Chart your observations and record your nursing care.

▲ Care for patients with respiratory problems. Look at their charts to find diagnostic test results and compare them with the written observations of the patients' progress in the nursing and medical notes. Ask doctors about additional tests if ordered on their patients.

▲ Observe in a pulmonary function lab while tests are being done on patients. Find out how the test results will affect the patient's medical treatment. Take a pulmonary function test yourself if possible.

▲ Look for patients who are collecting sputum specimens. Look at the date on their lab slip. How old is it?

▲ Read about the reason for their needing a specimen and what medication and treatment they are receiving that might help or hinder their being able to cough up a specimen. What system is used in your clinical agency to cover when an antibiotic is started and stopped? How is this information recorded?

▲ Determine how you might help patients expectorate more easily when having trouble obtaining a specimen. Would forcing fluids help? Evaluate the patient's attitude toward the subject. Write a NCP showing ways of meeting basic needs.

▲ Look at lab slips that have been returned from the lab on sputum specimens. How long does it take to receive a culture and sensitivity report? What information does the sensitivity test give you? What information did the nurse give to the lab along with the specimen?

▲ Care for patients who require pulse oximetry measurements continuously or on a routine basis. Learn how the oximeter works. Who can use it? Who cannot? What do you do when the O_2 Sat drops below an acceptable level?

▲ Observe ABG specimens being drawn. What special procedures are required?

▲ Look at lab slips of patients who have had ABGs. Look for abnormal tests and figure out why they are abnormal. Read the charts to find out what is done to assist patients to adapt and return to normal.

Relieving Respiratory Distress

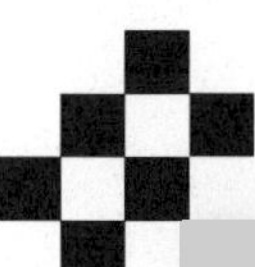

LEG VI-C

O b j e c t i v e s

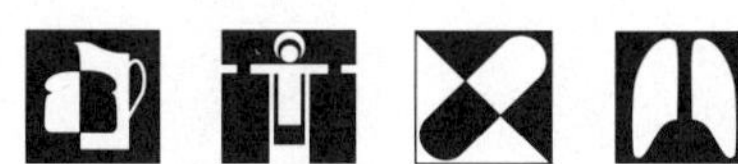

10. Describe the purpose for each of the following medical orders for patients with inadequate pulmonary ventilation due to obstruction, secretions, and/or infections: oxygen, hydration, at least 1500-calorie diet, elevate head of bed, postural drainage, breathing exercises, cold humidification, sputum specimen, and aerosol therapy.

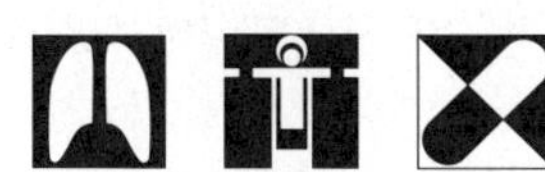

11. Demonstrate and/or describe in writing teaching a person self-administration of an aerosol medication and nose drops in order to obtain the maximum benefit.

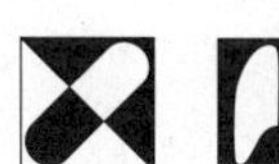

12. For each of the following drug classifications, state the action/use for respiratory problems, method of administration, a major side effect, and the nursing implications: emetic, sedative, bronchodilator, antibiotic, antitussive, expectorant, narcotic, antihistamine, steroid.

■ A. What's It All About?

1. Think about the desperate feeling you would have if you were unable to get adequate breath. Simulate the agony and discomfort. Try breathing with shallow breaths. Use a thick cloth over your mouth. Hold your breath. Imagine the relief medication or treatment could give. Anxiety and fear increase the agony. Patients who have trouble breathing need your help.

2. Talk with people who have chronic breathing problems. What tips can they give you to help your patients? Listen to and observe them as they take their medications and treatment.

3. Read about *COPD,* such as *asthma, emphysema, cystic fibrosis,* and *bronchitis* and about *drugs that affect the respiratory system* in pharmacology, medical-surgical, pediatrics, and geriatrics nursing references. Drug information is packaged with nebulizers containing bronchodilating medication sold over the counter in drugstores. Good instructions on use of nebulizer usually accompany these. Look at the different brands and read what medications they contain. See how many generic names you recognize.

4. View audiovisuals and read articles and books from a list given you by your instructor or read the following:

"Breaking Bronchospasm's Grip with MDIs." *AJN,* March 1990, pp. 34–39.

LEG VI-C

5. Write the answers to these questions as you read articles and chapters in your medical-surgical textbooks on adults and children with respiratory problems.

(a) How are each of these treatments helpful to patients with COPD?

oxygen
hydration
elevate head of bed
at least 1500-calorie diet
postural drainage
breathing exercises

(b) List the reasons patients need humidity and/or intermittent positive pressure breathing (IPPB) and all the possible ways they could receive humidity in the right-hand columns. Then apply this information to the patients in the left-hand column by filling in the number and/or letter from the right-hand columns.

Patients Needing IPPB	*List Reasons for IPPB*	*List Ways to Provide IPPB in the Hospital*
adult with emphysema	1.	a.
adult with atelectasis	2.	b.
	3.	c.
	4.	d.

Patients Needing Humidity	*List Reasons for Humidity*	*List Ways to Provide Humidity in the Hospital*
child with larnygo-tracheobronchitis	5.	a.
	6.	b.
patient with tracheos-tomy	7.	c.
		d.
patient with asthma		e.
child with bronchitis		f.
		List Ways to Provide Humidity at Home
		g.
		h.

B. Putting It into Action!

1. Practice in campus lab.

- Practice postural drainage, clapping, and vibrating for all lobes of the lung.

  Remain in the basic drainage position at the end for 10 minutes. Time yourself and see how long the entire procedure takes. How does the treatment make you feel?

  How will this procedure differ according to the age of the patient? Where will you find information on this procedure in the hospital? Who does it?

- Practice teaching breathing exercises to another person, preferably a smoker. Ask him to assume the role of patient and to ask you questions. What problems do you encounter when teaching someone who has not asked for information or help? Do you need to spend some time just talking about what good will come from doing the exercises and listening to the person's excuses or delaying tactics? Yes, this first step may be the most important in helping a person learn new skills that may help him remain in a better state of health and out of the hospital longer. Think it through now so that you will be ready to go when you have a real patient.

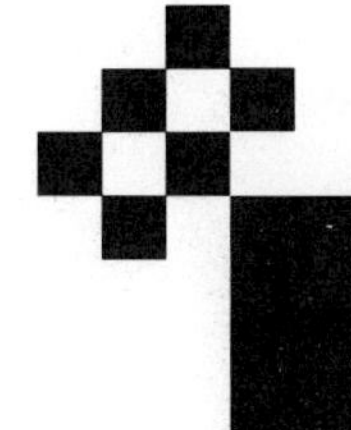

■ Role play teaching a person to use a medihaler or aerosol spray. What problems can arise from the use of bronchodilators? How can you prevent them? How would you recognize them?

If your patient uses both a bronchodilator and a steroid inhaler, which would be used first? How long would you wait to use the second one?

■ Role play teaching a patient with COPD how to cough effectively.

■ Check out self-practice materials "Respiratory Medications." You will find samples of nebulizers like those used in your hospital. Examine them and learn how they work. Practice instructing another person in their use. Become familiar with all the medications and their form. How will each be administered?

2. Plan for a clinical experience.

▲ Find a patient who is experienced with an inhaler and ask to be shown how it is used and how the medication makes the patient feel.

▲ Give medications to patients with respiratory distress.

▲ Accompany a respiratory therapist who is giving inhalation treatments and doing chest physiotherapy. Observe patients with respiratory problems; see how they are instructed about their treatments and how they tolerate them. While you are with the patients, practice your assessments for Objective 2; find out why they have their problems (Objective 1); notice the results of their treatment and what medications are used in the nebulizer (Objective 10). Make the best use of your time to see a variety of respiratory problems. Find out the responsibilities of the respiratory therapist. Make a video or audiotape of the therapist's demonstrations if possible. Find out what hazards are associated with nebulization, humidification, oxygen therapy, and positive pressure ventilation.

▲ Teach abdominal breathing exercises to a patient and family members. Discuss pulmonary irritants that should be avoided and ways to prevent infections and other complications that result from impaired respiratory function.

Respiratory Alterations

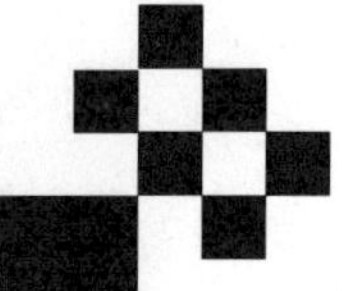

O b j e c t i v e s

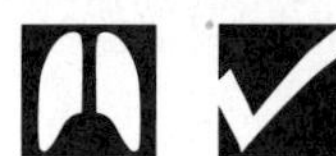

13. Describe respiratory problems that people with chronic obstructive pulmonary disease (COPD) experience, write a nursing diagnosis, and list nursing interventions for each problem including the physiologic cause of the problem.

14. Given a description of a child or adult with an alteration in respiratory function caused by one of the following disorders, explain the pathophysiology of the disorder and describe the nursing process, which includes teaching and discharge planning: influenza, asthma, pneumonia, cystic fibrosis, emphysema, bronchitis, tuberculosis.

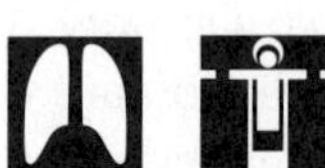

15. Describe the effects of aging on the respiratory system and identify ways to adapt nursing care.

16. Given medications and treatments and descriptions of patients showing respiratory distress, state the best action the nurse could take in each situation and include your rationale and charting.

■ A. What's It All About?

1. Think about how nice it is to be able to breathe automatically, without thinking. Any damage to the lungs increases the work of breathing, so it becomes more noticeable and worrisome as well as increasing susceptibility to infection. Understanding how the lungs are damaged and the effect on oxygen and carbon dioxide levels can help the nurse choose more effective treatments and medications to relieve the patient's distress. Spend some extra time on this section. It will pay off for your patients.

2. Read about *acute and chronic alterations in the respiratory tract, obstructive and restrictive diseases,* and *normal changes with aging* in medical-surgical, pediatrics, and pharmacology references.

3. View audiovisuals and read articles and books from a list given you by your instructor or read from the following:

Madsen, L. "Tuberculosis Today." *RN,* March 1990, pp. 44–51.
Orsi, A. J. "Asthma—The Danger Is Real." *RN,* April 1991, pp. 58–63.

4. Preview:

LEG IX-A Chronic Illness

LEG XII-C Acute Respiratory Problems

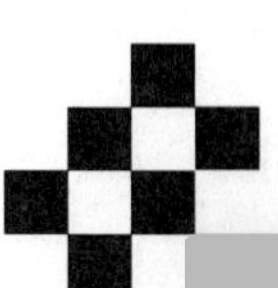

LEG VI-C

5. Answer these questions and bring to your group discussion.

List some characteristics of respirations that would make you believe they were symptoms of respiratory distress.

What is the difference between dyspnea and acute respiratory insufficiency or failure? State the nursing measures you would take for each and why.

6. List some normal alterations of the following types in the respiratory tract that occur with aging.

mechanical

structural

gas exchange

7. Talk with people who have had acute respiratory distress at some time, possibly an uncle with emphysema, a student with asthma, a friend with pneumonia, a mother whose child had an infection. Learn what the person was feeling during the acute period of distress and what actions on the part of others were *helpful:* Maybe having someone around but not talking, maybe playing a radio softly, or maybe being positioned comfortably in order to remain upright for an hour or more were helpful actions. Try to find out what were *harmful* actions, such as someone fussing with the covers and standing around awkwardly, staring at you. Use these bits of information to improve your approach to people in respiratory distress.

8. Look at the patient profiles for the patients described below. Why do you think each medication and treatment is ordered? Name some expected outcomes from the medications. What side effects or untoward effects will you be alert for? What equipment is needed to administer each? Know the answers to these questions before attending the group discussion.

How do the actions of codeine, ammonium chloride, and ipecac change when the dosage is increased? What side effect will codeine have on the intestinal system? How can you prevent this problem? What must you keep in mind when giving bronchodilators to the elderly?

Mrs. Paula Darvy, age 34, became extremely ill at home one evening with chest pains, temperature of 103, and a painful cough. Her husband brought her to the emergency room where she was given oxygen; blood and sputum cultures were taken. She was given an injection of an antibiotic and transferred to her room with a portable oxygen tank and mask.

Patient:	Paula Darvy
Diagnosis:	LLL pneumonia
Orders:	O_2 2–4L prn
	ultrasonic nebulizer tid
	Alupent 0.3 cc in 2 cc NS q4h prn
	D-5-0.45 at 100 cc/h
	Theophylline level, sputum C&S
	Tylenol 600 mg po T >101
	Diet as tol

LEG VI-C

Mr. Anthony Paoli, age 62, was admitted for the fifth time with chronic emphysema. He found it increasingly difficult to climb stairs without becoming extremely short of breath. During his office visit today, the physician suggested he be admitted to the hospital for respiratory monitoring and care.

Patient: Anthony Paoli
Diagnosis: pulmonary emphysema
Orders: Theodur i po 300 mg bid
Lasix 40 mg po bid
ABGs on room air
CXR, PA & lat, chem 16
O_2 2L prn
Albuterol (Ventolin) spray 2 puffs 4 × /d
Teach breathing exercises
Lo salt soft diet
I&O q8h

Tommy Stewart, age 4, has cystic fibrosis. He has been under treatment since he was a few months old. His mother supervises his respiratory treatment at home and is quite adept in helping him perform his postural drainage exercises. He has developed a respiratory infection and is hospitalized for its treatment and prevention of further complications. He is placed in a croupette upon admission.

Patient: Tommy Stewart, age 4
Diagnosis: cystic fibrosis
Orders: Hi cal, hi prot, mod fat diet
Encourage fluids
croupette with humidity
ultrasonic nebulizer 10 min qid with Mucomyst followed by postural drainage qid
sweat test, throat culture
Pancreatin 300 mg po with each meal
Vidaylin gtt 1 cc/d

Darlene Thomas, age 17, has had asthma all her life. She has been hospitalized twice before for acute episodes, associated with infection of her upper respiratory tract. She is angry at being hospitalized as she wants to go away to college in a few weeks and gain more independence from her parents. Now she sees herself as more dependent than ever.

Patient: Darlene Thomas, age 17
Diagnosis: acute asthma, URI
Orders: allergic to dust, feathers
PFT, WBC and diff
Alupent medihaler q3–4h prn
Sus-phine 0.3 cc sq prn dyspnea
Decadron 2 mg po tid × 5da
Cromolyn 20 mg/inhaler q6h
Cefzol gm i q8h IV
Tedrol-25 tab.i po q4h prn dyspnea
Dalmane 30 mg po hs prn

Jane Andrews was hospitalized and, after an AFB sputum culture, was diagnosed as having tuberculosis of the lung. She is being discharged home to her husband and two children, ages 4 and 8. She has been told that she will be taking INH and Rifampin for at least 9 months.

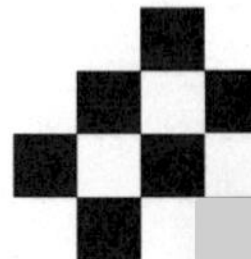

■ B. Putting It into Action!

1. Attend a small group discussion on "Nursing Process for Patients with Respiratory Problems," to simulate actual clinical experiences with the patients described above. Decide what action you would take when each of the following situations occurs and be able to state your rationale.

Chart to include your nursing assessments (using the correct terms), your actions, and the outcomes. Write the charting on the blackboard or below. If your group is large enough, break into six small groups for 10 min and each take a situation to problem solve and write charting for.

It is 10 A.M., and you are in Mr. Paoli's room. He appears to be sleeping quietly, but when you try to waken him for his medications, you cannot arouse him.

It is midnight, and Mr. Paoli is unable to catch his breath. He is sitting up at the edge of the bed gasping for air and coughing.

It is 4 P.M. and Miss Thomas's light goes on. When you arrive, she is leaning over the overbed table wheezing and in obvious distress. She is holding her nebulizer and has just used it as you walk in the door.

It is 8 A.M., and you are in Miss Thomas's room. You notice that she is wheezing slightly and ask her if she has used her nebulizer. She says no. You recall the day before when she required Sus-phrine for a severe attack and are wondering if you should encourage her to either take her Tedral or use her nebulizer now to prevent an attack.

You are to begin Tommy's postural drainage exercises at 9 A.M. The inhalation therapist will be up at 9:30 A.M. to give the IPPB treatment. It is now 7:30 A.M. You are also to help Tommy with his breakfast and give him a bath and care for the bed and croupette. How will you organize your activities? How and when will you offer fluids between 7:30 and noon?

It is 2 A.M., and as you pass Mrs. Darvy's room, you hear a dry, hacking cough. When you go in, you find her sitting upright in bed coughing. She says she is hot and asks you to turn the air conditioning up.

Charting:

LEG VI-C

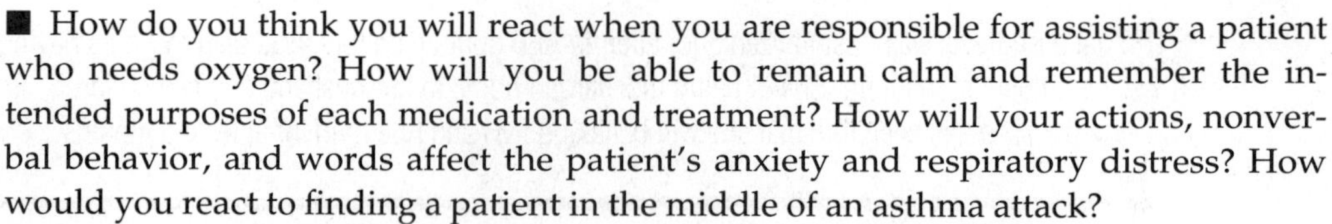
■ How do you think you will react when you are responsible for assisting a patient who needs oxygen? How will you be able to remain calm and remember the intended purposes of each medication and treatment? How will your actions, nonverbal behavior, and words affect the patient's anxiety and respiratory distress? How would you react to finding a patient in the middle of an asthma attack?

LEG VI-C

■ Which of the patients could be safely placed in a room together? (Disregard age and sex for a moment and think about infection precautions.)

■ What abnormal breath sounds do you think you would hear with each patient?

■ Imagine that Paula Darvy is an 8-year-old with pneumococcal pneumonia. How would the symptoms differ? What major problems would be present and what assessments would you expect to make? Which nursing goals and interventions would be the same and which different because of age?

■ What are the major areas of teaching that would be important for each patient with disease conditions listed in Objective 14?

■ What economic, social, and emotional pressures are these patients and their significant others having to cope with? How could discharge planning help them?

■ Role play assessing the learning needs of Mr. Paoli, Tommy Stewart's mother, and Jane Andrews (described on page 101). Make a teaching plan and practice teaching about one of the identified needs. Be sure to set expected outcomes for them.

■ Discuss the nursing care of a patient with COPD.

What learning needs may be present?

Who will initiate teaching abdominal breathing and resistive breathing exercises? Should the wife or husband be present for the teaching sessions?

How will you explain the value of walking and breathing exercises to the patient and spouse? Role play some examples of teaching.

Anticipate the nursing care you would give to this patient between 7 A.M. and 3 P.M. Use a blackboard, listing in time sequence your nursing actions, rationales, and observations for the day. Take turns adding to the list.

2. Plan for a clinical experience.

▲ Care for patients with the alterations in respiratory function listed in Objective 14. Write a nursing care plan for your patient that includes teaching and discharge planning. Include family members; assess learning needs, including any prior instruction in pulmonary hygiene, medications, and what advice is given if an emergency occurs in the home.

▲ Care for a child with cystic fibrosis. Talk with the family and find out what health measures are being followed at home to prevent infections and provide for respiratory drainage. What medications are being administered either orally or by aerosol to thin the secretions? How is the family coping emotionally with this problem?

▲ Care for a patient with COPD. Complete a data base form and nursing care plan that includes teaching and discharge planning. Use forms in "To the Student" or one provided by your instructor. Include the family if possible.

▲ Look for, study, and care for patients with a diagnosis of asthma, chronic bronchitis, COPD, cor pulmonale, croup, emphysema, pleural effusion, and tuberculosis.

C. Extra Added Attraction!

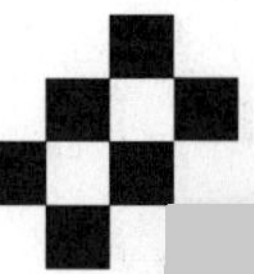

1. Give two examples of each of the following alterations in respiratory function.

(a) ventilation-perfusion mismatch

(b) shunting

(c) impaired diffusion

(d) depression of CNS

(e) neuromuscular disorders

(f) chest wall abnormalities

(g) obstructive disease

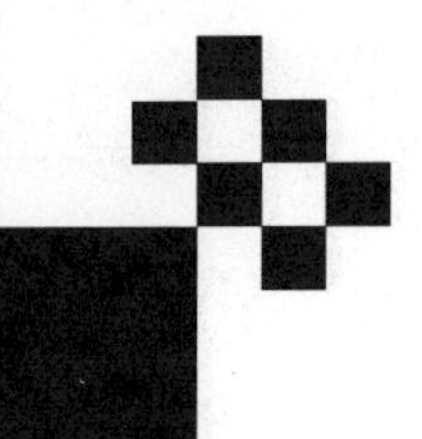

LEG VI-C

Using the Nursing Process for Common Problems Occurring with Respiratory Alterations

Objectives

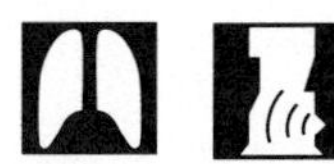

17. Describe how emotions affect respiratory distress.

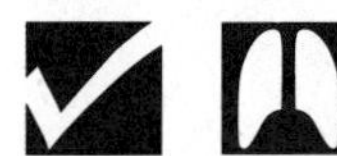

18. List measures that will increase the productivity of a cough or that will help control an irritating, nonproductive cough.

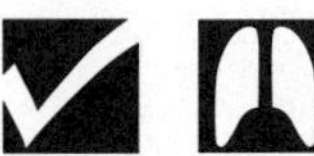

19. Given a situation in which a patient expectorates abnormal sputum, select from a list of possible actions the best ones to take and state your rationale.

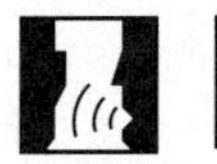

20. Describe positive interventions a nurse could use with a patient with hostility related to impaired respiratory function.

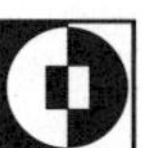

21. Given a patient experiencing fatigue related to dyspnea, demonstrate or describe in writing teaching the patient and family ways to save energy while enabling the patient to meet his own daily needs and maintain the highest possible level of wellness.

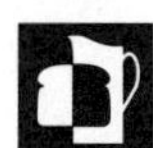
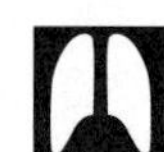

22. Given a patient experiencing anorexia related to dyspnea, coughing, and expectoration, describe two measures to increase interest in food and intake of food and fluid.

■ A. What's It All About?

1. Think about how you'd feel if you were dyspneic. Ask some people who have had asthma or emphysema to describe their feelings. Try these for starters: fear, anxiety, fatigue, worry, anger, and hostility. You have much to do to help a person who is overwhelmed with respiratory problems. Anticipate the feelings and take whatever nursing actions are indicated. These patients should not have to ask for help.

How many kinds of coughs have you heard? Dry, hacking, deep, productive, nonproductive? All are tiring and unpleasant for both patient and contacts. The trick is to help the patient get rid of the cough and its cause as quickly and as efficiently as possible. Your goal is to increase the productivity of the cough and yet prevent fatigue and irritation from it.

2. Read about nursing care of patients with *dyspnea, cough, fatigue, anorexia,* and *hostility* in medical-surgical, pediatrics, psychiatric nursing, psychology, and pharmacology references.

3. View audiovisuals and read articles and books from a list given you by your instructor or read the following:

Antai-Otong, D. "Dealing with Demanding Patients." *Nursing89*, January, pp. 94–95.

4. Answer the following questions:

(a) List the changes that occur in your breathing when you become anxious.

(b) List actions a nurse could take to:

Help a patient have confidence that a nurse will be available when assistance is needed.

Reduce anxiety during acute respiratory distress.

(c) How does taking a deep breath affect the bronchi? What effect does pursed-lip breathing have on the bronchioles and the respiratory rate? Which breathing exercises include pursed-lip breathing?

(d) List all the measures you know that will help to liquefy a patient's secretions and increase expectoration. Which can be used at home and need to be taught to the patient and family members? Which involve special equipment?

(e) List all the nursing measures you can find to help a patient who is experiencing a constant, unproductive cough that is exhausting him and irritating his family when he is at home. What measures can be taught and used at home?

(f) List all the nursing actions you might take when discovering any of the following types of sputum. Then write the numbers of the actions you would take with each type of sputum.

Sputum	*Nursing Actions*
rusty-colored, thick ________	1. *Example:* Observe patient for dyspnea, color, skin, temperature.
purulent, light-green ________	2.
thick yellow ________	3.
thin, frothy, excessive streaks of bright red ________	4.
dark-red clots, bright-red liquid ________	5.
	6.

5. List the problems that you imagine a patient, as described in Objectives 21 and 22, would have with daily needs (e.g., dry mouth, which might decrease appetite). Across from each problem briefly state the nursing interventions that might alleviate each problem. For example:

Problem	*Nursing Solutions*
Difficulty bending over to tie his or her shoes.	Exhale first, then bend down.

List additional problems that would be present if the patient were an infant or toddler.

Why would an asthmatic person, after experiencing dyspnea all night, complain of nausea, vomiting, and abdominal discomfort?

Why is dyspnea likely to be increased for the malnourished patient?

What are the "dyspnea positions"?

Imagine you were caring for an infant in a croupette with an IV going in the scalp vein, restrained on his back. You are instructed to feed the child. What precautions do you take? What if the infant begins to vomit?

List some long-term and short-term goals to use when caring for a patient expressing hostility.

Long-Term Goals	*Short-Term Goals*

Which goals are for the patient? Which are for you? What behaviors should the nurse use?

How can the patient achieve the goals listed above?

Comments on Patients Expressing Hostility

Many people with COPD are difficult to understand and cope with. The following guidelines may help you to assist patients in meeting their basic needs for acceptance and love.

The physical handicap causes feelings of hostility, fear, anger, anxiety, depression, and grief. These feelings are often focused on the nurse. Examples of feelings:

Fear of suffocation when difficult breathing occurs, especially at night or when alone.

Feelings of sadness, helplessness, and loneliness accompany depression.

Speech is slow, hygiene is neglected, eating and sleeping are affected.

Several losses have actually occurred: the patient's role in the family, employment, company of loved ones, self-sufficiency, and power.

Attitude of withdrawal, which in turn causes the family to also withdraw.

Guidelines for the Nurse

Look beyond the behavior and meet the real needs. Listen to the patient's anxieties so he or she can, in turn, relax and breath better.

Set limits while always providing support. Avoid overindulgence and punishment.

Depression is replaced by anger as the patient improves. Don't withdraw your attention too soon. Explain the change to the patient's family.

Family members may expect too much from the patient because they don't understand the disease.

Encourage the patient to develop interest in a hobby or some area that will occupy the mind and prevent the patient from constantly focusing on the disease.

Help family members to accept the need for changing family roles and the limitations that the patient's disease imposes.

B. Putting It into Action!

1. Attend a small group discussion on "Caring for and Teaching Chronically Ill Respiratory Patients."

Act out the following play between a patient and the two different nursing students. Stop the play as directed and discuss the questions.

Scene: Patient lying flat in bed with breakfast tray untouched. Nurse standing beside bed.

Nurse 1: Let me help you sit up to eat. [*nurse is timid and sweet.*]

Patient: I don't want to eat. [*cough, cough*] I'm too winded.

Nurse 1: You must eat!

Patient: Leave me alone!

Nurse 1: Your food will get cold.

Patient: I'm still coughing. It tires me out so. I'll eat later.

STOP . . . . Is coughing to be expected of this patient? What observations should the nurse be making of this patient? What is the patient talking about? The nurse? How do you think the nurse feels? What would you do now?

Scene: Ten minutes later. Same nursing student plus another enter room. Patient still flat in bed.

Nurse 1: Any better now? [*still timid*]

Patient: No. Still too tired to eat.

Nurse 2: Doing a lot of coughing this morning? [*spoken with concern*]

Patient: Yes. Can't eat. Too tired to sit up.

Nurse 2: You don't want to eat because you are too tired to sit on the edge of the bed or in the chair?

Patient: Yes.

Nurse 2: How would it be if we rolled the head of the bed up and propped you with pillows. I'll get you some mouth wash; then a little hot coffee and cereal might help loosen that phlegm.

Patient: O.K., as long as I don't have to sit on the side of the bed.

STOP . . . . Why did the patient agree to eat for this nurse and not for the first one? What did the nurse do differently? Did you recognize any therapeutic communication? Give an example.

Scene: Patient sitting up in bed eating cereal. Nurse 2 at side.

Nurse 2: Let me get you a straw for the coffee. Then you won't have to lift the cup each time to drink it.

Patient: Fine.

Later: After breakfast. Patient flat in bed again. Nurse 1 at side.

Nurse 1: How about a bath now? [*still apologetic*]

Patient: Let me rest. I'll bathe later.

Nurse 1: But it will make you feel better.

Patient: I can't. Leave me alone.

STOP.. What do you think about the nurse's actions? How do you think she feels? What should she do now? What would you have done in this situation?

Thirty minutes later. Same scene as above. Nurse 1 has clean linen in arms.

Patient: Why do you keep bothering me? I can't get any rest.

Nurse 1: I'm going to begin your bath now. I will do most of it and will work quickly so you can have a long rest period afterward. [*firmly*]

[Nurse 1 assembles equipment, puts bath blanket on patient. Is unbuttoning pajamas.]

Patient: All right. If you insist. Don't take off my pajamas. I haven't had them off since I came here. I'll get a cold. Just wash my hands and face. I'm not dirty.

Nurse 1: I've covered you with this thick cotton blanket so that you will stay warm while I wash you. I've also turned the air conditioning off in the room. The water is hot, and I'll work quickly. Let's try with just the top off.

Patient: O.K.

STOP.. What limits has this nurse set for this patient? What effect has it had? Why?

Scene: Nurse has soapy washcloth in hand.

Patient: I'll wash my face and arms if you just give me the rag.

Nurse 1: Fine.

Patient: That hot water feels good. [*Silence—washing*]

Patient: You from around here?

Nurse 1: Yes—and you?

Patient [*continuing with bath*]: No. I'm from Vermont. Worked up there until this thing crippled me up so. Was a sergeant in the police force. Doc said a warm climate would do me more good, so here I am. Third time I've been here in the hospital.

Nurse 1: You've been here twice before?

Patient: Yes, I can only stay home so long, then I get so I can't even make it to the bathroom without getting completely winded. Then the doc puts me in here for a week [*pause for breath*], gives me the breathing machine, and that helps. But each time it's worse. Each time I wonder if it's the last and if I'll ever go home again. [*pause to breathe—nurse looking at patient with interest showing in eyes*] But you don't want to hear about my problems. You've got enough to do if all your patients are as nasty as me.

Nurse 1: It gets discouraging for you, and you get irritable because you feel so bad.

Patient: Yes, I spend all my energy just to breathe, and I'm always tired.

Nurse 1: We know that, and the other nurses and I are going to try to plan the activities so that you have an hour of rest without interruption between them. I will wait to change the bed now until you need to get up to the bathroom. Ring and the aide or myself will help you and change your sheets. How does that sound?

Patient: Fine.

Nurse 1: I'd like you to drink this glass of water now. Every time we come in I'd like you to drink something. All the liquid will help to loosen that phlegm and make it easier for you to cough it up. What things do you especially like to drink?

Patient: Coffee, black, and ginger ale. Also cold pineapple juice.

Nurse 1: Fine. I'll see that we have some on the floor with your name on it. I will be back in an hour with your medicine.

Patient: Don't bother to bring that liquid stuff. I won't drink it.

STOP.. What would you do? Can you list the nursing care this patient received? Did you recognize any therapeutic communication skills? What was the result? What teaching occurred?

LEG VI-C

Nurse 1: You don't want the liquid medicine?

Patient: It makes me sick to my stomach.

Nurse: I'll see if I can find out why. See you in an hour.

Scene: Nurse looking in *PDR.*

Nurse [*to herself*]: This expectorant he is taking may be irritating his stomach. Since he is on a regular diet, I think I'll try giving it to him with milk and see if that helps.

STOP.. What would you chart in the nurses' notes for the morning?

LEG VI-C

2. Plan for a clinical experience.

▲ Care for patients with respiratory problems. Begin a nursing care plan before beginning to care for the patient.

Record your conversation with your patient whenever you feel you need to explore the dynamics of the interaction. Use the process recording form from Volume I or one supplied by your instructor. Recognize your own feelings of frustration, anger, discouragement, and disgust as well as your positive feelings. All feelings affect your behavior toward the patient. Chart on your patients. Include examples of behavior.

▲ Attend postconference and share your experiences. Discuss avoidance and other methods of treating patients that cause unpleasant or uncomfortable feelings in the nursing staff.

▲ Accompany a therapist from a respiratory service in your community. Find out what services are supplied: teaching, evaluation of learning or health care, and so on. Find out the qualifications of people supplying the services.

▲ Interview patients about measures they use to increase the productivity of their cough and how they reduce irritating, unproductive coughs. Inquire about how they feel emotions affect their respiratory problems and what they do to relax. If it is appropriate, teach some of the effective coughing and relaxation techniques you have learned. Listen to their breath sounds before and after coughing to determine if secretions are removed and lungs reexpanded.

▲ Visit pulmonary rehabilitation centers. Find out what services are available and how patients are referred. Accompany therapists on home visits. If a patient is to go home with respiratory treatment, where can the equipment be obtained? Who will assist the patient and family in the home? What signs and symptoms should alert the patient to seek medical help?

▲ Visit your local chapter of the American Lung Association. Find out what educational programs are available for patients with COPD and tuberculosis. Imagine that a good friend or your friend's father was diagnosed as having advanced emphysema or tuberculosis. What community resources are available for education, rehabilitation, and treatment in your area?

▲ Go with home health nurses to visit patients with chronic respiratory problems. How have they adapted their homes and lifestyle to meet their health and illness needs? Listen to the home health nurses as assessment is performed and teaching occurs.

Patients Receiving Oxygen and Humidity

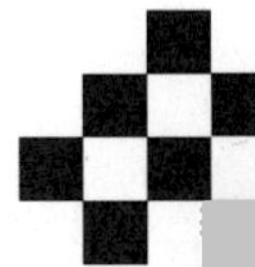

LEG VI-C

O b j e c t i v e s

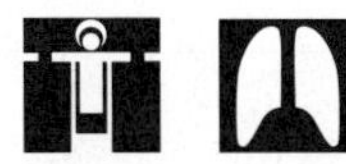

23. Demonstrate caring for a patient receiving oxygen and/or humidity via mask, cannula, hood, tent, mist mask, trach mist, T-piece, or isolette, taking measures to ensure that the patient is receiving the prescribed amount of oxygen and that the equipment is not causing the patient discomfort or injury.

24. Demonstrate caring for a child in a croupette, including turning the patient, changing the linen, and maintaining the optimum moisture and temperature control.

A. What's It All About?

1. Think about people who need oxygen or humidity or both. What a relief it must be to receive the needed treatment. Each method has its own problems, for example, skin irritation from the plastic or loneliness and dimming of visibility and sound within the croupette. Take time to make these treatments as comfortable as possible for each patient and go back to be sure your comfort measures really work.

2. Read about *oxygen therapy, humidification, croupette,* and *isolette* in medical-surgical and pediatrics references.

3. View audiovisuals and read articles and books from a list given you by your instructor or read the following:

Bolgiano, C. S., K. Bunting, and M. M. Shoeberger. "Administering O_2 Therapy: What You Need to Know." *Nursing90,* June, pp. 47–51.

4. Answer the following questions.

(a) List three ways to liquefy a patient's respiratory secretions other than with medications, and state why secretions need to be liquefied. (Review Objective 10.)

(b) Imagine that you were working in the emergency room and an unconscious patient was admitted with broken bones, dyspnea, and cyanosis. Oxygen is ordered. What clues would make you suspect COPD? (Try to make use of all the information you studied in the earlier Objectives in this LEG.)

(c) List the principles or guidelines that a nurse would follow in giving oxygen to a patient with COPD.

(d) List the dangers of oxygen therapy.

(e) When and why is hyperbaric 0_2 therapy used?

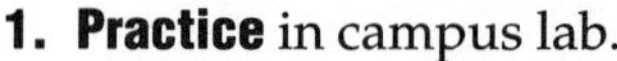

■ B. Putting It into Action!

1. Practice in campus lab.

■ Examine the various devices for O_2 administration. Fill in the chart below as you look at and read about them.

Method of Delivery	Advantages	Disadvantages	O_2 Delivery (L/M)
nasal cannula			
face mask			
Venturi mask			
nonrebreathing mask			
tent, incubator, or isolette			
trach collar			
T-piece			

■ Make a list of problems that may occur when a patient is receiving O_2 therapy. For three of the problems, write a nursing diagnosis, expected outcomes, and nursing interventions. Share your lists and discuss.

■ Check out for self-practice "Oxygen Equipment."

Practice wearing a mask at home for an hour. Draw the elastic tight enough for it to stay secure. How does it feel over the ears? To get the proper feeling if your hair is long, pull it back from the ears so that the hair is not padding the skin around the ears. This is where patients, especially men with short hairstyles, develop skin irritations. Try padding with cotton balls, then with gauze squares, and see how the ears feel.

Develop skill in placing the mask and padding it on another person. In actual practice you would encourage the patients to keep their hair over the ears for padding.

Try the same thing with the cannula. How does it feel in the nostrils? The prongs may be too long for some patients and require trimming by the nurse or the respiratory therapist. Become observant and look at the fit of the cannula on your patients.

Try it on different family members and see the difference. How does the skin feel under the mask? Hot, sweaty? What might you use on the skin to keep it cool and dry?

2. Attend a small group discussion on "Caring for a Child Requiring Oxygen Therapy." Imagine that 10-year-old Paul Harvey with asthma described in the nursing care plan below is your clinical assignment for tomorrow. Using the nursing process, plan together how you would care for him, what problems you would anticipate, and what approaches you would take with both the child and the mother. Compare your ideas.

Date	*Medical Orders*
3/27	Clear liquid diet.
	Encourage fluids.

Complete bed rest.

Elevate head of bed.

Special back care.

I&O.

IPPB with Bronkosol tid and prn for acute distress.

VS q2h until stable.

O_2 per cannula prn.

Medihaler prn q4h for acute distress.

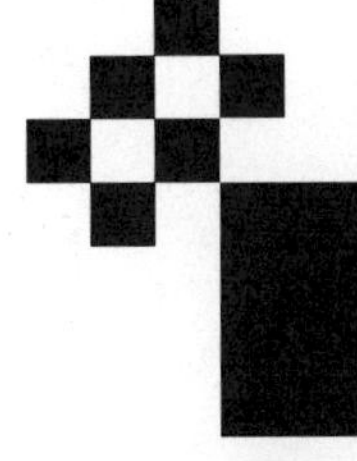

LEG VI-C

Date	Nursing Diagnosis	Nursing Interventions
3-27	Anxiety R/t unfamiliar surroundings	Explain all procedures before beginning.
	Fluid volume deficit	Offer fluids frequently; likes ginger ale.
	Alteration in family process: overprotection	Strive to gain mother's confidence and assure her that patient will be well cared for in her absence. Encourage independence of patient.
	Short-Term Goals: To relieve acute resp. symptoms.	
	Long-Term Goals: Help mother and child to accept this condition and achieve independence and normal lifestyle in home and community.	

List on a chalkboard some additional problems that would probably be present and the approaches you would take.

3. Plan for a clinical experience.

▲ Observe or give care to adults and children receiving oxygen or humidity or both. What types of problems do each of the patients have with each type of equipment? What are the advantages and disadvantages of the tent over the cannula or mask, the mask over the cannula, and so on? How do you prevent the patient in the tent from becoming chilled? How do you recognize oxygen-induced apnea? Who is most likely to become apneic and why?

Find out how the wall humidifier works. Who has the responsibility of maintaining temperature and humidity, and how is it done? Check the policy in your hospital. Practice your fingertip skills in adjusting the rate of flow. How is ultrasonic equipment used to supply humidity? What is the advantage of a Venturi-type mask?

▲ Observe patients recently removed from oxygen and/or humidity. How will you evaluate whether they need to return? Review Objective 2.

▲ Find out how the croupette works. If it uses ice, who has the responsibility of adding it? How is the drainage tubing connected? What is your responsibility? Become thoroughly familiar with this apparatus so that you can adjust it easily and spend more time with the child.

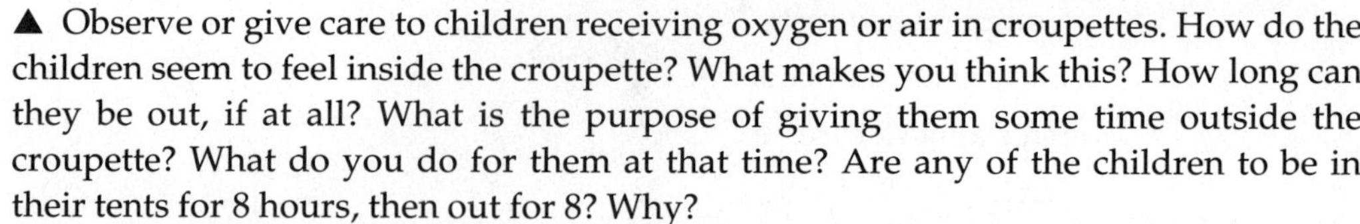

▲ Observe or give care to children receiving oxygen or air in croupettes. How do the children seem to feel inside the croupette? What makes you think this? How long can they be out, if at all? What is the purpose of giving them some time outside the croupette? What do you do for them at that time? Are any of the children to be in their tents for 8 hours, then out for 8? Why?

What would you do with a 2-year-old patient with croup who continually crawls out of his tent?

What safety measures must be taken in caring for a child in a croupette with oxygen? Include toys, call bells, TV remote controls, propped bottles, sharp objects, side rails.

▲ Check the oxygen concentration in an isolette with an oxygen analyzer. Why is it necessary? Without a doctor's order, you must always keep the concentration below what percentage? Why?

▲ Observe the use of ultrasonic nebulizers or micromists. What are the dangers of overhydration in infants? In your hospital, what would the nurse's responsibility be if the doctor ordered Ultrasonic 10 min q1h?

▲ Observe in a pediatric ICU. You will study more about children in acute distress in LEG XIII-B.

▲ Look for children on apnea monitors or using oximetry to monitor O_2 needs.

Observations for an Obstructed Airway

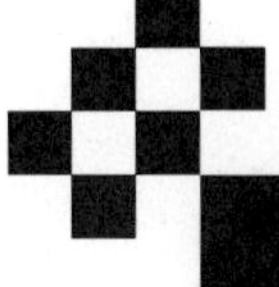

LEG VI-C

Objectives

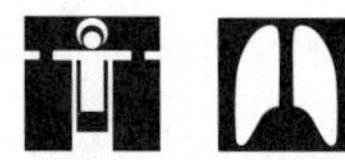

25. List four symptoms that would alert you to suspect an obstructed airway and chart the symptoms.

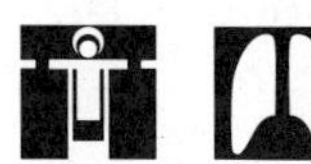

26. Given an end-of-shift report on a child with acute inflammation and infection of the larynx, trachea, and bronchial area, identify and list any missing information you would require in order to determine changes in the child's respiratory distress.

A. What's It All About?

1. Think about how you feel when your throat constricts over a piece of pepper or food. A moment of panic occurs before you can say to yourself, "Relax and it will ease up." Your eyes water, and you reach for a glass of water.

Compare these feelings with those of a child who becomes extremely apprehensive when unable to breathe. Your facial expressions and calm actions will do much to eliminate the fear.

2. Read about *respiratory obstruction* and *acute inflammation and infection of the upper respiratory tract* in medical-surgical and pediatrics references.

3. List the signs and symptoms that would alert you to a possible respiratory obstruction for each of the following patients. Describe the best position to place the patient in to prevent obstruction and state why. (If you know *why* the obstruction occurs, you will know how to position patients.)

Patient	Symptoms	Position
Child with laryngotracheobronchitis		
Anesthetized adult immediately after surgery		
Elderly person with a stroke (semiconscious)		
Patient with status asthmaticus, any age		
Patient with tracheostomy, any age		
Patient having anaphylactic reaction to a drug		
Person eating in a restaurant		

Describe nursing care indicated specifically in relation to positioning, oxygen need, fluids, and relief from symptoms.

■ B. Putting It into Action!

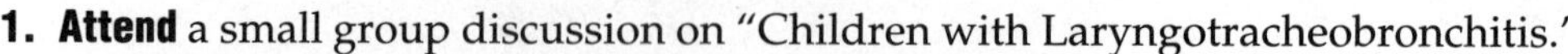

LEG VI-C

1. Attend a small group discussion on "Children with Laryngotracheobronchitis."

To prepare for this discussion, write the clinical manifestations and pathophysiology of a patient you have cared for with laryngotracheobronchitis (or create a situation from a patient chart). Describe the treatment and goals and the nursing responsibilities and rationale. What breath sounds would you expect to hear? What is *inspiratory stridor?*

■ Write out an end-of-shift report on a child with laryngotracheobronchitis, including the following information: voice and color, TPR, type of respiration, activity. Would you want to see this child, or would a verbal report be sufficient? Why?

■ What information would need to be included in the nurse's notes? How often would you chart on the patient? What legal implications are present?

2. Plan for a clinical experience.

▲ Care for a child with acute upper or lower respiratory infection. Write a nursing care plan.

▲ Review your **Clinical Performance Expectations** for Level Six.

Tracheostomy Care

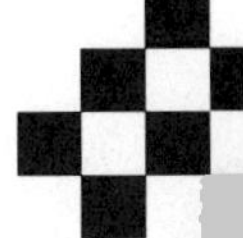

LEG VI-C

Extra Added Objectives

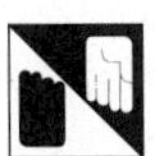 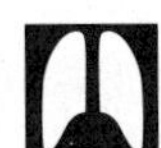

27. Demonstrate and/or role play suctioning a tracheostomy without causing injury to the mucosa or hypoxia to the patient and preventing growth and/or spread of pathogens.

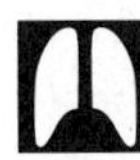

28. Demonstrate and/or role play caring for a patient with a tracheostomy including cleaning the inner cannula, changing the dressing, and giving oral hygiene.

Note: In Volume IV, LEG XII-C you will have required Objectives on tracheostomy care, including inflating and deflating cuffs and positioning the patient for effective suctioning.

A. What's It All About?

1. Think about how scary it must be to be dependent on a small tube for air and a nurse to assist in keeping the tube clear! When the nurse is not sure about how to suction and clean a tracheostomy, the delay can cause the patient much discomfort. Practice until you feel skilled, fast, and secure in this procedure so that you can intervene promptly to provide relief and decrease the anxiety of your patient.

2. Review:

LEG I-A Medical Asepsis

LEG V-A Surgical Asepsis Techniques

3. Read about *tracheostomy care* and *throat irrigations* in medical-surgical, pediatrics, and hospital nursing procedure references.

4. View audiovisuals and read articles and books from a list given you by your instructor.

5. Preview LEG XII-C Care of Patient with Laryngectomy.

6. Make a chart to compare medical and surgical aseptic technique for suctioning a tracheostomy. Write the purpose, equipment, advantages, and disadvantages of each.

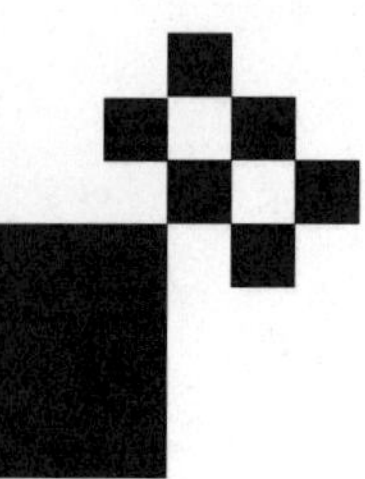

LEG VI-C

	Medical Aseptic Technique	Surgical Aseptic Technique
Purpose		
Equipment		
Advantages		
Disadvantages		

■ B. Putting It into Action!

1. **Practice** in campus lab.

   ■ Check out self-practice materials on "Tracheostomy Care and Cleaning." Handle the equipment, identify each part of the cannula, and take it apart. Practice cleaning the inner cannula with the gauze and pipe cleaners. Find out what works best for you before you are with an actual patient. A used inner cannula can be slippery. How will you keep from dropping it or keep the patient from coughing it out?

   ■ Describe your actions and state your rationale to an observer as you do the following:

   Suction "Mrs. Chase"

   Clean an inner cannula, and change the dressing

   Turn a tracheostomy patient with humidified air apparatus attached

   Throat irrigation

2. **Plan** for a clinical experience.

   ▲ Observe or care for a patient with a tracheostomy. Observe how activity affects the need for suctioning.
   Find out what procedure is being used for maintaining asepsis in the tracheal area during suctioning and dressing change.
   Evaluate the patient's reaction to the tracheostomy.

Intradermal Injections

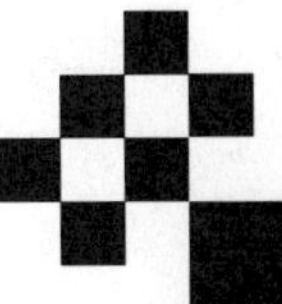

E x t r a A d d e d
O b j e c t i v e

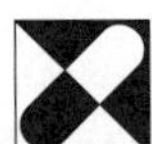 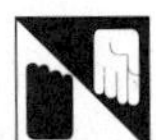

29. Demonstrate giving an intradermal injection.

Note: This will be a required Objective in LEG X-B.

■ A. What's It All About?

1. Think about what you would do if you were caring for a respiratory patient and the doctor asked you to give a tuberculin skin test! Would you know what to do? Learn this skill now. You will find many uses for it later: skin testing before giving medication, allergies, and others.

2. Read about *intradermal injections, skin testing,* and *allergy* in medical-surgical, pediatrics, and pharmacology textbooks.

■ B. Putting It into Action!

1. Practice in campus lab.

■ Practice giving intradermal injections. Develop skill in drawing up small amounts of medication (0.01 cc) accurately and injecting it under the skin. At what angle will you hold the needle? How will you prepare and hold the arm? What site will you choose? How is it recorded?

2. Plan for a clinical experience.

▲ Observe in an allergy or immunization clinic.

▲ Give intradermal injections when you are ready.

Have I Learned?

The following questions are for you to answer in order to find out if you have met the Objectives. All of the Objectives in LEG VI-C are covered in this series of questions. Pick a quiet time and answer them. Answers follow this selftest.

No space has been left for answering the questions related to the "doing" Objectives. Use a separate sheet of paper for your answers and then use the answers in clinical or campus lab for your own evaluation.

Objective	Question
1	**1.** What factors are present in each of the following situations that predispose the patients to respiratory problems?

(a) Stroke patient receiving tube feeding, lifted into a chair bid for 1 hour.

(b) Postoperative patient complaining of pain every 3 hours and receiving morphine regularly. Complains of pain when asked to move and refuses to cough. Tries to deep breathe.

(c) Patient was to receive oxygen by nasal cannula. The nurse lubricated the cannula with mineral oil and inserted it.

(d) Patient had a tracheotomy done. A humidifier is to be used at all times; patient was restless and kept pulling it off. Had difficulty swallowing and had a low fluid intake.

Objective	Question
2	**2.** Mr. Lucky, a patient with emphysema, was admitted and was sitting upright on the edge of the bed. His color was dusky, and he was coughing vigorously, expectorating thick yellow sputum. His chest was "barrel-shaped." With each breath you could see the neck muscles pulling tight as all his energies were concentrated on breathing. He called you Annie and asked where your mother was. BP 180/90; P 115. List the signs that could indicate hypoxemia and hypercapnea.
2	**3.** You are caring for Rachel, age 4, with pneumococcal pneumonia. She has been nauseated and vomiting, complains that her chest hurts, her cheeks are flushed, and her temperature is 39.4°C. Which of the following changes would make you suspect increasing hypoxemia?

(a) Increased restlessness, increased pulse rate, cyanosis, and irritability.

(b) Diarrhea and abdominal cramps, loss of appetite.

(c) Coughing up pink-tinged sputum.

(d) Dyspneic and unable to eat her breakfast.

Objective	Question
3	**4.** Demonstrate the nursing assessment of a patient with a respiratory problem. Use the criteria established by your instructor.
4	**5.** Choose from the following list one nursing diagnosis for the NCP of Mr. Lucky (Question 2).

(a) Ineffective airway clearance related to excessive thick secretions

(b) Ineffective breathing pattern related to pulse rate of 115

(c) Impaired gas exchange related to mechanical obstruction

(d) Alteration in respiration related to pneumonia

5 **6.** How can Rachel (Question 3) spread her respiratory infection? List two ways.

How can the nurse prevent this spread of microorganisms to himself or any other person in the vicinity? List three ways.

6 **7.** Match the following tests with the purposes at the right.

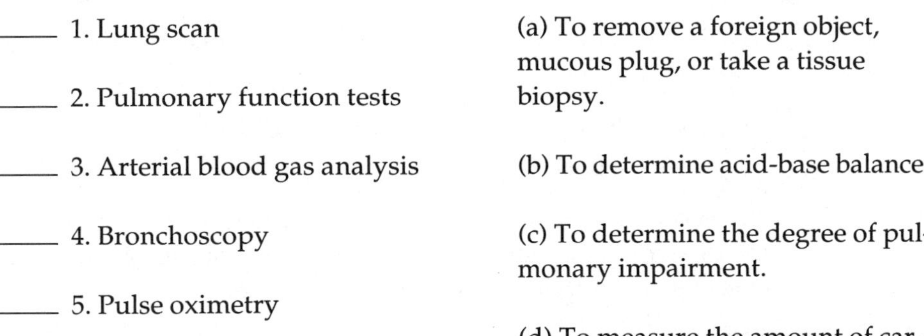

_____ 1. Lung scan

_____ 2. Pulmonary function tests

_____ 3. Arterial blood gas analysis

_____ 4. Bronchoscopy

_____ 5. Pulse oximetry

(a) To remove a foreign object, mucous plug, or take a tissue biopsy.

(b) To determine acid-base balance.

(c) To determine the degree of pulmonary impairment.

(d) To measure the amount of carbon dioxide accumulating in the blood.

(e) To show ventilation and/or perfusion patterns in the lungs.

(f) To measure arterial hemoglobin saturation.

7 **8.** State the nurse's primary responsibility to the patient before a bronchoscopy and after it to prevent complications, and describe what complications are being prevented.

8 **9.** From the following list, add, delete, or change the actions to correctly describe each step in collecting an early-morning sputum specimen in correct sequence.

1. Fill out lab slip and post.
2. Take container to patient and leave at bedside.
3. Start antibiotic.
4. Remove the patient's water at midnight.
5. Collect specimen before breakfast.
6. Attach lab slip to specimen and send to lab.

9 **10.** The arterial blood gas analysis results for Mr. Lucky (see Question 2) are as follows:

pH 7.33 (normal 7.35–7.45)

$PaCO_2$ 65 (normal 38–42)

HCO_3 32 (normal 22–26 mEq/1)

Is he in danger of developing respiratory acidosis or respiratory alkalosis?

9 **11.** When you go into Mr. Lucky's room to remove his breakfast tray, you discover that he has fallen asleep without eating. What is the best action for you to take next and why?

(a) Remove the tray and keep the food hot in the kitchen.

(b) Wake him up and try to get him to eat.

(c) Lower the head of the bed and position him for sleeping.

(d) Try to wake him up and assess his level of consciousness and vital signs.

10 **12.** Briefly describe the purpose for each of the following orders for a patient with impaired respiratory function caused by asthma, emphysema, or pneumonia:

oxygen	postural drainage
hydration	cold humidification
elevate head of bed	breathing exercises
1500-calorie diet	

11 **13.** Write the steps you would include when teaching another person to use a medihaler. Ask another person to evaluate your teaching, using the steps as a checklist. Be prepared to state your rationale.

12 **14.** State the classification, action/use, and one major side effect of bronchodilators and two nursing implications.

13 **15.** Describe four respiratory problems that develop in people with impaired gas exchange due to COPD and state why. Write a nursing care plan based on your problems including goals and interventions, rationale, and outcome criteria.

14 **16.** Write a nursing care plan for a patient with one of the disorders listed in Objective 14 (or one assigned by your instructor). Include the pathophysiology of the disease and teaching and discharge plans. Be prepared to role play your teaching or discharge plan.

15 **17.** Normal alterations of aging seen in the respiratory system include:

(a) Increased alveolar surface area

(b) Decreased vital capacity

(c) Residual volume decreases

(d) Respiratory muscles are weaker

15 **18.** Nursing care for the aged includes:

(a) Continuous bed rest to improve pulmonary blood flow

(b) Careful use of sedation to prevent respiratory depression

(c) Routine use of oxygen therapy to improve the O_2 saturation

(d) Strenuous activity to improve exercise tolerance

16 **19.** Refer to the patient profile of Darlene Thomas on p. 100. At 10 P.M. Darlene took her bedtime sedative and went to sleep. At 1 A.M. she awoke with dyspnea. She used her medihaler and sat on the edge of the bed for 20 minutes trying to catch her breath with very little relief obtained. After that time she turned her light on to call the nurse. If you were the nurse answering the light, which of the following actions would be the best one to take and why?

(a) Assess the skin color, if diaphoretic, use of accessory muscles, and flared nostrils.

(b) Find out medications given during the last 4 hours and the past 24 hours.

(c) Offer Tedral if situation is unchanged after 3–5 minutes.

(d) Give Sus-phrine sq as ordered.

17 **20.** Describe two effects of anxiety on respiratory distress.

18 **21.** List three measures that will increase the productivity of a cough.

18 **22.** While caring for Mr. Lucky, you learn that he is coughing frequently and unproductively during the night. What is the best reason for finding ways to reduce his coughing?

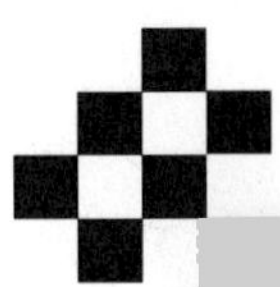

- **(a)** It uses up his energy and creates fatigue.
- **(b)** It keeps the other patients awake.
- **(c)** It makes his throat sore.
- **(d)** It spreads infectious organisms.

18 **23.** List three measures that will help control his cough.

19 **24.** Refer to p. 99 for Mrs. Paula Darvy. The morning after her late night admission she is receiving her IPPB treatment and begins coughing before it is through. She coughs up thick yellow sputum. She complains that this treatment always makes her cough, and does she have to finish it? You look at the sputum and reply:

List two actions you will take related to the sputum.

20 **25.** A nurse walked into the room to find out how the medication was helping a patient having dyspnea from an asthmatic attack. Upon seeing the nurse the patient said in a sarcastic tone of voice, "If it's not too much trouble, would you hand me some tissues?" After doing so, the nurse asked if the medication was helping. The patient replied, "Not much. Nobody here knows how to help me. Then they send in some young punk like you who has probably never even seen anyone with asthma before. A lot of good you'd be if I really needed help!" Describe two approaches that the nurse might use at this point, to be helpful to this patient.

21 **26.** Role play teaching a patient with COPD ways to save energy and to improve muscle strength and efficiency.

22 **27.** Jerry, age 3, was admitted at midnight with acute laryngotracheobronchitis. His orders are:

encourage fluids
take TPR q3h
check color, pulse, and respirations q15 min
croupette with high humidity
full liquid diet

You are assigned to his care in the morning. He is obviously tired, with a moderate amount of respiratory distress. Describe three nursing interventions you will take to meet some of his daily needs without tiring him further.

22 **28.** Refer to the patient profile of Mr. Paoli (p. 100). Mr. Paoli says his food has no taste and that he is not hungry. He drinks hot coffee in the morning and takes a little soup at noon. Describe two actions you would take to try to increase his food and fluid intake.

23 **29.** Prepare a list of the actions you would take to provide a patient receiving O_2 with minimum discomfort and maximum safety—or use your school's skill list. Ask another student to evaluate you, using the list as a checklist.

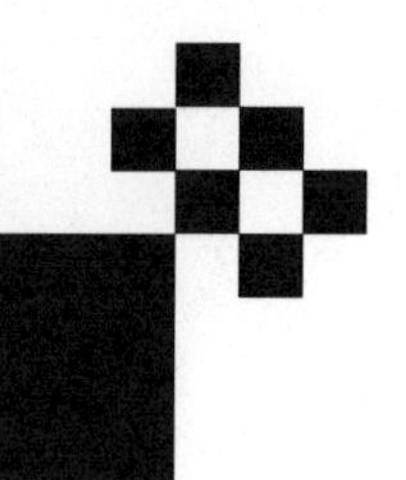

24 **30.** Prepare a list of the actions you plan to take to provide a child in a croupette minimum discomfort and maximum safety—or use your school's skill list. Ask another student to evaluate you, using the list as a checklist.

25 **31.** List four symptoms that indicate an obstructed airway.

26 **32.** You receive the following report on Jerry. (See Question 27.)

> He slept on and off during the night. His rectal temperature is 101.8, pulse 110, respirations 32. He wouldn't drink much fluid for me last night. I just changed the ice in the back of the croupette. His mother spent the night in the room. She may go home this morning.

What additional information do you need on this child to be able to intelligently assess for a change in his condition?
How will you obtain this information?

27 **33.** Write the steps you plan to take in order to suction a tracheostomy or use your school's skill list. Use a real patient or "Mrs. Chase" and ask another student to use your checklist as you are observed. Be prepared to defend your actions.

28 **34.** Write the steps you plan to take to clean the inner cannula, change the dressing, and give oral hygiene—or use your school's skill list. Use a real patient or "Mrs. Chase" and ask another student to use your checklist as you are observed. Be prepared to state your rationale.

29 **35.** Demonstrate preparing and giving an intradermal injection.

Answers to Have I Learned?

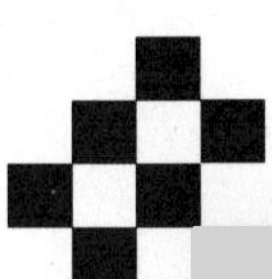

LEG VI-C

LEG VI-C

1. **(a)** *Immobility* and lack of exercise cause fluid to collect in lung, decrease expansion of lung tissue, decrease removal of bronchial secretions, encourage venous stasis in lower extremities, and formation of emboli. *Tube feeding* causes mucus and bacteria to collect on tube that can drop into trachea causing pneumonia. *Improper feeding methods* can accidentally introduce formula into trachea, causing pneumonia.

   (b) *Morphine* depresses respiration. *Immobility* after surgery causes mucous plugs to form and if not removed by coughing, can cause atelectasis to occur. Venous stasis also occurs in legs.

   (c) *Mineral oil* as a lubricant in the nares can cause oil droplets to fall into the trachea, causing aspiration pneumonia. *Always* use a water-soluble lubricant, not mineral oil.

   (d) *Lack of humidity* in the air will dry out the secretions and cause mucous plugs to form rapidly. *Lack of body fluid* will aid in the drying out of secretions.

2. Sitting upright to breathe; dusky color; barrel-shaped chest; use of accessory neck muscles to breathe; high BP and rapid pulse; confusion.

3. **(a)**

4. Attend a GES. Be prepared to demonstrate the correct procedure for a total lung sounds assessment. Identify why you might listen to various areas in the lungs and what you would expect to hear normally and for any specified respiratory problem.

5. **(a)**

6. By droplets **(a)** in the air and **(b)** in the sputum she is expectorating.

   (a) Teach patient to cover mouth with tissue when coughing.

   (b) Supply receptable for used tissues and empty frequently.

   (c) Turn your face away from patient when she coughs.

   (d) Wash your hands when leaving patient.

7. 1**(e)**, 2**(c)**, 3**(b)**, 4**(a)**, 5**(f)**.

8. *Before:* Sign consent, nothing by mouth for 6–8 hr to avoid vomiting and aspiration. *After:* Nothing by mouth until patient can cough and swallow reflex returns to avoid aspiration. *Observe for* hemoptysis (report excessive bleeding), dyspnea, subcutaneous emphysema around face and neck, SOB and laryngeal stridor from edema.

9. 1. add: label container with patient's name and room number.

   2. add: instruct patient about what you want, why you want it, and when you want it.

   3. start antibiotic after collecting specimen as it interferes with identification of organisms.

   4. delete and change to: offer fluids to liquefy secretions.

   6. add: check specimen to see if it contains food or other contaminants that would make it unacceptable to the lab.

   Correct sequence: 1, 2, 4, 5, 6, 3

10. Respiratory acidosis.

11. **(d)** Somnolence and decreased attention span can be signs of hypoxia. It needs to be treated immediately before he drifts into respiratory failure. You should also consider the possibility of hypercapnea (CO_2 narcosis). Check the O_2 flow meter rate of delivery.

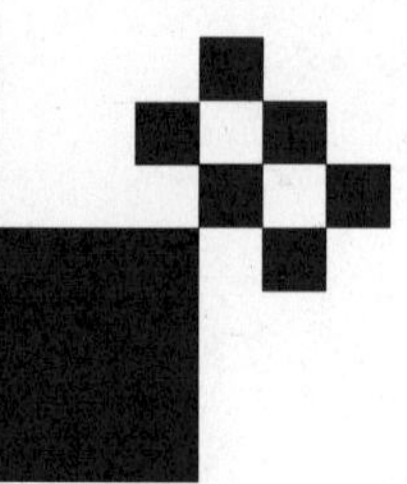

12. *Oxygen* to increase concentration in blood and decrease respiratory efforts to obtain it; *hydration* to liquefy secretions; *elevate head of bed* to expand thoracic cavity and decrease dyspnea; *1500-calorie diet* to maintain respiratory muscles for work of breathing; *postural drainage* to aid in the removal of secretions from all lobes of the lung; *cold humidification* to liquefy secretions, and reduce temperature; *breathing exercises* to relax and get maximum ventilation with less energy and increase muscle strength.

13. Compare what your observer saw you do and what you planned to do.

14. A bronchodilator relaxes the bronchioles and may cause gastric irritation. Teach the patient to report side effects and to watch young children for signs of increased CNS stimulation such as irritability, insomnia, headache, or twitching.

15. Your four problems might include:

> ineffective airway clearance related to excessive and tenacious mucous secretions
>
> fatigue or activity intolerance related to decreased oxygen and decreased nutrition
>
> potential alteration in nutrition related to fatigue and dyspnea
>
> potential alteration in health maintenance related to lack of information about respiratory infections and how to prevent them
>
> anxiety and fear or powerlessness related to dyspnea
>
> potential complication: pulmonary hypertension

Share your plans during a postconference or discussion time or as directed by your instructor.

16. Attend a GES to share your plans and role play teaching and preparing patients for discharge and home care.

17. (d)

18. (b)

19. All of the answers could be acceptable nursing actions. However, **(c)** is better than **(d)** unless the distress is severe. During an asthmatic attack the smooth muscles of the bronchi contract and go into a spasm. Then edema of the mucous membranes occurs and the thick secretions increase. Nursing actions should be aimed at relaxing the spasm. Tedral contains two ingredients that have sympathomimetic actions and are bronchodilators. A third ingredient is phenobarbital, which will sedate and decrease anxiety, another factor that increases bronchial spasm. Another consideration is route of administration, how fast relief can be obtained, and how severe the distress is.

20. Anxiety, fear, and hostility increase oxygen consumption and thus the heart rate and the respiratory rate. They can aggravate an asthmatic attack. The patient is unable to maintain sufficient gas exchange to meet the increased energy expenditure that occurs with the emotions. The patient will adapt by using obsessive-compulsive behaviors and rituals or internalize emotion to decrease the response. This reaction can lead to increased energy expenditure again.

21. Your answers might include the following: increasing humidity, offering fluids, instructing how to cough effectively, postural drainage and clapping, and using expectorants.

22. (a)

23. Your answers might include the following: raise the head of the bed, provide a beverage to be sipped, help patient relax, teach coughing techniques that remove secretions if present (if rhonchi are heard in the lungs), reduce irritants such as smoke in the room.

24. *Reply:* The purpose of the IPPB is to help you cough up this thick sputum, so it looks like it is doing the job.

(a) Find out if there is a requisition for a sputum specimen or if the doctor might like to see the sputum, in which case you would save it in a sputum container with her name, the date, and the time on it.

(b) Chart the description of the sputum in the nurse's notes.

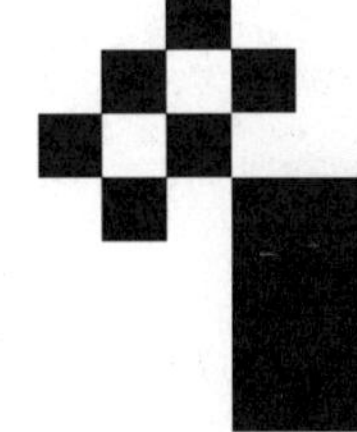

25. **(a)** Help patient to clarify feelings. Give information about the medical orders you have if needed. Involve patient in making decisions about treatment.

(b) Excuse yourself from the room and talk with another staff member if you find you are feeling hurt or angry and are unable to listen objectively to the patient's complaints. Discuss patient's reasons for feeling anxious and behaviors that could be expected. Then return to the patient and say you are still concerned about how he is feeling. Try not to become insulted or defensive. Maintain control of your own behavior. Discuss with patient alternative ways to express emotion. If you are unable to return to the patient, then see that another person does.

LEG VI-C

26. Attend a GES. Your teaching should include a schedule of a day's activities to allow for regular exercise as well as for periods of rest. Encourage breathing out with pursed lips when exerting; for example, when going up stairs or lifting a heavy object.

27. *Activity:* Turn him from side to side every 2 hours.

Nutrition: Offer him small amounts of fluid frequently in whatever container is easy for him to drink from. Avoid carbonated drinks.

Environment: avoid chilling from wet linen. Change as necessary.

28. **(a)** Find out special food and fluid preferences.

(b) Offer fluids q2h.

(c) Mouth care 6 × /da.

29. Compare your actions with the checklist.

30. Compare your actions with the checklist.

31. Increased restlessness; rapid weak pulse; increased retractions; increased noise of breathing; cyanosis.

32. Color, degree of retracting, exact fluid intake and output, noise and voice, any sign of restlessness.
Assess the patient with the nurse reporting off.

33. Compare what your observer saw you do with the skill list.

34. Compare what your observer saw you do with the skill list.

35. Attend a GES. Complete a demonstration as required by your instructor.

Why Should I Study?

In Level Six you were introduced to some basic concepts, attitudes, and knowledge that will be applied to a variety of nursing situations in Levels Seven and Eight. It will be your responsibility to return to the related Objectives in Level Six whenever you need to review.

The LEGs in this Level are organized into the same three components of care: **A. Crisis, B. Regulatory,** and **C. Body Systems.** Continue to route yourself through the flow chart in your own way so that you know which LEG is next in your plan.

In Level Seven you will be expected to perform at an increased level of clinical proficiency. Look at:

- how you organize your information before giving patient care
- the questions you ask
- the amount of skill you display in carrying out both old and new procedures
- the attitude with which you seek new solutions and additional information

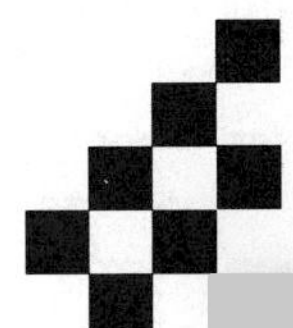

Level Seven

All of these will indicate whether you are learning and applying your knowledge to actual patient care, which is your ultimate goal.

The following statements describe your specific **Clinical Performance Expectations** for Level Seven. By the end of this level you should be able to:

1. Carry out with ease and confidence nursing skills learned in Level Six (for example, collecting sputum specimens).
2. Find information on preparation for diagnostic tests in the health agency with less direction than in Level Six.
3. Display increased self-confidence when working with patients, staff, and instructors.
4. Apply the principles of asepsis to more-complex problems with less guidance from your instructor.
5. Make more complete assessments of patients in less time than in Level Six.
6. Seek information about patients in addition to what is given to you in report.
7. Care for multiple patients with problems according to priority of care.

Look for relationships, listen, and think when other students are describing their experiences in group conferences. Ask for clarification if you do not understand their descriptions. Try out ideas on the group for discussion; use each other for stimulation, evaluation, moral support, empathy, sympathy, encouragement. Nursing is working with people. If you can be successful in communicating with your peers and your instructors, you will be successful with patients and staff members.

What Will I Learn?
LEG VII-A Surgery

In this LEG you will be studying the preoperative and postoperative care of patients of all ages. Surgery is a **Crisis** event.

Objectives 2, 3, and 6 will build on your communication skills as well as your knowledge of the crisis and the grief process. With children you will learn the techniques of play therapy. With adults you may have your first opportunity to do some planned teaching, either individually or in small groups, as you explain postoperative exercises and care.

Objectives 7 and 8 will add to your knowledge of nutrition. Patients undergoing surgery have their nutritional status severely taxed, and you can help.

When does preoperative preparation begin? On admission? The evening before surgery? At home when packing the suitcase? Or in the doctor's office when the decision to have surgery is made? Who helps in the preparation? The family? The doctor? The nurse? When is postoperative care completed? When the patient starts eating? When the last dressing comes off? When the patient goes home? Or goes back to work?

Your hospital contact with patients represents only a part of their entire surgical experience. You will wish to find out what preconceptions, what worries, what expectations patients bring with them, and what responsibilities and living conditions they are returning to after discharge. The perioperative experience can be life-threatening or lifesaving. For all, it is an energy-consuming experience. The body takes many weeks to return to normal function even though the exterior may appear to be healed and intact. Patients need help in reaching this goal in order to make practical plans after discharge and not make unreasonable demands on or expectations of themselves.

As you move through this LEG, try to identify when information falls into the categories of **Regulatory** and **Body Systems,** on the basis of knowledge learned in Level Six.

What's Ahead in Later LEGs

LEG VIII-C Gastrointestinal Problems
LEG IX-B Care after Orthopedic Surgery
LEG IX-C Care after Urinary Surgery
LEG X-A Convalescence and Rehabilitation Following Radical Surgery for Cancer
LEG XII-B Neurosurgical Nursing Care
LEG XII-C Intensive Surgical Nursing Care
LEG XIII-B Intensive Pediatric Nursing Care
LEG XIII-C Intensive Medical Nursing Care Including Endocrine Imbalances

■ Overview of Learning Experiences in LEG VII-A

Objectives	Campus Lab/ Self-Practice	Group Discussions/Lectures	Clinical Lab Focuses
Emotional Preparation for Surgery **1,2.** Emotional preoperative preparation **3.** Preparing for change in body image			**B2.** Talk with postoperative patients about preoperative feelings Talk with patients preoperatively Write a process recording Observe a nurse using play therapy with a child Read charts of surgical patients
Preoperative Teaching **4.** Factors influencing perioperative experience **5,6.** Preoperative teaching	**B1.** Preoperative teaching	**B2.** Assessing and teaching preoperative patients	**B3.** Try out teaching approaches for children Observe anesthesiologist talking with a child before surgery Talk with adults before surgery Assess a patient; make a teaching plan Observe in x-ray
Physical Preparation for Surgery **7,8.** Assessing risks and providing nutritional support **9.** Preoperative lab tests **10.** Skin preparation **11.** Preparing a patient for surgery using a checklist **12.** Preparing room for a postoperative patient	**B1.** Moving patients on and off stretcher Skin prep	**A6.** Laboratory reports and their implications for surgical patients **B3.** Preparing patients for surgery GES Objective 11	**B4.** Observe preoperative medications being prepared Observe in the OR Accompany person doing skin preps Care for patients preoperatively Prepare a postoperative bed and room Accompany a dietitian on rounds Help move patients on and off stretchers
Preoperative Medications **13,14.** Preoperative medications **15.** Pediatric calculations	**B2.** Preoperative meds	**A6.** The autonomic nervous system	**B3.** Give preoperative meds

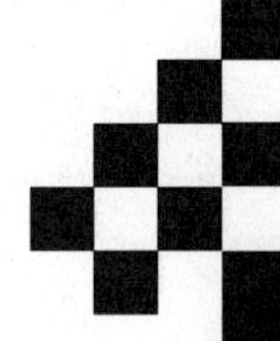

LEG VII-A

■ Overview of Learning Experiences in LEG VII-A (cont.)

Objectives	Campus Lab/ Self-Practice	Group Discussions/Lectures	Clinical Lab Focuses
Immediate Postoperative Period **16,17,19.** Early postoperative assessments and actions **18.** Suctioning mouth and nose		**B3.** Care of the patient recovering from anesthesia	**B4.** Care for patients in the recovery room or short-stay unit
Using the Nursing Process for Postoperative Care **20.** Preventing postoperative complications **21.** Using drugs for postoperative problems **22,23.** Using the nursing process to care for postoperative patients **24.** Wound care	**B1.** Assisting with a dressing change	**B2.** Planning postoperative care	**B3.** Care for a postoperative patient Give nursing care to elderly surgical patient Write a nursing care plan **C1.** Care for wounds with drains
Planning Care for Two to Four Patients **25.** Organizing preoperative care for two to four patients **26.** Involving a relative in care of a surgical patient			**B1.** Prepare two or three patients for surgery Care for patients who have visiting relatives

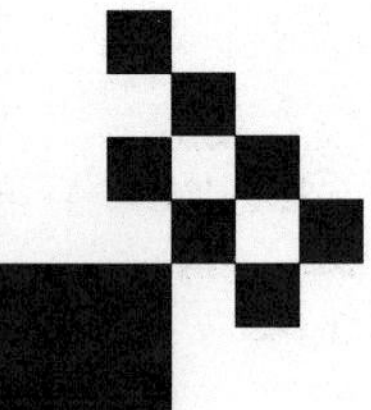

New Terms

dehiscence
-ectomy
elective
evisceration
intraoperative
laparotomy
laryngospasm
-oscopy
-ostomy
perioperative
photophobia
-plasty

Abbreviations

D & C
EKG
LASER
OR
RBC
RR
T&A
TUR
WBC

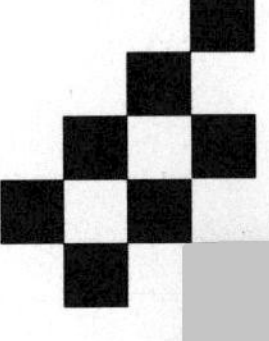

Emotional Preparation for Surgery

Objectives

 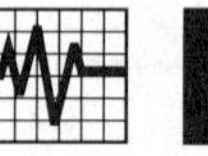 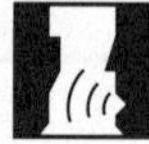

1. State the benefits of helping a preoperative patient cope emotionally with an impending surgical experience.

 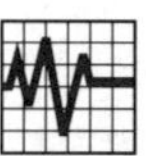 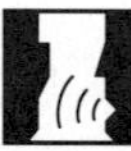

2. Given a sample conversation between a nurse and a patient, identify the clues that the patient is giving the nurse about preoperative fears, and state whether the nurse's responses are encouraging or discouraging the patient to explore and express those fears.

 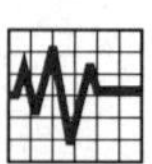 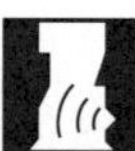

3. Demonstrate by role playing how a nurse can assist a patient to become emotionally prepared for a change in body image related to surgery.

LEG VII-A

■ A. What's It All About?

1. Think about fear of the unknown. Apply it to:

A teenage boy going into a hospital to stay without his family, surrounded by strangers, new smells, sights, sounds, and noises.

A woman knowing that she will be anesthetized and strangers will cut and probe. She wonders if they will find a cancer growing.

You yourself going into a new patient's room to talk with him about his surgery tomorrow morning.

A 3-year-old girl having her crib pushed into the operating room and watching a mask being placed over her face.

A man wondering how much pain he will have and if it will be more than he can tolerate without crying out.

A young woman wondering what her life will be like after her hysterectomy.

You yourself admitting a 6-year-old boy and his parents to a pediatric unit for your first time and the child's first hospital stay.

■ What do all these situations have in common? Could it be the feeling of not knowing what will happen, the unknown?

■ What can be done in each situation to reduce the stress to manageable amounts? Why is it so important to reduce stress?

■ Why do the elderly respond poorly to stress?

■ How can each person be better informed and *know* more and *fear* less? What type of *knowing* is necessary in each case? Is *telling* a person what will happen enough to alleviate fear and anxiety? Is *showing?* Would trying a "dry run" help?

■ Which situations can be considered **crises?**

■ How does surgery cause a change in body image? What problems can be expected to occur? Emotional? Sexual? Occupational? Social?

■ Can you think of two surgeries that cause a structural change in the body? Two that cause a change in body function? A surgery that does both?

2. Review:

LEG III-A Patient Admission
LEG III-C Anxiety and Defense Mechanisms
LEG VI-A Crisis Intervention

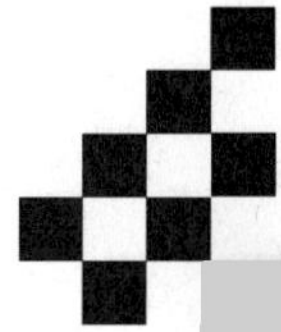

3. Read medical-surgical, pediatrics, growth and development, and psychiatric nursing references. Look in the index under *preoperative preparation, admission procedure, body image, fear, stress, play therapy.*

4. View audiovisuals and read articles and books from a list given you by your instructor or read the following:

Sweeney, M. L. "Your Role in Informed Consent." *RN,* August 1991, pp. 55–60.

5. Preview LEG XIII-B Play Therapy.

6. Describe briefly how each of the following responds to surgery (stress) and what behaviors or symptoms will be seen.

	Response	Behaviors or Symptoms
sympathetic nervous system (SNS)		
aldosterone		
antidiuretic hormone (ADH)		
glucocorticoids		

■ B. Putting It into Action!

1. Write nursing goals for the patients in each of the following situations to prepare them for surgery. Write opening statements you would make with each patient.

> *Your niece*, age 5, is going into the hospital for a tonsillectomy next week. She lives nearby, and you are able to visit her easily. Her parents look to you for advice in how to prepare her for the hospital experience. When you go to their home, you take your nursing cap and scissors. You ask your niece if she would like to play "hospital" with her favorite doll. She sees your cap and asks if she can be the nurse. [You take it from here.]

A woman, age 46, is admitted for a breast biopsy and a possible radical mastectomy. You are assigned to her care before surgery. She is talking about the new fashions, her family, and so on. Not a word has been mentioned about the forthcoming surgery. You wonder what you should say. The following possibilities pass through your mind:

"You haven't mentioned one word to me about your surgery."
"I wonder if you have any questions about your surgery that I might help you with."
"Is this the first time you have had surgery?"
"Not knowing exactly what the outcome will be must be very difficult to face."

A man, age 23, is having a hernia repaired (herniorrhaphy). When you bring in his medication, you overhear him telling his visitors how he hopes he will be "out of it" for several days so he won't "feel" anything. You wonder if this patient is afraid of appearing unmanly if he complains of pain and needs to express this concern. You wonder if he knows about the orders the physician leaves for pain medication. You make a note to spend a few minutes talking with him later.

An elderly man and his wife are visiting together the evening before surgery. When you come into the room, they ask you exactly what the events will be in the morning and when he is expected to come back to the room. The patient says, "I don't want my wife waiting here at the hospital all day. If anything should happen to me during the operation, I want her at home. We both know that the risks are greater when you get to be my age."

While on the pediatric unit, you are asked to admit the 3-year-old girl who is coming in for elective surgery. You are asked to get a urine specimen; take a rectal temperature, apical pulse, weight, height; make general observations; and get her settled in the room. You quickly start to think of those things you have learned about 3-year-olds: how the separation will affect the child; how you can help the parents understand the child's change in behavior; how you can find out about the child's habits, vocabulary; what explanations will need to be given to the parents about meal time, visiting hours, obtaining information about their child from the nursing staff.

After you have clearly identified your nursing goals for each of these patients, how will you attempt to meet those goals? List specific nursing interventions you would take to avoid adding *additional stress* to a patient before surgery. Be specific.

■ What will you do and say if parents ask to stay with their children? (You must know your hospital's policy to answer this honestly.) How do you feel about this policy and why? What facts do you know to support a decision for or against it? Would age affect it?

■ Who is experiencing a crisis event when a child is hospitalized?

■ Are any of the patients above expressing preoperative fears? Who are they? What are their fears?

2. Plan for a clinical experience. Select one or more of the following activities.

▲ Talk with postoperative patients about preoperative feelings.

■ Encourage them to recall and tell you what concerns, worries, fears, and thoughts they had before going to the operating room (OR). Include family members in the conversation if they are present.

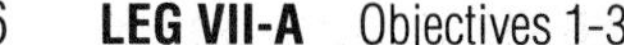

■ Find out what sources of help were made available to the patients preoperatively for getting information and helping them clarify their thoughts and feelings.

Record the information immediately upon leaving each patient's room for later sharing with other students in conference.

Note: This activity is not intended to be aimed as a criticism of the staff but rather is an aid to help you find out what actions, behavior, or words reach patients and how to let them know that you care and want to listen and help.

▲ Read about several patients' postoperative courses and make some assumptions about the effect of their preoperative preparation on their postoperative behavior.

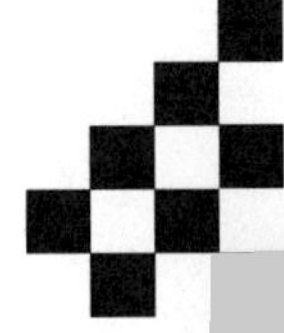

▲ Talk with patients (adults or children) preoperatively. Listen to them. Assess verbal or nonverbal clues that reveal their attitude, fears, concerns. Be aware of how you feel and are responding. Are you:

_____ Uncomfortable and relieved when a patient says very little about the surgery and changes the subject?

_____ Afraid you will be asked a question that you won't be able to answer? (Never be afraid to admit you do not know but you will find out.)

_____ Elated when he gives you a clue and you have a chance to help him put down his barrier for a little while and talk honestly with you?

_____ Able to apply and use some of your communication skills learned last term?

_____ Convinced that talking out a patient's fears now will really help the postoperative course?

▲ Observe a nurse preparing a child for surgery by using play therapy, puppets, picture books, tours, and so on.

Preoperative Teaching

O b j e c t i v e s

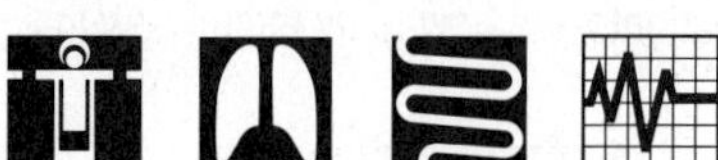

4. Given a patient situation, state how each of the following will help or hinder a patient's ability to withstand the stress of anesthesia and surgical trauma: age, weight, normal activity, respiratory function, cardiac function, kidney, and hepatic function.

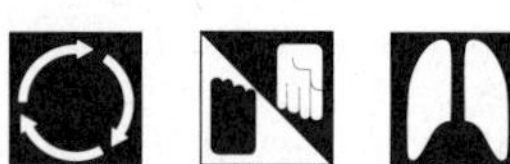

5. Demonstrate explaining to a patient why and how to move in bed, ambulate, deep breathe, and cough soon after surgery, using the criteria of preventing undue strain and discomfort on the operative site.

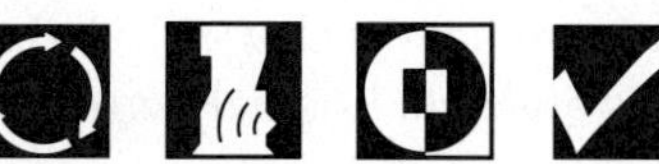

6. Given a description of a patient, state what specific preoperative explanations and teaching would help the patient's postoperative progress and state in what way it would help.

■ A. What's It All About?

1. Think about the times you have heard someone say, "It's just minor surgery," or "She's going to have an exploratory laparotomy." What is the difference between minor and major surgery? Is one safe and one dangerous? How should a patient view each surgical procedure that involves receiving anesthesia? What are the risks?

2. Read about *preoperative preparation* and *teaching, postoperative complications and care,* for the surgical patient.

Read a "Consent to Treatment or Operative Procedure" (operative permit) from your local hospital.

3. Answer the following questions:

(a) How does the stress of surgery affect the fluids and electrolytes and hormone secretion in the body?

(b) What are the differences between the following types of surgery:

diagnostic	ablative
exploratory	reconstructive
cosmetic	constructive
curative	palliative

Find examples of each of the above types of surgery on your surgical unit.

c) List examples of health problems that might occur because of each of the following pathologic processes and describe what can be accomplished through surgery to alleviate the problem:

obstruction	erosion
perforation	tumor

(d) What postoperative complication would you be especially alert for in each of the following patients?

A heavy smoker has a history of heart disease and is 40 pounds overweight, age 49.
Is 2 months old.
Has a history of hepatitis and kidney disease (no albumin in the urine), age 20.
Has slightly elevated liver enzymes, age 9.
Is 74 years old and had a mild stroke 5 years ago.

The nursing care a patient receives before surgery has a major impact on how he tolerates surgery and recovers from it. How would your preoperative teaching differ for each of the patients above and why?

4. List five potential postoperative complications and describe the nursing interventions that are aimed at preventing them. Underline those measures that need to be taught to the patient preoperatively.

Potential Complication	**Nursing Interventions**

How many of these complications are listed on the operative permit? Why?

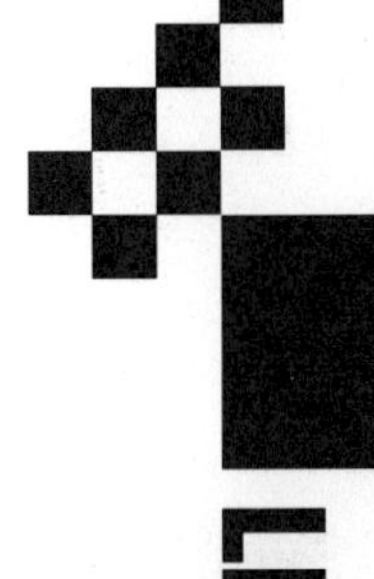

LEG VII-A

■ B. Putting It into Action!

1. Practice each of the following activities with another nursing student:

■ Explain to a patient how to move in bed, exercise legs and feet, how to cough with the least amount of pain, yet effectively, and how to deep breathe.
Splint the "incisional area" with the nurse's hands, then the patient's hands, and then try a pillow.
Reverse roles.

What position should the patient be in to cough? In what order will you proceed when you have an order to turn, cough, and deep breathe the patient? How are deep breathing and coughing different when a patient has COPD? How do you know a cough is effective? What do you chart about a cough?

■ Explain to a patient how to use an incentive spirometer.

2. Attend a small group discussion on "Assessing and Teaching Preoperative Patients."

■ Think about how you get information, whether through an interview or from the chart. What kinds of information would you expect to find on the chart? What information can you obtain by interview? What questions will you ask?

■ What health problems decrease the body's ability to withstand stress?

■ List examples of stress responses that can occur postoperatively.

■ Why are the elderly poor surgical risks? List at least three reasons.

■ Discuss the reason for the operative permit, the responsibilities of the nurse, and legal implications for the doctor, nurse, and hospital.
What does informed consent mean? Who provides the information needed by the patient? What must be included?
When the nurse witnesses the patient signing the consent, what does it mean?
What do you do when the patient is a minor? When the patient is unable to sign his name? In an emergency? When the patient says she doesn't understand what the doctor said? When the patient says she doesn't want to have the surgery?

■ List at least four principles of teaching that you should be aware of when teaching a preoperative patient. Practice teaching each other using these principles and the preoperative teaching topics listed below.

Topics for Preop Patient Teaching

Explanation of surgical procedure

Explanation of surgical consent

Importance of early activity (deep breathing and coughing, splinting incision, moving in and out of bed)

Preoperative preparation

Recovery room and immediate postoperative care

How family can be kept informed

Postoperative equipment and routines (IVs, tubes, monitors)

Postoperative limitations

Expected postoperative discomforts, pain; how to handle them

Any expected procedures related to surgery (tracheostomy care)

■ How does your teaching plan change because your patient is elderly? What kind of graphics could you create to make your explanations especially clear? How can you make your instructions clear and uncomplicated with frequent repetition, without making them appear childish? This is not easy and takes practice.

3. Plan for a clinical experience.

▲ Try out some teaching approaches for children.

▲ Observe an anesthesiologist talking with a child and the parents before surgery. Find out what information is given to them and what facts determine the choice of an anesthetic.

▲ Talk with adults before surgery. Find out what they know about the recovery room (RR) and about their postoperative care. Then plan what information you could give them to help them better cooperate during their postoperative period.

▲ Complete a preoperative patient assessment based on admission information. Interview the patient and review the chart. After talking with the patient, write a teaching plan for that patient.

▲ Observe patients in the x-ray department before surgery. Accompany the technician as the patients are x-rayed; look at the films with the radiologist. Observe the patient's signs of stress, discomfort, fear, fatigue, hunger, and dehydration.

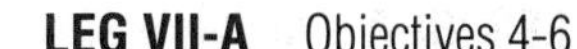

Physical Preparation for Surgery

O b j e c t i v e s

7. Identify nutritional conditions that increase the risk of postoperative complications.

8. Identify preoperative and postoperative nursing actions that support the nutritional needs of the surgical patient.

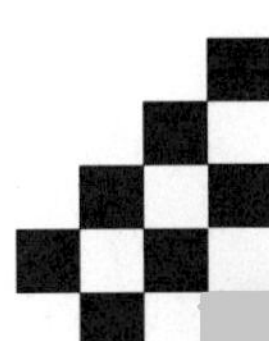

LEG VII-A

 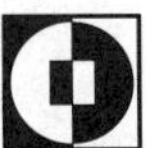

9. Given a patient situation and a list of laboratory reports for white blood count, hemoglobin, hematocrit, bleeding and clotting time, and urinalysis and their normals, state which would need to be called to the physician's attention preoperatively and might prevent surgery.

10. List the equipment needed and the actions you would take to complete a skin prep on a patient before surgery.

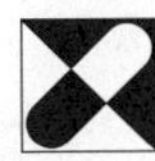 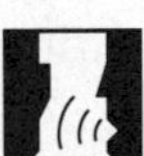

11. Demonstrate or describe in writing preparing a patient for surgery on time, using a preoperative checklist.

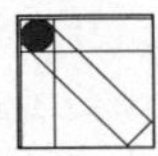

12. Demonstrate making a surgical bed and preparing the room to receive a patient from surgery.

Comments on Viewing Operations

It is difficult to view films that show incising the skin and exploring the internal organs without identifying with the patient being operated on. Blood is shown freely, and we assume the patient must be feeling pain, although our reasoning tells us that the patient has been anesthetized and is asleep. Think this through before viewing the films at this Level and you may find yourself better prepared to view operations both filmed and live.

A. What's It All About?

1. Think about the last 12–14 hours before surgery. It is 8 P.M. and the visitors have left. Now the patients get their skin preps, enemas, and showers. Try to imagine what your patients' feelings and thoughts are. How can you complete your schedule of work and still meet their needs? What will help them sleep a little better?

How can the needs of a patient who is not admitted until the morning of the surgery be met? What must it be like for that patient at home alone or with a loved one?

How do foods and diet affect the patient who needs surgery? Remember how the reward of ice cream is promised to a young patient after a T&A (tonsillectomy, adenoidectomy)? You will learn the implications of diet therapy for surgical patients.

2. Review:

LEG I-B	Listening to and Observing Communication
	Nutrition and Nutrients
LEG II-C	Nutritional Needs and Basic Diets
LEG III-A	Nutritional Needs
LEG III-C	Body's Response to Physical Injury
	Infection Control
LEG IV-A	Therapeutic Communication Skills
LEG IV-B	Calculating Parenteral Medication Dosages
	Preparing Parenteral Medications
LEG IV-C	Special Diets
LEG V-A	Surgical Asepsis Techniques

3. Read about *preoperative preparation, nutritional needs of surgical patients,* and *laboratory tests* in medical-surgical and nutrition references and hospital procedure manuals.

4. Answer the following questions:

(a) Why is the period before, during, and after surgery sometimes called a time of limited starvation? How does the burning of fat tissue for energy relate to metabolic acidosis? What routine therapy prevents this condition? How?

(b) What is the importance of the following nutrients for the surgical patient: iron, vitamins C and K, protein, carbohydrates? How could these nutrients be given to a postoperative patient who is NPO?

(c) What is the main purpose of preoperative meals? What are five reasons that it is important to make a nutritional assessment of a surgical patient? If your assessment of a preoperative patient indicates that dehydration is present, what nursing actions should you take? Why?

(d) List foods that provide the following nutrients:

carbohydrates

protein

vitamin K

vitamin C

vitamin B

calcium

iron

zinc

LEG VII-A

5. Write a nutritional plan for a postoperative patient. Include the patient and family members in this plan. Remember to consider religious and cultural customs. If the diet plan does not fit in with the culture and religion of the patient, it will not be followed.

6. Attend a lecture on "Laboratory Reports and Their Implications for Surgical Patients."

■ B. Putting It into Action!

1. Practice in campus lab.

■ Help someone on and off a stretcher from a bed. Give your "patient" different physical limitations, such as a painful abdominal incision or the inability to move the left side. Then add the various types of tubing that might be present, such as an IV in one arm, a NG tube, and a urinary catheter and drainage bag (any or all of these). You may find that you need to organize your plan of attack before starting.

When the patient returns to the room, several people are involved in the transfer. Don't be embarrassed by having a stool, chair, or congested bedside stand in the way. Be sure your patient's room is ready. Try it in campus lab without preparation.

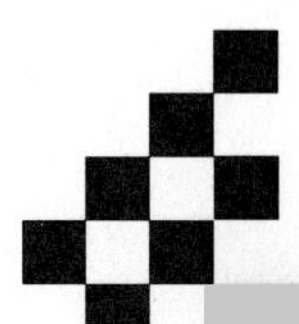

■ Check out self-practice materials "Skin Prep" after you have viewed a demonstration. Examine its contents. Is the soap supplied? The razor? Go through the steps as if you were going to complete a skin prep. How can you see if you have removed all the hair? What is the harm in leaving a few hairs, nicking the skin, or scraping the skin? Have you ever had tape applied to scraped skin and then pulled off again? Ouch!

Because of the skill involved and the importance of the prep being done properly, some hospitals designate one person to do all the preoperative preps, or it may be done in surgery. However, if a patient needs to go to emergency surgery, you may be the one to prepare the patient, so it will be to your benefit to be familiar with the equipment and have some practice in shaving another person, be it patient or friend.

LEG VII-A

Comments on Giving Instructions

What is very clear to you may not be clear at all to the patient. As an example, an RN in a large teaching hospital had the following experience. One of her patients was scheduled for abdominal surgery the next morning. After visiting hours, she went to the patient and explained that the doctor wanted him to shower before going to bed. She handed the patient three ounces of liquid soap, a washcloth, and a towel and told him, "Take this and have a good shower." The patient returned from the shower a short time later and told the nurse, "That stuff tasted awful! But the shower felt good." (He thought he was supposed to drink the soap, and did.)

Fear, anxiety, and apprehension affect your patients' comprehension of instructions and seemingly simple things like the soap. Be very careful to make sure that your patients understand.

2. Obtain three preoperative checklists from your hospital or instructor, three sheets of nurse's notes, and medication records, and do the following:

■ Record preoperative care on your checklist, nurse's notes and medication records. Record according to your local policy. Bring them to your clinical lab.

■ Write *nursing diagnoses* in order of priority for two of the following patients; then write a plan of care for each. Be sure to include rationales. Include what physical and emotional care you will give each patient before surgery, including giving medications. Compare your plans with another student's.

Discuss how the plan of care would be different for patients admitted early in the morning before surgery than when one is admitted a day or two before surgery.

Mrs. Greene, age 30, had been having vaginal bleeding between her regular menstrual periods. Her physician decided to examine the uterine lining to determine the cause. A D&C and biopsy of tissue were done in the doctor's office. On the basis of his findings, he decided to perform a hysterectomy. The Greenes have one child and had hoped for one or two more. They are disappointed but willing to accept the doctor's decision.

Mr. Serch, age 66, has been having difficulty with urination for the past few years. His physician had told him that his prostate gland was enlarging and one day he would need to have surgery to remove the tissue encroaching on his urethra. His difficulties did increase, and now he has to get up three and four times during the night to void. He is admitted to the hospital one day before surgery for a TUR (transurethral resection).

Alice Tunsel, age 7, has had repeated attacks of tonsillitis and ear infections. The doctor has advised having her tonsils and adenoids removed when she is free from infection. Her parents have never had a child in the hospital and are uncertain of exactly how to prepare her for this experience. The doctor gives them a booklet to read. She is scheduled for admission the morning of surgery.

3. Attend a group discussion on "Preparing Patients for Surgery" after you have completed B.1 and B.2.

■ Assume you are the morning nurse and are responsible for preparing your patient (select one of the patients in B.2) for surgery. It is 7:15 A.M. Surgery is scheduled and you are waiting for a phone call to give the "on call" medications. You have between *3 and 5 minutes* after the phone call before the patient will be taken to the OR.

■ If your patient is admitted the day before surgery, how can you make sure the patient is well hydrated before surgery?

■ Many doctors do not use any preoperative sedation. What is their rationale?

■ Organize your nursing actions so that your patient is completely ready for surgery on time without feeling rushed or anxious. What rationale will you use to organize your actions?

■ When do you check the lab reports? How do you check for allergies? How are allergies called to the surgeon's attention?

■ What additional care will your patient require other than what is included on your checklist?

■ What safety precautions do you take if an adult or a child receives medication preoperatively?

■ Look back at the descriptions of Mr. Serch and Mrs. Greene. How will you help them onto the stretcher preoperatively and off postoperatively? How do their ages make a difference in their care? What if Mr. Serch were 84 instead of 66?

■ Which of the following assessments would need to be reported to the physician and might cause the surgery to be canceled?

elevated temperature

elevated white blood cell count (WBC)

low Hgb

abnormal EKG

runny nose and cough

■ When might an abnormal report be expected and not need to be reported?

■ In many hospitals, children and adults are admitted 2 or 3 hours before surgery; therefore, the preoperative assessment is important. What if:

the admitting temperature is 101°?

the patient is coughing and/or has a rash?

the mother admits to giving her child "just a little breakfast" before coming to the hospital?

a toddler is found clutching another child's bottle and the nurse is unable to determine whether the child drank anything?

you are unable to obtain a urine specimen?

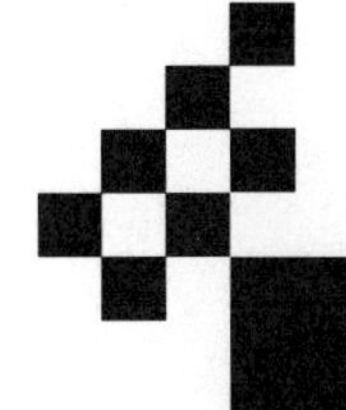

LEG VII-A

■ What charting will you be doing and when will you do it? Once you have decided on a plan of action, role play it, with another student acting as the patient. Include preparation of the medication with a practice syringe, needle, and vial. Time yourself. Did it take longer than you expected? Evaluate your plan and make changes as necessary.

4. Plan for a clinical experience.

▲ Observe the preparation of preoperative medications in the morning. How long does it take the staff nurse to prepare, give, and chart a medication?
Look closely at the various medications so that you will know exactly how to prepare them when you have an opportunity to do so.
Read some of the preoperative orders for patients waiting to be "called" and think through exactly how you would draw them up and where you would chart them. Practice drawing up and giving medications in preparation for the next Objectives on preoperative medications.

▲ Accompany the person doing skin preps. Observe the technique and the finished skin area. What would your strengths and weaknesses be if you were doing this procedure? Is your hospital using a dipilatory? How does the procedure change? What safety measures would you need to take? Would you check for possible allergies before the prep was done? Why?

▲ Observe an admission procedure for a patient going to surgery. As soon as you feel comfortable with your skills and organization, admit a patient for surgery. You will not have much time, so you will need to be organized.

▲ Care for patients preoperatively in the morning or evening and assume as much responsibility for their surgical preparation as you are able. Accompany them to the OR and observe the surgery if possible.
Take notes of their behavior and appearance after receiving their preoperative medications. If arrangements have been made ahead of time, stay to observe the patient

receive anesthesia and the operative procedure. (If you know the purpose of the operative procedure ahead of time and have done some reading about it, you will learn a great deal more while in the OR and will be able to ask intelligent questions.)

▲ Look up the preoperative medication orders for different children. Write them down. Look at the medications on the unit and write down how each medication is supplied (for example, 10 mg tablets or gr ss per cc or 50 mg per suppository).

▲ Attend postconference to share your experiences. Discuss these questions:
Which patients have bleeding and clotting times done before surgery? Why?
How can you assist the preoperative medications to achieve their desired effect?
What side effects did you observe?

▲ Accompany a dietitian making rounds on a surgical floor. Observe and listen for questions from pre- or postoperative patients.

▲ Help move patients on and off stretchers.

▲ Prepare a room to receive a postoperative patient.

Preoperative Medications

Objectives

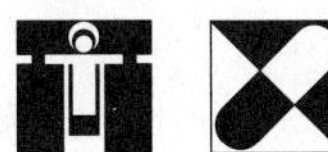

13. Given a list of desired and undesired effects of drugs in the following classifications, select those for which you would be observant when giving each drug to a patient: narcotic, analgesic, anticholinergic, benzodiazepines, and barbiturates. A drug list will be provided by your instructor.

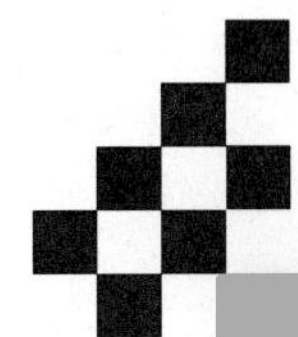

 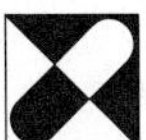

14. Demonstrate safety while giving a preoperative medication exactly on time.

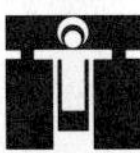 

15. Given an order for a preoperative medication in a pediatric dosage, describe how you will prepare the medication, how much you will administer in cubic centimeters or minims, and how you will administer it to the child.

LEG VII-A

■ A. What's It All About?

1. Think about medications and their effect. What can you tell your patient to make the unpleasant effects such as dry mouth or dizziness less bothersome and frightening? Fear of an injection and actually receiving the injection may be worse for a child than the fear of the unknown waiting in the operating room. Prepare your patients of all ages for their medications. They will be relieved to know the reaction is expected and has purpose.

2. Review:

LEG IV-A Effects of Drugs on the Older Adult
LEG IV-B Calculating Parenteral Medication Dosages
Preparing Parenteral Medications

3. Read about *pediatric dosages, anatomy and physiology of the autonomic nervous system,* and *preoperative medications* in medical-surgical, pediatrics, geriatrics, and pharmacology texts, and in the following:

Reiss, B., and M. Evans. *Pharmacological Aspects of Nursing Care,* 4th ed. Albany, NY: Delmar Publishers, 1993.

Spratto, G., and A. Woods. *RN's NDR-93 Nurse's Drug Reference.* Albany, NY: Delmar Publishers, 1994.

4. List in the chart on p. 148 the desired preoperative effect and the undesired actions that might occur for the preoperative drugs on a list given you by your instructor. Group the drugs according to the classifications in Objective 13. Find drugs on patients' charts and in reference books. Look up and write down the normal dose for an adult and a child. The first listing is an example. You may want to use drug cards instead.

Which of the following medication dosages would be safe for children and which for adults? Select your answer from the column at the right and write it in the blank.

Children (under 90 lb)	**Choice of Answers**
Demerol ______________________	Demerol, 25 mg
Atropine ______________________	Demerol, 75 mg
Vistaril ______________________	Demerol, 150 mg
	Vistaril, 2 mg
	Vistaril, 25 mg
Adult (150 lb or more)	Vistaril, 75 mg
Demerol ______________________	Vistaril, 150 mg
Atropine ______________________	Atropine, gr 1/500 (0.12 mg)
Vistaril ______________________	Atropine, gr 1/200 (0.3 mg)
	Atropine, gr 1/150 (0.4 mg)
	Atropine, gr 1/20 (3 mg)
	Atropine, gr 1/5 (12 mg)

Classification	Drug	Desired Action/Use	Undesired Action/Use	Dosage Adult	Dosage Child	Nursing Implications	Drug Interactions
anticholinergic	atropine	reduces secretions and salivation	causes excitement; talkativeness;dilates the pupils causing blurred vision; reduces sweating; causes flushing	0.4 mg	0.12 mg	explain flush caused by vasodilation note signs of tachycardia	

5. Answer these questions:

(a) What group of drugs mimic the sympathetic nervous system? What effect do they produce? Name one such drug.

(b) What group of drugs mimics the parasympathetic nervous system? What effect do they produce? Name one such drug.

(c) What do cholinergic blocking agents do? Name one such drug.

(d) What do adrenergic blocking agents do? Name one such drug.

6. Attend a lecture on "The Autonomic Nervous System."

■ B. Putting It into Action!

1. **Work** the following dosage problems and state how much medication you will give each patient in cubic centimeters or minims.

> Tommy, age 4, 40 in. tall, 38 lb, is to receive 25 mg of Vistaril IM. The Vistaril is supplied 50 mg/cc.
>
> Cindy, age 7, 50 in. tall, 58 lb, is to receive atropine gr 1/500 IM. The atropine is supplied gr 1/300/cc, 1/200 per cc, and 1/150 per cc.
>
> Susan, age 6, 48 in. tall, 48 lb, is to receive Demerol, 25 mg IM. The Demerol is supplied 100 mg/2 cc, 50 mg/1 cc, and 75 mg/2 cc.

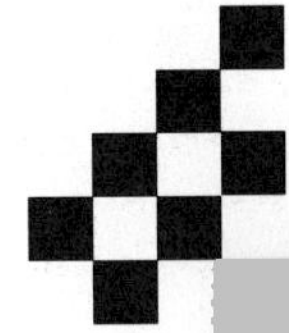

LEG VII-A

2. **Practice** in campus lab.

- Role play how you would prepare the following preoperative medications:

  Demerol, 25 mg, and scopolamine, 0.25 mg IM to a 4-year-old.

  Morphine sulfate, 4 mg, and atropine, 0.15 mg IM, to a 2-year-old.

  Scopolamine, 0.15 mg IM to a 1-year-old.

- Which of the above dosages and medications would you give without question and which would you not give without verification by the physician and why?

Note: You are mixing two medications in one syringe. The dosage is very small and your need for accuracy is very important! Practice!

- What differences might you find in dosage for an elderly adult? Why?
- Practice preparing preoperative medications. Be sure you can draw up two medications in one syringe without contaminating the second vial. Try drawing up a colored solution first and a clear solution second.

Problems for Solving

> You were preparing atropine for a patient and accidentally got some on your finger. You failed to wash your hands and later rubbed your eyes.

What effect will it have on your vision? What effect could be seen by an observer?

> You are admitting a patient and inquiring about allergies. The patient states he is allergic to morphine. You ask him what symptoms occur when he takes it.

What might he tell you? How do allergic manifestations differ from side effects?

> A physician inquires about a patient's history of heart disease and glaucoma before writing her preoperative orders.

Why?

After receiving an injection of medication, the patient becomes quite apprehensive and tells you he feels "peculiar." He throws off the bed covers and rubs the palms of his hands together and sits upright. He seems to be having difficulty breathing.

What could be happening to this patient, and what is the best action for you to take?

A physician orders a child to receive codeine gr $\frac{1}{6}$ (10 mg) and you know you have codeine gr $\frac{1}{4}$ and gr ss in the narcotic cupboard. You decide to tell him this, and he changes his order to gr $\frac{1}{4}$ and tells you he'd rather have you spend your time with the patient than figuring out drug problems in the medication room and that the difference between gr $\frac{1}{4}$ and gr $\frac{1}{6}$ is negligible for this patient.

How did you approach the problem? Think about the problem above and what you, the nurse, said and did that influenced the outcome.
Role play it with another student assuming different attitudes and observe the effect.

3. Plan for a clinical experience.

▲ Give preoperative medications within 5 minutes after patient is called from the operating room.

Observe patient reactions to medications.

Complete checklist and charting.

Immediate Postoperative Period

O b j e c t i v e s

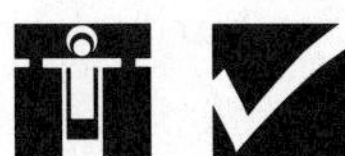

16. Describe the expected behaviors of patients including the child and the elderly patient in the 2- to 3-hour period after surgery with general anesthesia or spinal anesthesia and list three safety precautions required in caring for them during this period of time.

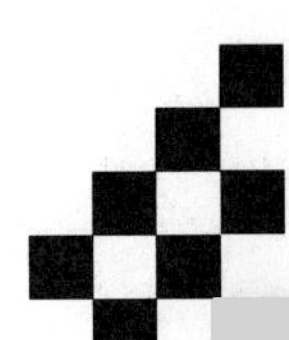

 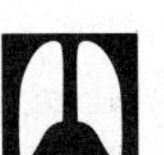 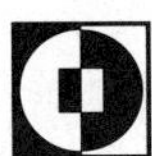

17. List assessments that would make you suspect a patient was bleeding or going into early shock after surgery.

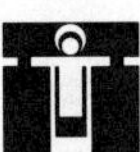 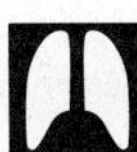

18. Demonstrate suctioning a person's mouth and nose to maintain a patent airway and to facilitate gas exchange.

 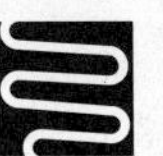 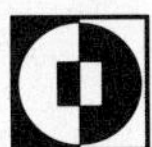 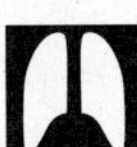 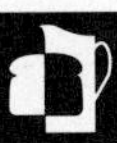

19. Demonstrate caring for a patient during the immediate 1- to 3-hour period after surgery with a general anesthetic, making assessments and planning nursing interventions for the following:

patent or obstructed airway

level of consciousness and reflexes

IV absorption, type, and amount

restlessness

discomfort

amount and type of wound drainage

early signs of shock

vomiting and aspiration

■ A. What's It All About?

1. Think about patients coming out of anesthesia immediately after surgery. These people are absolutely unable to care for themselves; they are totally dependent on the observations and care of the recovery room nurses. Can you meet their every need? Can you anticipate their needs? With time you will be able to. Observe and assist as much as possible. Prepare yourself well so that you know what assessments to make and are familiar with the equipment used in the recovery room.

2. Review:

LEG IV-C Assessing Fluid and Electrolyte Balance
Parenteral Fluid Administration

3. Read in medical-surgical, pediatrics, and geriatrics nursing references about *care of the patient during and immediately after surgery, types of anesthesia, oxygen, suctioning, early shock, recovery room nursing, intraoperative nursing, care of the unconscious patient.*

4. View audiovisuals and read articles and books from a list given you by your instructor or read from the following:

Burden, N. "Post-Anesthesia: When the Patient Is Unconscious." *RN,* April 1988, pp. 34–39.
Burden, N. "Post-Anesthesia: When the Patient Wakes Up." *RN,* April 1988, pp. 40–44.
"Post-Op Care after the Patient's Had a Spinal." *RN,* September 1990, p. 93.

5. Preview LEG XIII-A, Shock.

6. Fill in this chart in order to help you understand and remember the stages of shock. Shock is a very complex condition, and unless treatment is started early it becomes very difficult to reverse the chain reaction effect in the body. Always be suspicious of early symptoms. Don't wait for the late stage to occur.

SHOCK		
Symptoms	**Early/Compensatory Stage**	**Late/Noncompensated Stage**

LEG VII-A

■ B. Putting It into Action!

1. Prepare for a group discussion by organizing your assessments and postoperative care of the three patients on p. 144.

- Find out about the surgery that was done.
- List the observations you will make of these patients postoperatively.

2. Answer the following questions.

(a) List the postoperative assessments and precautions you should take when each of the following types of anesthetic agents is given to patients.

Inhalation Agents	**Intravenous Agents**
Fluothane	Ketamine
Ethrane	Innovar
Nitrous oxide	Versed
Regional Anesthesia	**Topical Anesthesia**
Spinal	Lidocaine
Epidural	Procaine

(b) What is conscious sedation and when is it used? Name one drug or a combination of drugs that may be used.

3. Attend a group discussion on "Care of the Patient Recovering from Anesthesia." Bring your completed answers to A.6, B.1, and B.2.

■ Discuss the following situation.

You are one of the nurses in the recovery room. You are assigned two patients who have just arrived from the OR. One has had a spinal anesthetic and the other a general anesthetic. Organize your data under the following headings:

	Description of Expected Patient Reactions, Response, or Behaviors	**Safety Precautions**
Spinal anesthetic	1. 2. 3.	1. 2. 3.
General anesthetic	1. 2. 3.	1. 2. 3.

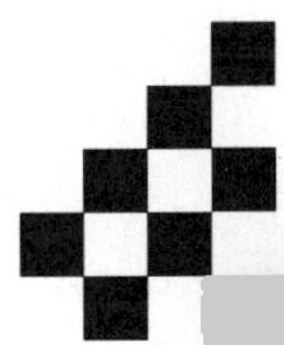

Describe an assessment of each patient that might indicate that one of the following major complications is occurring and state why the patient is at risk.

hypoventilation
hypoxia
hypovolemia

What positions should these patients be in when admitted from the OR to the recovery room?
What positions should they be in during the recovery period? Why?
How often are their vital signs taken? Why?
What observations might make you suspect your patient is bleeding or going into shock?
List other things that you as the nurse must check for during the recovery period. Consider priorities. Beside each item state how you might check for it.
Which anesthesia can cause a hallucinogenic reaction? What will be the nursing approach to a patient experiencing such a reaction?
Would you say anything to your patients during this period? Why? Or why not?
How would you recognize pain in the unconscious patient? List the assessments you would make before giving the first analgesic medication postoperatively.
Would you give your patients any medications during the recovery room period? Which ones and why?
How long would these patients remain in the recovery room?
What would their behavior be like by the time they were ready to be returned to their rooms?
Assume that your patient who had a general anesthetic is a child, 4 years old. How does age influence safety precautions, vital signs, and your observations?
How would your observations and care differ if the patient were elderly?
Describe the progression of motor and sensory loss that occurs with spinal anesthesia. How does function return?
You have returned your patient to her room. As you move her into her bed, she tells you she hears ringing in her ears. What should your next action be and why?

Mrs. Catherine O'Farrell is admitted to the same-day-care surgery unit at 6:00 A.M. and is scheduled for (L) cataract extraction at 9:00 A.M.

Discuss how each of the following would be different from a patient who was admitted the day before a surgery.

Preoperative teaching

Lab studies

Physical status

Postoperative care

Discharge

Home care

Follow-up care

Frank Phillies is having a laser procedure.

How is he prepared for laser surgery? How is the equipment prepared? What is the nursing care after the procedure? What should the nurse keep in mind for safe laser use?

4. Plan for a clinical experience.

▲ Care for patients in the recovery room. Take vital signs. Observe behavior of patients, signs of shock and bleeding, respiratory distress. Assist with admission of patient, connecting drainage tubings, giving medications, setting up IV solutions, absorption of IV solutions, positioning of patients, suctioning mouth and nose, inserting nasal cannulas, checking for drainage.

▲ If you are unable to have an experience in the recovery room, select a postoperative patient to study. Read his recovery room nursing record and list the nursing actions that you would have carried out if you had been his nurse in the recovery room.

▲ Read your agency's procedure manual for what is routinely expected of the nurse caring for patients intraoperatively. Read several patient records. Review the preoperative checklist, the operative record, and the recovery room record. Look at the assessments and nursing actions that have been taken.

▲ Go to a short-stay surgery unit. Observe and assist with preoperative and postoperative care. How does the nurse decide when to discharge a patient? Listen to the discharge directions and home care instructions provided by the nurse. Notice whether the nurses make follow-up calls the day after surgery. What kinds of questions do they ask?

▲ Care for patients in the same-day care center. Look for patients who have had cholecystectomy, lithotripsy, cataract extraction, hernia repair, arthroscopy, breast biopsy, laser surgery.

C. Extra Added Attractions!

1. **Describe** the stages of general anesthesia.
2. **Define** malignant hyperthermia.
3. **Describe** the care of a patient with hypothermia.
4. **Write** a paper about how basic asepsis principles are applied in the operating room.
5. **Talk** to 25 patients who have had surgery. Make a list of the five most common fears. Make another list of the four most important actions a nurse could take to relieve those fears.
6. **Describe** concerns for the elderly patient undergoing surgery and tell how you would adapt your nursing care.

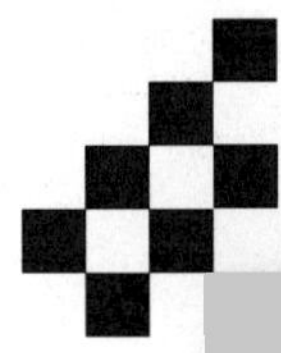

Using the Nursing Process for Postoperative Care

O b j e c t i v e s

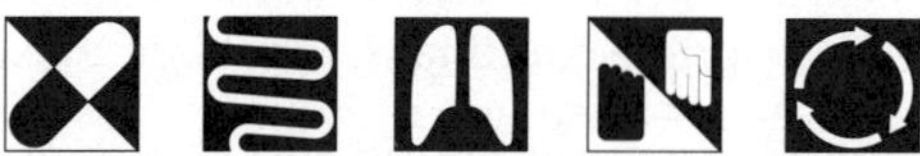

20. Given a list of actions, select those that will help to prevent atelectasis, thrombophlebitis, and wound infection and state how they may help.

21. Describe how tranquilizer, narcotic, narcotic antagonist, cholinergic, and anticholinergic drugs contribute to or relieve the following postoperative problems: distension, urinary retention, vomiting, pain, constipation, and respiratory depression.

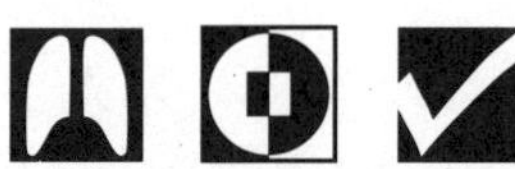

22. Care for a postoperative patient during the first 24 hours after surgery, including planning, writing, and implementing a nursing care plan using the steps of the nursing process.

23. Care for a surgical patient more than one day postoperatively and write a nursing care plan that includes both long- and short-term goals.

 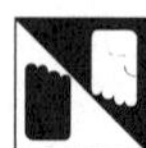

24. Demonstrate changing dressings and giving wound care following the principles of surgical asepsis and charting your procedure and observations.

■ A. What's It All About?

1. Think about a person's recovery from surgery. The answer to "How did it go?" or "How was the operation?" can be drastically changed for the worse if careful assessments aren't made for early signs of complications and reporting and nursing care given. The nurse sees the patient the most and must always be on the lookout to prevent complications.

Discomfort, although not always a complication, need not be great. You are the one responsible for easing discomfort. Your patient should not have to ask. Observe, check the records, and take action. Seeing a patient with numerous attachments such as a nasogastric tube and IV, knowing that the patient has an incision, and hearing the patient say, "Please do that later," may be enough to convince you to actually leave your patient alone. What will happen if you do?

2. Review:

LEG IV-C Irrigating a Nasogastric Tube
LEG V-A Surgical Asepsis Techniques

3. Read about *postoperative care* and the *effect of drugs* in medical-surgical, pediatrics, and pharmacology references.

4. Preview LEG VIII-C Irrigating a Wound.

5. Write how you would assess the postoperative patient upon that person's return from the recovery room. You must begin immediately. The nurse does an assessment that includes:

What Is Assessed	What the Nurse Is Looking For
Airway	
BP, P, R	
Urine output	
Catheters, drainage tubes, drainage	
IVs	
Dressings	
Level of consciousness	
Color and temperature of skin	

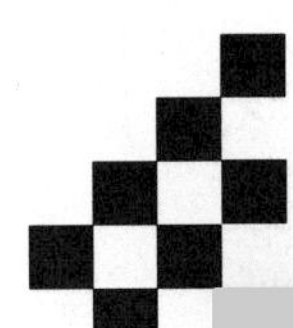

LEG VII-A

Note: The responsibility for care of the immediate postoperative patient begins as soon as that person is returned to the room. All of the conditions listed above should be of concern to the nurse receiving a postoperative patient. Be sure that you know how to do this checking and assessing for your postoperative patients.

6. List a narcotic antagonist that is effective in respiratory depression. What are the nursing implications? The common dosage?

7. Write your answers to the questions below and bring them to your discussion. What steps of the nursing process did you use?

You have been assigned to a surgical floor for an evening shift. The patients you will be caring for are in a four-bed room or two two-bed rooms:

Mr. Thoms, age 60, had a suprapubic prostatectomy yesterday. He has a Foley catheter to straight drainage; an IV running (5% D/NS 1000 cc per shift); an abdominal dressing is in place.

Mr. Williams, age 76, had a laparotomy 4 days ago. He has not had a bowel movement since his surgery but does have bowel sounds.

Mr. Stevens, age 45, is in the OR.

Mr. Roberts, age 29, had an appendectomy this morning. It is now 4:30 P.M. and he has not voided. He returned to the floor at 10:30 this morning.

Write (and then be prepared to discuss) some expected patient outcomes. What will your first actions be when you come on duty? Remind yourself of the priorities of care. What nursing actions will you make as a result of each patient's problems during the course of the evening?

What drugs might be useful for each of these patients? For their specific problems? Give specific examples of drugs.

Mr. Stevens returned to the room at 5:00 p.m. after a bowel resection. What actions will you take immediately? He is complaining of severe pain and will not deep breathe and cough or move.

What will you do?

Write a sample of the charting you would do on Mr. Stevens as he returned to the room and after your initial assessment.

You are caring for a patient who has had a hysterectomy and is being discharged on the third postoperative day. List some potential postoperative complications (both physiologic and psychologic) that can occur after she goes home. Write out what instructions you would give the patient before discharge.

LEG VII-A

■ B. Putting It into Action!

1. Practice in campus lab, assisting a physician to change a dressing.

Your student "physician" will not know all the special needs, but you should be able to anticipate the needs and have supplies and instruments ready for use.

■ Which of the following actions would you take *before* the physician gets into the room? Why? In which order?

______ Remove the soiled dressing
______ Expose the soiled dressing
______ Explain to the patient what will happen
______ Set up a sterile field
______ Check your supplies
______ Arrange a bag to receive the soiled dressing
______ Focus a light on the dressing
______ Screen the patient for privacy

2. Attend a small group discussion on "Planning Postoperative Care" of Mr. Serch, Alice Tunsel, and Mrs. Greene (p. 144). Bring and take turns presenting your nursing care plans.

■ List on the chalkboard the physiologic changes and influencing factors that occur during the phases of postoperative recovery. Discuss the related nursing care and assessments to prevent complications and discomfort for a patient, 24 hours, 48 hours, 3–7 days, and 7 days after major surgery and a general anesthetic. You may want to make a chart of this exercise. Bring as much as you can to the group session and add and share.

- What is a temperature of 101.6°F likely to mean during the first 24–72 hours after surgery and then later? Why does a surgical patient frequently have a low-grade temperature?
- Discuss the increased need for protein during the postoperative period. How can you be sure that this need is met? What is the usual progression from IVs to a regular diet for a postoperative patient? Why should a patient remain NPO until bowel sounds are heard and the bowels begin working?
- Discuss the major fluid and electrolyte problems the patients might have. List assessments you would make and how you would know a problem exists.
- List the signs and symptoms of the following wound complications: hematoma, infection, evisceration, and dehiscence. Discuss the likely timing of each. What action would you take if you suspected one of these complications? Which complications lead to wound infection?
- Discuss postoperative complications and elderly patients. What differences would you expect to find in their susceptibility to infection and the symptoms they present?
- What would you do to involve the parents in Alice's care? What if other members of the family or friends called and wanted to help? What would you do or say? What growth and development expectations do you have for Alice?

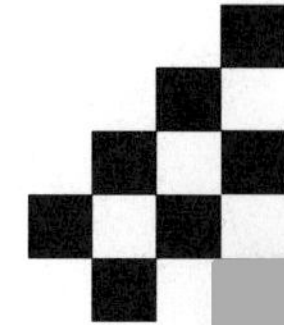

You will have more opportunity to practice these skills in later LEGs when children are hospitalized for a longer time. Begin now. Think about developmental tasks for a 4-year-old.

LEG VII-A

Problems for Solving

> The evening after surgery, Mrs. Greene's blood pressure is 100/66, P 94.

You check to see what her blood pressure was before and after surgery. Where do you find this information?

> Her normal BP is 126/84, P 76, and postoperatively she has been running between 118/80 and 112/72. You decide to call the doctor and report the blood pressure.

What additional information do you want to know before calling the doctor to help decide whether the patient may be bleeding? (There are at least three additional observations you should make.) Why?

> On the third day, Mrs. Greene's doctor asks you if there was any brown drainage on the dressing when you changed it the day before. You don't remember, and so the two of you look in the nurse's notes. The notes read "Dressing changed. Small amount of drainage."

How do you feel now? What information should have been included besides color and type of drainage? What does "small" mean to you—one 4 × 4 or five 4 × 4s, or one-half of an ABD pad?

> The afternoon after surgery, Alice asks you for a soda.

You have both Coke and ginger ale in the kitchen. Which will you give her and why? What observations must be made to determine if she is bleeding?

> Alice wakes up crying at 3 A.M. and has a large tarry stool. Her color is paler, according to her mother.

What would you do now if you were the nurse in charge?

3. Plan for a clinical experience.

▲ Care for a postoperative patient. Begin a nursing care plan (NCP) before caring for the patient.

Note: It will be necessary to read about each patient's surgical condition and special postoperative needs ahead of time until you have gained experience and knowledge. Keep the care plan after you have completed the lab and make comments on it to guide you when you care for your next patient with similar needs.

▲ Care for an elderly postoperative patient. Be alert for signs of confusion that might be caused by stress, trauma, anesthesia, drugs, and alteration in environment and lifestyle associated with the surgery. Be prepared to share in postconference what you did to prevent confusion from occurring or how you intervened if confusion was present. *Confusion is not effectively treated by sedation and restraint: it may be necessary for you to act as a patient advocate to avoid such measures.* Discuss how you might speak on behalf of a confused patient.

▲ As you care for patients, think about why certain nursing interventions are needed. What discomforts are you preventing? Easing? What nursing actions can you take to either assist the action of the drug groups in Objective 21 or require less of the drugs? Work at it. There is no magic. A really good nurse takes action because of learned rationales.

■ C. Extra Added Attraction!

1. Look at and learn how to care for and empty wound drains used by doctors in your area. Learn how they are used, how they work, and your responsibility for their care.

Planning Care for Two to Four Patients

O b j e c t i v e s

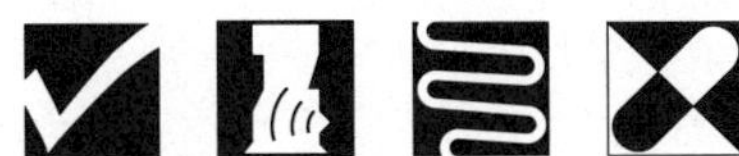

25. Given two to four patients to prepare for surgery during a specified period of time, state how you would organize your time and implement care without forgetting any details, completing the preoperative checklist and assessing patient needs.

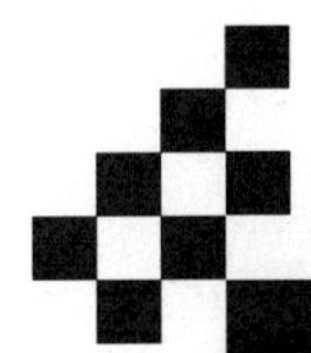

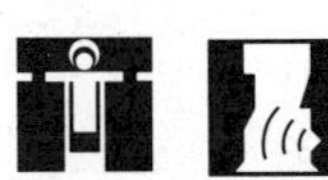

26. Describe two ways a family member or a friend could assist a patient both pre- and postoperatively in a positive manner and how the nurse could facilitate this.

LEG VII-A

■ A. What's It All About?

1. **Think about** what you hear patients say when returning home after surgery. For example, "Oh, it was really O.K. except that I was so sick from the anesthesia." "I just couldn't get going even though I didn't really hurt." Family members can be a great help. Observe and learn how to help patients and families cope. You can do this even when you have several patients to prepare and care for. But it takes effort and organization. You can do it!

2. **Read** about *planning patient care* in medical-surgical references.

■ B. Putting It into Action!

1. **Plan for** a clinical experience.

▲ Find out how many patients are going to surgery in the morning and when they are scheduled. Read their preoperative orders and look at their checklists. Write out exactly how you would proceed if you were going to prepare them all for surgery.

▲ Prepare two or three patients for surgery and be available to continue their care until they are taken to surgery. (A same-day-care surgical department would be a good place to observe and participate in giving preoperative care to groups of patients.)

▲ Care for patients who have visiting relatives. Plan ahead of time which assessments and/or actions could be accomplished by a relative in attendance and try to determine if the relative would like to be involved. Helpful areas are mouth care, offering fluids, recording intake, observing for side effects of medications, giving a back rub, checking color, and circulation. Try one or two areas and see how the relative likes being involved. Don't desert the patient because someone else is there.

Examine your own feelings during this experience. How do you like someone else caring for "your" patient? How do you like having to consider the relative's needs as well as your patient's? How do you determine whether the relative really wants to be involved but is afraid or would rather not be asked to participate? How do you explain treatments and routines to the visitor? Can you avoid using medical terminology?

Have I Learned?

The following questions are for you to answer in order to find out if you have met the Objectives. All of the Objectives in LEG VII-A are covered in this series of questions. Pick a quiet time and answer them. Answers are found at the end of this selftest.

No space has been left for answering the questions related to the "doing" Objectives. Use a separate sheet of paper for those answers, and then use the answers in clinical or campus lab for your own evaluation.

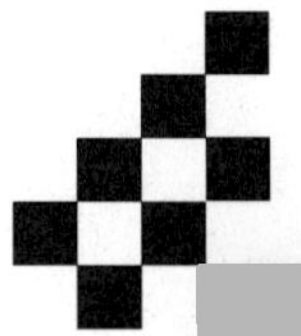

LEG VII-A

Objective	**Question**
1	**1.** How can a patient's postoperative discomforts be affected by preoperative *emotional preparation?* List two ways.
2	**2.** What clues is the following patient giving the nurse about preoperative fears? What effect does *each* of the nurse's responses have on the patient's willingness to explore thoughts and express fears?

(a) P: I sure hated to have to come in the hospital at this time. It's the busiest time for us at work.

N: Oh, what type of work are you in?

(b) P: I'm a salesman. Sell home-cleaning equipment. I visit homemakers during the day in their homes. Strictly a commission job. Sure hate to miss the business for this next month, and who knows how much longer after that. But the doc said I shouldn't put it off. The surgery, that is. Said it's pretty rare, but there's always the chance it's malignant. Course he doesn't think so in my case.

N: I'd believe your doctor if I were you. Your doctor is a well-respected surgeon in this hospital.

(c) P: Oh, I do.

N: But you can't help that little nagging possibility in the back of your mind, can you? It's not easy to wait and not know.

(d) P: That's exactly it. I'm willing to go through with it and really don't mind missing the work if it just turns out not to be cancer.

N: You've probably read a lot about cancer in the papers and seen programs about it on TV. But facing the possibility of it happening to you seems so remote.

3 **3.** Mrs. R is going to surgery in 2 days for a colostomy. You know that a colostomy is an artificial opening in the abdominal wall for the purpose of emptying the intestine and can be permanent or temporary, depending on the cause. In either case, the patient will undergo a change in body image.

Ask another student to take the part of the patient, and you take the part of the nurse preparing the patient for her change in body image. Ask a third student to write down what is said during the role playing. Evaluate the written recording for evidence of "helpful statements" you made to the patient.

4 **4.** How will the following patient's age and physical condition affect him while he is having surgery?

> Mr. Steel, age 45, is a moderate to heavy smoker with a history of having had hepatitis. He is 20 lb overweight and has a desk job. The only physical exercise he gets is playing golf on the weekends. He is on an antihypertensive medication. He has no history of kidney or heart disease.

5 **5.** Demonstrate explaining to Mr. Striker why and how to ambulate, deep breathe, and cough, and then help him to carry out these instructions while another student observes.

Mr. Striker, age 56, had a laparotomy done. This is his second postoperative day. These are his postoperative orders for today:

NG to suction, clamp to amb.
D/5/0.45 IV/125cc/h
tcdb q2h
incentive spirometer 6 × /d
amb qid
NPO
TED hose

You go into the room and he is looking sleepy. He says, "Oh, please don't bother me now. I'm so tired. I didn't sleep at all last night." What will you say and do?

6 **6.** Mr. Steel (see Question 4) is having surgery to repair a peptic ulcer. His postoperative orders will include:

NPO
Gastrostomy tube to straight drainage
Intake and output
Turn, cough, deep breath q2h
Vital signs q4h after stable
PCA Demerol with basal rate of 1 cc/h and self-administered dose of 1 cc/dose, a 15-min delay and 1 hour maximum limit of 40 mg/h (10 mg/cc)
D/5/0.45 saline at 125 cc/h
Ambulate this pm and at least qid

What preoperative teaching, explanations, and actual practice will this patient need?

7 **7.** List three nutritional conditions that increase the risk of postoperative complications.

8 **8.** List three preoperative and three postoperative nursing actions that support the nutritional needs of the patient.

9 **9.** Select which of the following lab reports would need to be called to the physician's attention preoperatively.

(a) Hemoglobin 9 gm/100 cc
(b) Hematocrit 45%
(c) WBC 8000/cu mm
(d) Hematocrit 30%
(e) WBC 18,000/cu mm

10 **10.** List the equipment you would need to do a skin prep on a patient before surgery, and list the steps you would take to do it.

11 **11.** It is 5 A.M. You have a patient with the following preoperative orders:

Morphine gr ¼ (16 mg)
Scopolamine gr 1/150 (0.4 mg) } IM on call

List the actions you would take, in the order you would do them, to prepare the patient on time for surgery. (Use the preoperative checklist from your hospital.)

12 **12.** Demonstrate that you can make a surgical bed and prepare a room for a surgical patient.

13 **13.** Select the desired and undesired effect(s) from the list at the right for each of the drugs listed on the left, for use as preoperative medications.

Drug	**Drug Actions**
(A) morphine	(a) drowsiness
______ desired effect(s)	(b) nausea, vomiting
______ undesired effect(s)	(c) flushed, warm
(B) scopolamine	(d) excitement, restlessness
______ desired effect(s)	(e) depressed respirations
______ undesired effect(s)	(f) reduced anxiety and fear
	(g) dilated pupils
	(h) reduced respiratory and salivary secretions
	(i) reduced nausea, vomiting

14 **14.** Demonstrate giving a preoperative medication exactly on time. Write a list of steps you expect to take, including the time of starting preparation and completion of administration and charting.

15 **15.** You are to give atropine gr 1/500 (0.12 mg) IM to a child. You find the solution in the narcotic cupboard and it is labeled gr 1/200 (0.3 mg)/cc. How many cubic centimeters or minims will you give?

16 **16.** List three expected behaviors of a patient during the postanesthesia period after a general anesthetic, and list three safety measures taken to protect the patient during this period.

17 **17.** List six assessments that would make you suspect your patient might be bleeding or going into shock.

18 **18.** List the steps you would take to suction a patient's mouth and nose. How does the procedure differ when the patient has had a tonsillectomy?

19 **19.**

Mabel Jones, an 83-year-old patient in the recovery room, begins to get restless. She has an IV running and a catheter in place. She responds to your questions with mumbles.

Which of the following actions would you take to assess her condition and state why:

(a) Check catheter for patency and type of drainage.

(b) Calculate how fast the IV is running and how much fluid she has received.

(c) Check for bleeding at the wound site.

(d) Ask her if she is having any pain.

(e) Check her vital signs.

(f) Observe the rate and depth of her respirations.

19 **20.** Mabel Jones begins to vomit. What is the most important action you can take at this time and why:

(a) Call the doctor.

(b) Splint the incision.

(c) Get an emesis basin.

(d) Position patient on her side.

19 **21.** Patients in the recovery room can develop hypotension for which of the following causes?

(a) The effect of general anesthesia.

(b) The effect of spinal anesthesia.

(c) Being exposed in a cold room.

(d) Being turned and moved quickly.

19 **22.** How often are vital signs routinely checked immediately after surgery?

(a) Every hour until stable.

(b) Every half hour until stable.

(c) Every 10–15 minutes until stable.

(d) Every 5 minutes until stable.

19 **23.** You are caring for a child immediately after a T&A. The recovery room nurse shows you how to hold the child's jaw forward. Why is doing this important? Select the best answer:

(a) It keeps the tongue pushed forward and the airway open.

(b) It encourages the drainage to flow out of the mouth.

(c) It improves respiration.

(d) It prevents aspiration of vomitus.

20 **24.** Which of the actions in the right-hand column would help to prevent each of the postoperative complications in the left-hand column? Write the letters in the blanks.

_____ atelectasis	(a) aerosol therapy
_____ thrombophlebitis	(b) avoid pressure under knee
_____ wound infection	(c) coughing
	(d) apply elastic bandages or hose
	(e) deep breathing
	(f) preoperative skin prep
	(g) turning in bed
	(h) surgical aseptic technique during dressing change
	(i) walking
	(j) medical aseptic technique
	(k) sitting in a chair
	(l) forcing fluids

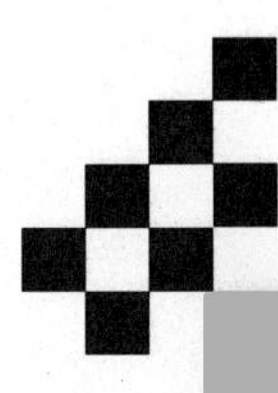

LEG VII-A

21 **25.** Fill in the blanks with "increase," "decrease," or "have no effect on."

(a) Morphine (a narcotic) will ______ the problem of distention and constipation after surgery and will ______ the problem of pain.

(b) Scopolamine (an anticholinergic) will ______ the problem of postoperative vomiting and will ______ the problem of urinary retention and constipation.

(c) Compazine (a tranquilizer) will ______ postoperative vomiting and will ______ the pain.

22,23 **26.** List two actions that a nurse could take to relieve each of the following postoperative problems other than giving medication.

(a) distention (gastrointestinal)
(b) urinary retention
(c) vomiting
(d) pain
(e) constipation
(f) respiratory depression

22 **27.** Write a nursing care plan for a patient during the first 24-hour period after surgery. Use a real patient or a case study provided by your instructor.

23 **28.** In the following situation, identify and state two problems, and list the nursing measures that you feel would lead to resolving those problems.

> Mr. R. is a 25-year-old football player who has had an appendectomy. The first postoperative day he stood to void, and was able to void, but he became dizzy and nauseous and required assistance to lie down. Later, he was assisted to sit up in a chair; he sat stiffly and requested that the nurse not leave him.

23 **29.** Mr. R. has an order for two types of pain medication: an injection of Demerol and an oral codeine tablet. List the actions you would take to determine which pain medication to give to Mr. R.

23 **30.** When writing your nursing care plan, identify at least one long-term and one short-term goal for Mr. R.

24 **31.** Write the steps you plan to take as you give wound care and change a sterile dressing, following the principles of asepsis. Ask another student to observe you, using your checklist, as you change a sterile dressing. What information must be included in your charting?

25 **32.** Look at the list of patients going to surgery during one morning in your clinical area. Imagine that you are either the night nurse or the day nurse. Plan how you would organize your actions so that two to four of the patients were prepared on time. The night nurse and the day nurse each do part of the preparation, depending on what time the patient is admitted and scheduled. List the actions you would take. Ask another student to do the same thing. Compare your lists.

26 **33.** Imagine that an elderly woman is being prepared for surgery for removal of gallstones. Her husband is anxious and always hovering over her. List three actions he could take to assist in her care before and/or after surgery and what the nursing action would be to make this possible.

Answers to Have I Learned?

LEG VII-A

1. The incidence of vomiting and the degree of pain are reduced in a patient who has reduced his preoperative fears by asking questions and expressing concerns. The amount of anesthesia required is reduced in a patient with decreased anxiety and is therefore safer.

2. *Clues to patient's fears:* "Hated to come in the hospital." "There's always the chance it's malignant."
Nurse's responses to patient:

(a) Directs conversation away from patient's feelings and toward his work.

(b) Denies the patient's right to worry.

(c); **(d)** Encourages the further expression of concerns by recognizing his feelings.

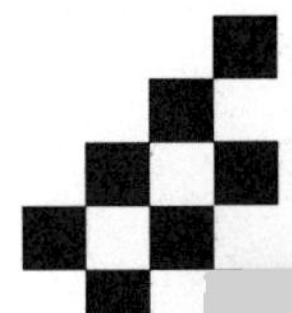

3. Did your observer hear you do the following?

Encourage the patient to talk about the forthcoming surgery.

Encourage the patient to express her feelings about the surgery and the change it will make in her appearance.

Accept her feelings regardless of what they are.

Use therapeutic communication skills to help the patient examine her feelings and concerns.

LEG VII-A

4. He is in a safe age range. His smoking will have decreased his respiratory function and increased the secretions in the respiratory tract. His hepatitis may have decreased his liver function and his ability to detoxify drugs. His kidney and heart condition should assure good elimination and circulation. The walking during golf will have benefited his respiratory and circulatory system. The burden of extra weight will place an extra strain on his heart. The antihypertensive medication to reduce blood pressure can cause further decrease (shock) during surgery.

5. Evaluate yourself with at least one other student.

6. *Explanations:* That he will have nothing to drink and IVs will be running; will have a drainage tubing in place for a few days, possibly an NG tube.

Teaching and practice: How to deep breathe and cough; how to do leg exercises in bed; how to splint incision; how to get out of bed without using abdominal muscles.

7. Obesity, malnutrition, nutritional deficiencies.

8. *Preoperatively:* Provide a high protein, vitamin C enriched fluid intake before the NPO order. Be sure the NPO time is correct for the time of surgery. Offer juice bars and lollipops to children as sources of fluid and glucose.

Postoperatively: Accurate assessment of total fluid intake in relation to total fluid output to prevent circulatory overload. Provide oral intake: IVs are a temporary measure and should be discontinued as soon as the patient can tolerate oral fluids. Help patients out of bed. Ambulation increases appetite as well as prevents many postoperative complications. Make mealtimes as appealing as possible; avoid treatments and dressing changes near mealtime. Encourage patients to eat and drink slowly to avoid swallowing air. Increase protein to correct negative balance and vitamin C to promote healing.

9. **(a)**, **(d)**, **(e)**.

10. *Equipment:* Container for water, soap, razor, gauze, scissors, bright light. Does your list include the following actions?

Explain procedure to patient and drape.

Remove long hair with scissors.

Scrub area with soap and water on gauze.

Shave area, being careful not to nick the skin.

Rinse area with water and gauze.

Check for any missed hairs.

Dry area.

11. Attend a GES to share your lists and review once more how to prepare the patient for surgery. Be sure you are ready for this when you get to clinical. Your actions will vary depending on when the patient arrived and how long you have before surgery calls. Your list may include admitting the patient to the unit. You will probably need to be well organized and work quickly in order to be on time. When you are ready, demonstrate giving care to an assigned patient.

12. Did you prepare the room so that the stretcher can easily reach the bed? Did you supply extra linen for the bed and equip the room with the necessary supplies?

13. **(A)** desired: **(a)**, **(f)**; undesired: **(b)**, **(c)**, **(d)**, **(e)**.
(B) desired: **(a)**, **(h)**, **(i)**; undesired: **(c)**, **(g)**.

14. Have your instructor or another student evaluate you according to your list. Be sure you know the reasons for your steps.

15. 0.4 cc or 6 minims.

16. *Behavior*

(a) Unconscious.

(b) Restless, eyes open, and may talk unintelligibly or groan.

(c) Reactive, appears fully conscious, understands your instructions, talks intelligibly, but does not remember.

Safety Measures

(a) Side rails up at all times.

(b) Constant observation of behavior; check vital signs every 15 minutes.

(c) Position to avoid aspiration.

(d) Airway in position until gag reflex returns.

(e) Geriatric patients may have decreased ability to ventilate and decreased kidney function for elimination of anesthesia.

17. Your answer might include normal to slight decrease in **(a)** blood pressure; **(b)** rapid, weak pulse; respirations rapid and shallow; decreased temperature; **(c)** pallor; **(d)** restlessness, feeling of apprehension; **(e)** cold, moist skin; **(f)** bleeding visible on dressings, emesis, oozing from nares (T&A), frequent swallowing (T&A); **(g)** dry mucous membranes; **(h)** thirst.

18. Does your list of steps include the following actions?

- **(a)** Wash your hands if time permits.
- **(b)** Turn on suction and fill cup with saline or water.
- **(c)** Insert suction catheter into nares or mouth with Y-tube open so suction not working.
- **(d)** Cover Y-tube opening to start suction after catheter in place.
- **(e)** Rinse suction tip in solution to clear as necessary.
- **(f)** Wash your hands when finished.

When suctioning following a tonsillectomy, avoid dislodging clots in back of mouth, so suction only front of mouth, and do that gently.

19. All of the actions should occur for these reasons:

- **(a)** The catheter may be plugged and the bladder distended.
- **(b)** There may be an overload of fluid on the circulatory system because of her age.
- **(c)** There may be bleeding and early signs of shock.
- **(d)** Pain can cause stress and shock symptoms.
- **(e)** She may be in early shock.
- **(f)** There may be respiratory obstruction from poor positioning.

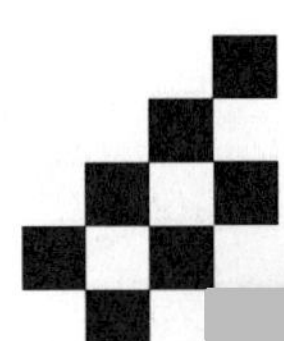

LEG VII-A

20. **(d)** To prevent the patient from aspirating her vomitus.

21. All of the answers are correct.

22. **(c)** or **(d)** depending on hospital policy and patient's condition.

23. **(a)** is the most complete answer.
(c) is correct but does not explain why.
(b) and **(d)** are incorrect.

24. Atelectasis: **(a)**, **(c)**, **(e)**, **(g)**, **(i)**, **(k)**.
Thrombophlebitis: **(b)**, **(d)**, **(g)**, **(i)**, **(k)**, **(l)**.
Wound infection: **(f)**, **(h)**, **(j)**.

25. **(a)** increase, decrease; **(b)** decrease, increase; **(c)** decrease, decrease.

26. **(a)** Avoid hot or cold liquids, decrease food intake; exercise, walk; expel gas with rectal tube or more privacy in bathroom, enema if ordered.
(b) Position on bedpan as close to normal position as possible, provide privacy, pour warm water over perineum or put hands in basin, run water, offer fluids, if not effective, catheterize.
(c) Have patient suck ice chips or sip tea or soda; provide restful environment; remove food.
(d) Remove cause of pain, use supports or splints; position change; back rub and conversation; allow patient to choose type of treatment to relieve pain.
(e) Increase fluid intake, hot liquids; increase roughage, food; privacy in bathroom; more exercise; enema if ordered.
(f) Encourage deep breathing q1h, use incentive spirometer, and turn and encourage activity as tolerated.

27. Share your care plan in postconference or as directed by your instructor.

28. May have pain related to surgical incision. Ask if he is having pain.
May have fears about too much activity causing harm. Explore with patient.
May not ask for pain medication, related to self-image. Accept patient and provide relief without his asking.
Unable to ambulate safely without assistance, related to pain, fear. Walk with patient until steady on his own.

29. Find out when and what he received last and determine its effectiveness.
Find out which he prefers. Explain the effect of each and how they differ. Assess the severity of his discomfort.
Investigate the possibility that his earlier nausea was related to receiving an analgesic.
Check his vital signs.

30. Compare your goals with at least three other students. Can your short-term goals be met in 1–2 days? Will your long-term goals be met while Mr. R. is still in the hospital?

31. Compare what your observer saw you do with what you actually did. Charting will include description of wound, care given, amount and color (and odor if present) of drainage, type of dressing applied.

32. Do your lists include charting of medications and signing of each checklist and chart? Which actions can be delegated to nursing assistants and which must the RN perform? What will you do if the orderly comes for the patient before the patient is ready?

33. He could help her with mouth care and hairbrushing the morning of surgery before she is medicated.
After surgery he can rub her back and shoulders.
He can remind her to take deep breaths every 20–30 minutes and to wiggle her feet and toes.

What Will I Learn?
LEG VII-B Fluid and Electrolyte Balance during Illness

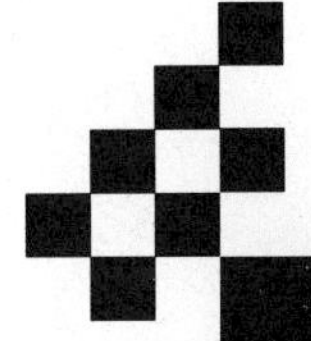

In LEG IV-C you learned how to measure fluid intake and output and to recognize some symptoms of *dehydration.* Many years ago this was all nurses needed to know. Since then, scientists have begun to recognize the importance of all the fluids in our body such as urine, gastric and intestinal juices, sweat, blood, and cellular fluids.

In the hospital, patients' fluid and electrolyte balance is often drastically altered when they are kept NPO and given IV fluids. We know now that patients can be critically influenced by imbalances in a very short time. Patients with nasogastric tubes connected to continuous or intermittent suction are in danger of fluid and electrolyte imbalance unless the *nurse is alert to early signs and symptoms!* You will learn about intestinal decompression tubes, what the various lumen allow you to do, where to get the equipment, and how to help with intubation.

In LEG VI-C you learned what arterial blood gas analysis measured and read about patients developing *respiratory acidosis* and *alkalosis.* In LEG VI-B you discovered that acidosis can occur from uncontrolled diabetes and then it is called *metabolic acidosis.* As all of these new terms come tumbling at you, you may wish to hide under a rock (denial?) or wish that you were nursing in an earlier era. Be that as it may, believe us when we say that we and your instructors understand because we've had similar impulses at one time or another. But fluid and electrolyte balance is a subject that will follow you relentlessly into every clinical area and every Level of LEGs. If you have already studied fluid and electrolytes in one of your science courses, review your notes before starting this LEG. You may need more help than usual from your instructor during this LEG because the majority of the reading resources are complex for a beginning student to understand completely. However, by the time you reach Volume IV and care for patients in intensive care, you will be able to understand them, and will want to use these readings again as references.

Many of the Learning Experiences in this LEG are "write" or "fill-in" exercises. At the completion of LEG VII-B you will have a reference LEG on the **regulatory functions** of fluids, electrolytes, and acid-base balance. Move this LEG along as you study other LEGs so that it is available for quick reference. Frequent review will make this information an integral part of your nursing knowledge.

What's Ahead in Later LEGs

LEG VII-C	Problems Due to Fluid Excess
LEG VIII-C	Caring for a Patient Receiving Hyperalimentation Therapy
LEG X-B	Blood Administration, IV Fluids, and Medications
	Problems with Hyperalimentation Therapy
LEG XI-A	Intubating and Feeding an Infant
LEG XII-C	Arterial Blood Gases
LEG XIII-A	Fluid Shifts Following a Burn
	Shock

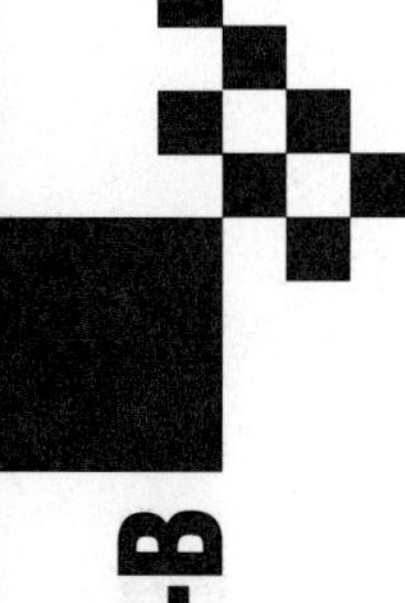

■ Overview of Learning Experiences in LEG VII-B

Objectives	Campus Lab/ Self-Practice	Group Discussions/Lectures	Clinical Lab Focuses
Fluid Balance and Imbalance **1.** Regulation of fluid and electrolyte balance **2.** Dehydration in all ages		**B2.** Normal fluid and electrolyte balance	**B3.** Look at lab reports and I&O records for fluid and electrolyte balance
Fluid and Electrolyte Imbalances **3.** Nursing care for fluid volume deficit **4.** Assessment of fluid and electrolyte balance **5.** Sodium, potassium, magnesium imbalances **6.** Nursing interventions for nausea, vomiting, and diarrhea		**B1.** Nursing patients with problems of fluid volume deficit, hyponatremia, diarrhea, and vomiting GES Objective 3	**B3.** Look for patients with signs of or at risk for dehydration Read charts Care for children with fluid and electrolyte imbalances Use fluid and electrolyte checklist
Acid-Base Imbalances **7,8.** Causes of respiratory and metabolic acid-base imbalances **9.** Recognizing when metabolic alkalosis might occur	**B3.** Lab report forms	**B1.** Acid-base imbalance	**B4.** Observe breathing exercises Look at charts and lab reports Care for patients with acid-base imbalances
Parenteral Solutions **10.** Using parenteral solutions **11.** Using a microdrip set **12.** Adding IV solutions to existing infusion **13.** Caring for venipuncture site **14.** Intervening when IV equipment fails to function properly	**B1.** Superimposing IVs Calculating and regulating flow rate Changing dressing at infusion site Troubleshooting IVs	**A7.** The nurse's role in hospital malnutrition with dietitian **B2.** More on fluids and electrolytes—parenteral solutions GES Objectives 11, 12, 13	**B3.** Observe IV therapy Care for infusion site Change IVs Use infusion monitors or pumps
Gastric and Intestinal Tubes and Feedings **15,16.** Insertion and use of gastrointestinal tubes **17.** Enteral feedings **18.** Inserting a nasogastric tube		**B3.** Nasogastric intubation and delaying tactics GES Objectives 15, 17, 18	**B5.** Observe patients with various nasogastric and decompression tubes Assist with insertion and removal of tubes Give special nose and mouth care to patients with NG tubes Observe for fluid and electrolyte imbalance Give enteral feedings

New Terms

active transport
anion
ascites
base
  deficit
  excess
bicarbonate
buffer
carbonic acid
cation
diffusion
edema
  dependent
  periorbital
  pitting
  refractory
electrolyte
extracellular
homeostasis
hyperosmolar
hypertonic
hypotonic
interstitial
intravascular
ion
isotonic
osmolality
osmolarity
osmosis
plasma
semipermeable membrane
specific gravity
tetany
third space
turgor

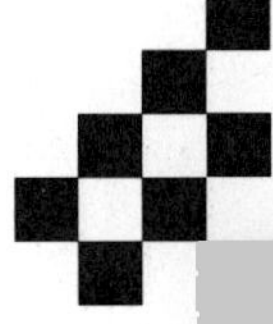

Abbreviations

BE
Ca
Cl
ECF
ECV
HCO_3
HPO_4
ICF
K
mEq
Mg
Na
pH

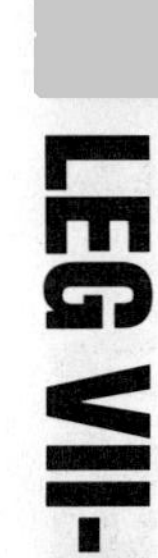

Fluid Balance and Imbalance

Objectives

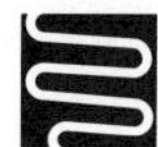
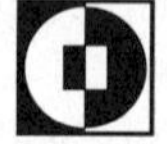

1. Describe the role of each of the following in maintaining fluid and electrolyte balance in the body: semipermeable membranes, plasma proteins, kidneys, gastrointestinal tract, nervous system, hormones, electrolytes.

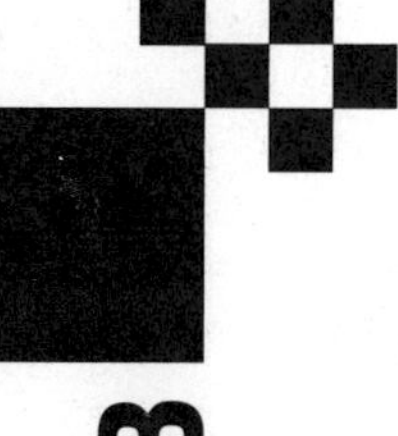

2. Describe orally or in writing why dehydration or ECF volume deficit is more common in infants and the aged than in young and middle-aged adults.

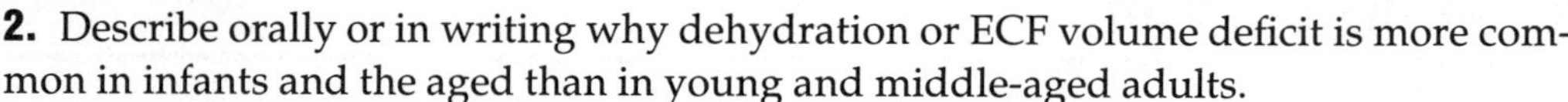

LEG VII-B

A. What's It All About?

1. Think about all the body parts and particles of food and fluid that work together automatically and normally to keep us alert, healthy, and happy. When opposite symptoms occur, your fluids and electrolytes may be mildly out of balance. Try this: drink a tall glass of water, Gatorade, or other soft drink after a long day at school, and notice the quick pickup in your feeling. Better yet, train yourself to take several sips of water every time you pass a fountain (at least eight times a day), and you may not need the big glass at the end so much.

Regulation of fluids and electrolytes is a fascinating and vital part of our physical ability to adapt and keep going. Learn it well, and observe your patients for signs of imbalances; then make the necessary interventions.

2. Review LEG IV-C, Assessing Fluid and Electrolyte Balance.

3. Read about *body fluids, electrolytes, gains and losses, homeostatic mechanisms, fluid and sodium imbalances,* and *dehydration.* Begin reading in a fluid and electrolyte reference recommended by your instructors. As you read, fill in the answers to the questions in A.4 and A.5. Continue to use your reference as you complete this LEG. With later Objectives you will also find some good journal articles that will supplement your basic reference. Don't expect to understand or be able to remember all the information the first time you read it. Read a chapter, attend a discussion, then reread the material.

4. Write your answers to these questions as you read and view audiovisuals.

(a) Body water contains cations and anions. Each cation is always balanced chemically by an anion. So, if cations increase, the anions also increase. In this fashion, electrolyte balance is maintained. Which of the following are cations (+) and which are anions (–)? Na____ K____ Cl____ HCO_3 (bicarbonate)____ Mg____ HPO_4 (phosphate)____.

Which of the above anions and cations might join together chemically? ________

Name the major cation found in the ECF (extracellular fluid)________________

Name the major anion found in the ECF ________________________

Name the major cation found in the ICF (intracellular fluid) ______________

Name the major anion found in the ICF________________________

Which of the following are contained in the ECF____; the ICF____?

1. plasma in blood vessels
2. tissue fluid in interstitial spaces
3. intracellular fluid

(b) List two ways that the osmolarity (the density of a fluid) of body fluids can be altered.

___

___

Which of the following can be actively transported across a cellular membrane: Na, K, Cl, protein ___

Why are people with edema often placed on a low-sodium diet? ___

___

(c) Why do people who work outdoors in a hot climate take salt tablets? ___

___

What changes in the osmolarity of the body fluids can cause thirst? ___

What are the major purposes of electrolytes in the body?

___

(d) List several food sources for each of the following:

Na ___

Cl ___

K ___

protein ___

Ca ___

Mg ___

(e) Describe briefly how the following work together to regulate the fluid and electrolyte balance in our bodies. What does each one do?

semipermeable membranes ___

plasma proteins ___

kidneys ___

gastrointestinal tract ___

nervous system ___

hormones ___

electrolytes ___

5. Answer the following questions on fluid imbalance in children and the aged.

(a) Describe how the amount of water a person's body contains changes with age and state one implication the amount of water has for each of the following age groups:

Infant

Aged

(b) Describe what fluid shift occurs between the ECF and ICF when the following situations occur.

A man is playing baseball on a hot day and sweats a great deal. ___

___

LEG VII-B

When the game is over, he is very thirsty and drinks a quart of water.________

____

When does the osmolarity of the ECF change, and how does the body compensate for this change?

(c) Describe the following types of dehydration and their causes:

Type of Dehydration	Description	Causes
Isotonic		
Hypertonic		
Hypotonic		

What is the difference between hypovolemia and dehydration?

(d) Describe in the space provided how each of the following could change because of dehydration in an infant and in an aged person.

	Infant	Aged
BP		
Respirations		
Pulse		
Skin turgor		
Tearing and salivation		
Mucous membranes		
Tongue		
Thirst		
Eyeballs		
Behavior and general appearance		
Crying		
Body temperature		
Pulse		
Urine output and concentration		
Urine specific gravity		
Stools		
Vomiting		
Hematocrit		
Body weight		

LEG VII-B

(e) Read about Luis, who is admitted with vomiting and diarrhea (p. 197). Which of the above changes did he have on admission?

(f) List the body sites where dehydration can best be observed.

(g) How do the following change with dehydration?

vital signs
hematocrit
urine specific gravity
serum sodium

■ B. Putting It into Action!

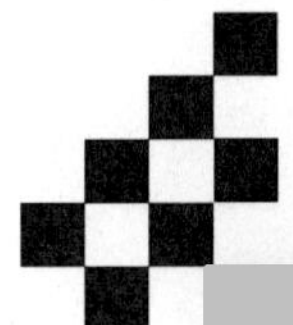

LEG VII-B

1. Fill in the blanks below. Cover the answers.

Na is a ________ ion; is a ________ electrolyte; is a cation.	++
Cl is a ________ ion; is a ________ electrolyte; is an anion.	−−
Sodium and water are excreted ________.	together
Ideally body fluids are ________.	isotonic
Extracellular fluid is composed of ________ and ________ fluid.	plasma interstitial
Fluid that occupies "spaces between" is called ________ fluid.	interstitial
Fluid passes from cells to spaces and back by ________.	osmosis
Body fluids have equal osmotic pressure that is called ________.	isotonic
To keep the ECF isotonic the kidneys must reabsorb ________ Na.	↑
Sodium combines with ________.	water
Therefore, the kidneys also ________ water.	reabsorb
A symptom that the body needs more fluid is ________.	thirst

2. Attend a group discussion on "Normal Fluid and Electrolyte Balance." Bring your completed answers and your questions.

3. Plan for a clinical experience.

▲ Look at lab reports and intake and output records. Review how you know there is a fluid and electrolyte balance.

Fluid and Electrolyte Imbalances

3. Given a patient with fluid volume deficit related to diarrhea, inadequate fluid intake, postoperative bleeding, or nausea and vomiting, use the nursing process to reach a solution.

4. Demonstrate completing the Fluid and Electrolyte Assessment Checklist on p. 186 as you care for a patient with a potential or existing fluid and electrolyte imbalance, and list three independent nursing actions you could take that are related to the imbalance.

5. List assessments that you would make and nursing interventions related to each of the following electrolyte imbalances: decreased sodium, increased sodium, decreased potassium, decreased magnesium.

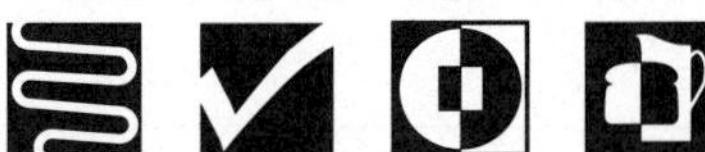

6. Given patients with problems of diarrhea or nausea and vomiting related to drug allergy, intestinal obstruction, vertigo, or postoperative course, describe why vomiting or diarrhea occurs with each and state two nursing actions specific for each.

A. What's It All About?

1. Think about your own symptoms: thirst following a ham dinner; polyuria after drinking several glasses of fluid; feel of your skin with fever. These are common signs of fluid and electrolyte regulatory actions by the body systems. Try to explain logically the signs and symptoms of fluid and electrolyte imbalances you observe. Learn what to do to help your patient.

2. Review LEG VI-B, Adaptation to Stress.

3. Read about *diarrhea, nausea, vomiting, hemorrhage, hypo- and hypernatremia, hypokalemia, hypomagnesemia,* and *fluid and electrolyte assessments* in fluid and electrolytes, medical-surgical, and pediatrics references.

4. View audiovisuals and read articles and books from a list given you by your instructor or read from the following:

Mueller, K. D., and A. Boisen. "Keeping Your Patient's Water Level Up." *RN*, June 1989, pp. 65–68.

Rowland, M. "When Drug Therapy Causes Diarrhea." *RN*, December 1989, pp. 32–35.

5. Preview:

LEG VII-C Problems Due to Fluid Excess
LEG XIII-B Acute Imbalance in Children
LEG XIII-C Calcium and Protein Imbalance

6. Describe risks and abnormal losses from the following:

gastrointestinal tract

skin

kidney

third space

altered intake

hemorrhage

Who is at risk for fluid imbalance?

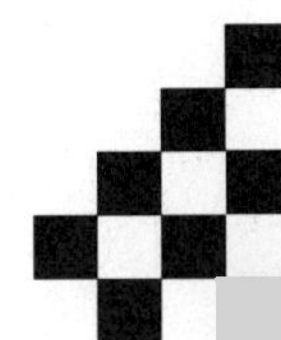

LEG VII-B

7. Fill in the blanks below.

Electrolyte Imbalance	Causes	Nursing Assessments
Increased sodium		
Decreased sodium		
Decreased potassium		
Decreased magnesium		

8. Match these terms:

_____ Increased magnesium	(a) hyponatremia
_____ Increased sodium	(b) hypernatremia
_____ Decreased potassium	(c) hypokalemia
_____ Decreased magnesium	(d) hyperkalemia
_____ Increased potassium	(e) hypomagnesemia
_____ Decreased sodium	(f) hypermagnesemia

9. Write the symptoms (for example, onset, type of stool) for diarrhea in the pediatric and adult patient related to the following causes:

Cause	What You Will Probably Observe
Drug allergy pediatric adult	
Impaction pediatric adult	
Diet pediatric adult	
Infection pediatric adult	

10. Write when each of the following interventions would be used for a patient who has just vomited. State whether this is effective for a pediatric or an adult patient.

Give water if allowed.

Give special mouth care.

Send the emesis to the lab.

Note the characteristics of the emesis.

Report the vomiting to the team leader, head nurse, or physician.

Give an antiemetic.

Stay with the patient for a few minutes.

Get the patient up in a chair.

Raise the head of the bed.

■ B. Putting It into Action!

1. Attend a lecture or small group discussion on "Nursing Patients with Problems of Fluid Volume Deficit, Hyponatremia (Na↓), Diarrhea, and Vomiting."

■ Discuss your immediate thoughts (observations and questions) if you found the following patients complaining of thirst. What more will you look for? Why? What action will you take? Why?

Mr. H. on his third postoperative day after major abdominal surgery.

Little Jane Feba, age 5, who has a high fever due to a generalized infection, says "I'm thirsty."

Jack Drie is admitted to the hospital at 3:00 P.M. He has had intermittent vomiting for 2 days and has retained little fluid. A pyloric stricture is diagnosed by x-ray. He is scheduled for surgery to repair the stricture at 8:00 A.M. tomorrow. What is your major role for this patient up until midnight the night before surgery? State your rationale.

Carol Ray has a possible small bowel obstruction.

Orders:
NPO
NG to suction
BP q2h
Check urinary output qh
To OR tomorrow A.M.

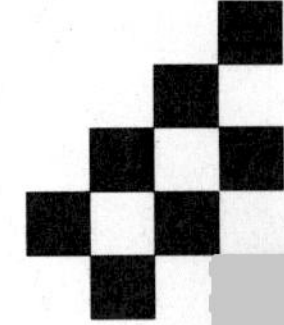

LEG VII-B

■ What do you expect to happen to the BP and P if there is an ECF↓? Why? What would anuria or oliguria preoperatively indicate to you?

If the patient is not voiding a minimum of 50 ml/h before surgery, what actions would you expect to be taken? How would you prepare for it?

■ Consider the following situation.

After surgery Carol Ray returns with an IV in place, also a nasogastric tube to intermittent suction. She is NPO. You allow her to rinse her mouth frequently. The second postoperative night she tells you she feels frightened, that she feels she is going to die, and asks you to please call her husband. It is 2:00 A.M.

What actions should you take and why? Call her husband? Call her doctor? Take her vital signs? Check her I&O? Give her sedation?

■ What nursing actions do the following patients need?

Gloria Young, 53 years old, postoperative TAH (total abdominal hysterectomy) receiving IV because of inadequate intake of oral fluids. She appears anxious, and her respirations are labored.

Bobby, with dehydration, is receiving IV fluids. You have not been able to get the child to void, and there is no record of voiding within the last 6 hours. You notice that his eyes are looking swollen, and his weight this morning has increased 4 1/2 pounds in 24 hours.

Hannah Griffin, age 82, exhibits behavior changes: confused as to time and place, drowsy, and has periods of being "out of contact." She has been hospitalized for 3 days following a left hip repair. She has taken no oral fluids and is taking about 2500 cc IV fluid per day.

Richard Lim had a paracentesis 2 days ago. You notice that he has a distended abdomen and is complaining of shortness of breath, and you note pitting edema of his legs.

■ How would you handle the following situation?
What observations would you make related to fluid and electrolyte imbalance?

Jimmy, 6 weeks old, is admitted to isolation with a diagnosis of gastroenteritis, manifested by nausea, vomiting, diarrhea, and irritability. The doctor orders:

IV therapy

NPO

Stool cultures × 3

The mother is standing outside the door while the baby is crying vigorously. As the nurse approaches, the mother becomes hysterical and states, "If you'll only feed him, he will stop crying. He's just hungry."

■ What observations will you chart at midnight about the following patient that might be related to a fluid and electrolyte imbalance?

Jack Hansen was admitted this afternoon for a possible bowel obstruction. You come on duty at 11:00 P.M. and are told in report that the new patient vomited twice and was given Phenergan. As you make rounds you notice his respirations are shallow but regular. He is sleeping and his foot is jerking under the sheet as if he is having a dream. When you wake him up at midnight to take his TPR he jumps and seems to have a hard time holding the thermometer in his mouth.

What decisions do you need to make?
What imbalance is he susceptible to?
What lab work might be ordered? Why?

■ What assessments would you make for the following patient related to fluid and electrolyte balance?

Bryan, age 38, has multiple wounds on his coccyx and ankles and is on a Clinitron bed.

■ Why do you think constipation may be a factor for the patient below?

Molly Green, an 83-year-old lady, has just been transferred to your unit because of symptoms of dehydration and electrolyte imbalance (verified by the lab report). Her physician tells you to be sure that the patient is not constipated and prescribes a stool softener and a cathartic twice a week.

How would you be sure the patient is not constipated?
What is the effect of her age on this condition?

■ What nursing diagnoses could be used for patients with fluid and electrolyte imbalances? List as many nursing interventions as you can think of for patients with vomiting, diarrhea, or dehydration. Give your rationale for each nursing intervention. Include how it will help correct the imbalance. Discuss the Fluid and Electrolyte Assessment Checklist on p. 186. Discuss related nursing interventions for each symptom described.

2. Complete the following chart for use now and as a reference with other LEGs. Use the chart as you observe patients this term and next year. Compare their problems, your assessments, and your chart.

Imbalance (Where Studied)	**Causes**	**Symptoms or How to Recognize**	**Corrective Nursing Interventions and Precautions**
ECF volume deficit (IV-C), (VII-B) (dehydration)			
Na deficit (VII-B)			
Na excess (VII-B)			
K deficit (VII-B)			
Mg deficit (VII-B)			
[The following imbalances will be studied later. You may wish to complete the chart now and use it for a reference.]			
ECF volume excess (VII-C) edema			
K excess (IX-C)			
Plasma to interstitial fluid shift (XIII-A)			
Interstitial fluid shift to plasma (XIII-A)			
Ca deficit (XIII-C)			
Ca excess (XIII-C)			
Protein deficit (XIII-C)			

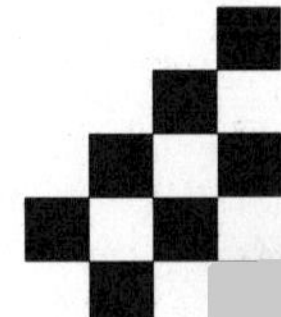

LEG VII-B

3. Plan for a clinical experience. Select at least one of the following activities:

▲ Look for patients who have signs of, or who are at risk for, dehydration related to: diarrhea (a child); inadequate fluid intake; postoperative bleeding; nausea, vomiting, and fever. Evaluate these signs in relation to their I&O, diet, level of consciousness (LOC), behavior, and lab reports.
Visit with these patients during their dehydrated state and/or after the dehydration has been relieved. Were they aware of their condition? What were their particular nursing needs?

▲ Look at these patients' charts. Compare the medical and nursing measures taken to relieve the symptoms. Make notes. What time elapsed between report of symptoms and initiation of therapy? What were the first symptoms noted? What was the first nursing action? Complete your Fluid and Electrolyte Assessment Checklist.
Look for abnormal lab reports of plasma Na, K, and Ca if possible.
Read the nurses' notes for signs and symptoms noted. Visit the patient and make notes, afterward, of your own observations.

▲ Care for children with symptoms of fluid and electrolyte imbalances. Chart your observations.

If possible, care for an infant or young child with diarrhea. As you make your assessment, be aware that it may change very rapidly. How do you assist the parents in caring for their child?

Fluid and Electrolyte Assessment Checklist

Circle assessments that are present in your patient. Add more. Use them in charting on your patients.

Subjective (information obtained from the patient)

thirst	cramps	weakness
fatigue	anorexia	poor coordination
nausea	paresthesias	lethargy
dizziness		

Objective (information based on a professional assessment)

Cerebral dysfunction (behavior)	apathy	restlessness	disorientation
	belligerence	hallucinations	depression
	twitching	confusion	agitation
	facial spasms	coma	hyperirritability
	plucking at bedsheets	tingling or numb fingers	seizures
	tremors		
BP change	hypertension	hypotension	shock
	postural change of more than 10 systolic (supine when seated)		
Pulse change	arrhythmia	full, bounding	weak, thready
		bradycardia	tachycardia
Temperature	fever over 100°F	subnormal	
Respiration	rapid	shallow	cough
	hyperactive	dyspneic	sputum frothy or pinkish
	labored	wheezing	
	slow	deep	rales
Intake, output	intake exceeds output	sugar in urine	vomiting
	output exceeds intake	increased respiration	constipation
	diarrhea	sweating	no bowel sounds
	concentrated urine		
Weight change	increase since admission	decrease since admission	change since previous day
Fluid collection	edema—pitting, dependent, refractory	ascites	

LEG VII-B

Skin	flushed	turgor poor	eyes sunken
	eyes puffy	cyanosis	odor
	decreased elasticity	cold, warm	moist
	dry		
Mucous membranes	dry	sticky	moist
Tongue	shrunken, dry	moist, swollen	breath odor
Neck veins	appear full or less full when lies flat		
Lab findings	serum Na	Hgb	$PaCO_2$
(↑ ↓)	serum K	serum Cl	arterial pH
	PaO_2	HCO_3	serum Ca
	serum albumin	serum Mg	S osmolality
	EKG	urinalysis	

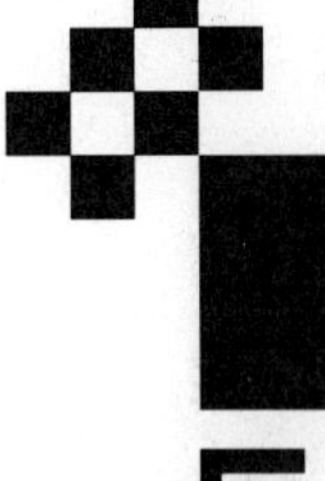

LEG VII-B

Acid-Base Imbalances

Objectives

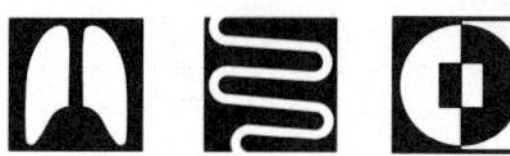

7. Describe, orally or in writing, how lung function, altered respirations, vomiting, and diarrhea can cause respiratory or metabolic imbalances and label each imbalance acidosis or alkalosis.

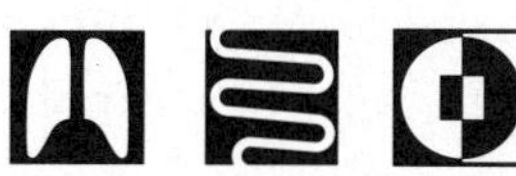

8. Explain, orally or in writing, the difference between respiratory and metabolic acid-base imbalance in terms of which body system causes the imbalance and how the body compensates for the imbalance.

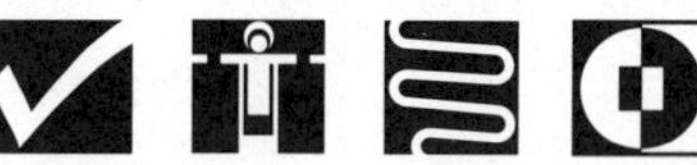

9. Describe two patient situations in which you would be alert for signs of increased base bicarbonate (metabolic alkalosis) and two assessments that you might chart.

LEG VII-B

A. What's It All About?

1. Think about the terms used in these Objectives. Compare them with common acids (vinegar), bases (soda), neutralizers, buffers, pH. Try to make them everyday terms as you work through some of the following learning experiences.

2. Review:

LEG VI-B Preventing Acute and Long-Term Complications of Diabetes
LEG VI-C Arterial Blood Gases Related to Respiratory Acidosis and Alkalosis

3. Read in medical-surgical, fluid and electrolyte, pharmacology and laboratory tests references about *acid-base balance, metabolic and respiratory acidosis* and *alkalosis,* the contributing conditions and resulting symptoms.

4. View audiovisuals and read articles and books from a list given you by your instructor.

5. Preview:

LEG VIII-C Conservative Medical Therapy
LEG XIII-C Acidosis and Alkalosis

6. Complete the following:

You will observe ______ respirations when the patient has respiratory acidosis.
You will observe ______ respirations when the patient has metabolic acidosis.
You will observe ______ respirations when the patient has respiratory alkalosis.
Failure to exhale sufficient carbon dioxide causes ______.
Vomiting or gastric suctioning may result in a loss of ______ ions and cause ______.
Diarrhea or intestinal suctioning results in a loss of ______ ions and causes ______.

Complete this chart.

Condition	Description	Causes	Assessment Findings	Nursing Care
Metabolic acidosis				
Metabolic alkalosis				
Respiratory acidosis				
Respiratory alkalosis				

7. Study the following diagram as you answer the questions that follow it.

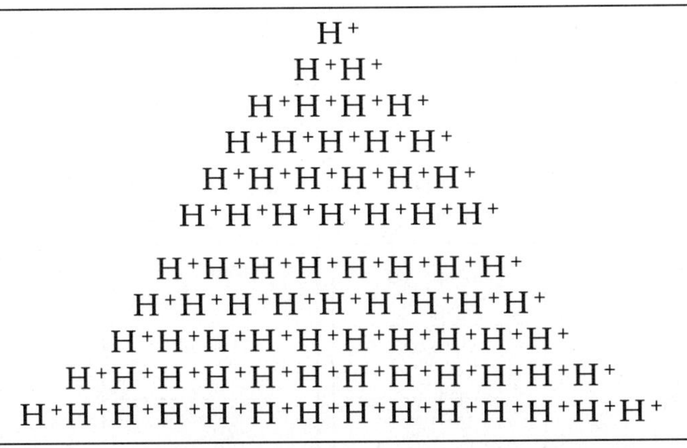

pH 14

↑

ALKALOSIS

pH 7.35 to 7.45 normal body fluids

ACIDOSIS

↓

pH 0

LEG VII-B

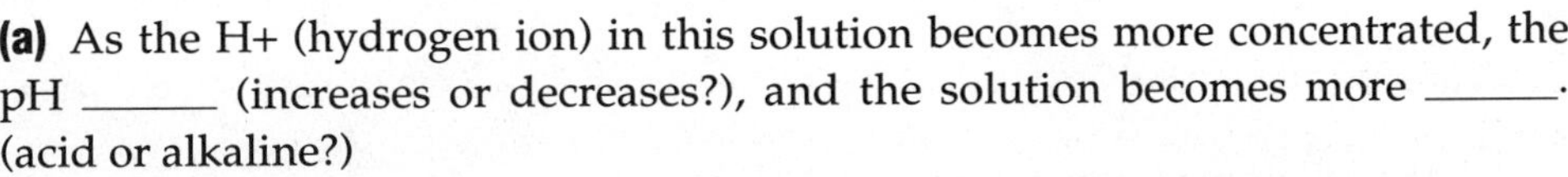

(a) As the H+ (hydrogen ion) in this solution becomes more concentrated, the pH ______ (increases or decreases?), and the solution becomes more ______. (acid or alkaline?)

(b) Our body solutions are normally slightly ______. (acid or alkaline?)

(c) Acidosis occurs when there are ______ (too few or too many?) H+ in the blood.

(d) Alkalosis occurs when there are ______ (too few or too many?) H+ in the blood.

Facts about Acidosis and Alkalosis

1. Acidosis is an imbalance in which the H+ concentration is above normal or the bicarbonate concentration of the body is below normal.

2. Alkalosis is an imbalance in which the H+ concentration of the body is below normal or the body base is above normal.

3. In H+ imbalance all the major signs and symptoms are the result of disturbances of the central nervous system.
In acidosis (either respiratory or metabolic), the major problem is depression of the CNS. Decrease in mental capacity, delirium, coma, and death may result.
In alkalosis, the major problem is overexcitability, and tetany results.

4. Compensatory mechanisms resulting from H+ imbalance include the following:

- **a.** The first line of defense is the dilution of H+ in the ECF and buffering.
- **b.** The second line of defense is the respiratory system.
- **c.** The third line of defense is the renal system.

5. The lungs regulate the H_2CO_3 level. If the basic failure is with the *pulmonary system,* the condition is called *respiratory acidosis or alkalosis.* In acidosis, hydrogen ions are being retained within the body fluids as excess carbonic acid. In alkalosis they are being excreted too rapidly in the form of CO_2 and water vapor.

6. The kidneys regulate the HCO_3 level. When the basic failure is renal in nature, the imbalance is called *metabolic acidosis or alkalosis.* In acidosis, excessive hydrogen ions are being retained within the body fluids, or bicarbonate is being lost in abnormally large amounts from the kidneys. In alkalosis there is either an abnormal loss of H+ or an abnormal gain in bicarbonate by the ECF.

8. Complete this chart on the information given in Facts about Acidosis and Alkalosis.

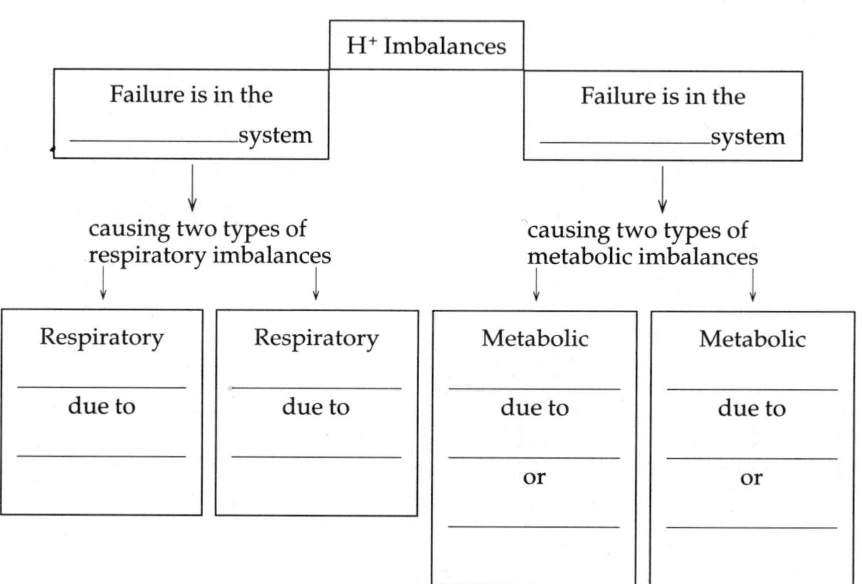

Match the following terms with the imbalances:

____ Metabolic acidosis	(a) Primary CO_2 excess
____ Metabolic alkalosis	(b) Nonrespiratory acidosis
____ Respiratory acidosis	(c) Primary CO_2 deficiency
____ Respiratory alkalosis	(d) Hypercapnea
	(e) CO_2 retention
	(f) Nonrespiratory alkalosis

Note: You may want to have all of your blanks and exercises filled in before attending a discussion group. If you have problems finding answers to your questions, request a resource teacher to sit in on these discussions.

LEG VII-B

■ B. Putting It into Action!

1. Attend a small group discussion on "Acid-Base Imbalance."

■ Work through the exercises. Electrolytes are normally found in gastric juice (for example, H, Cl, K, and Na). Imbalances in fluids and electrolytes result with loss of gastric juice.

■ Fill in the blanks. Cover the answers.

(a) What acid is present in gastric juice? ________	HCL
(b) Loss of hydrochloric acid results in an increase of the base bicarbonate as a compensatory measure (metabolic alkalosis). In metabolic alkalosis the plasma pH is ____. H and Cl are ____. In an effort to compensate for loss of Cl the ____ increases. In ____, when the carbonic acid is ____, the regulatory functions of the body attempt to retain carbon dioxide by ____. Other electrolyte and fluid imbalances that may occur along with metabolic alkalosis are decreased ____, ____, ____, and ____.	↑ lost base bicarbonate metabolic alkalosis ↓ slow, shallow respirations ECF, K, Na, Ca

■ Explain how the following nursing actions help the patient to combat metabolic alkalosis, and identify which are *independent* nursing actions.

Discourage oral water intake when on gastric suction.

Report vomiting early.

Give medications for vomiting prn.

Measure and estimate amounts of vomitus.

Weigh daily. (Record weight upon admission and note comparisons.)

Irrigate nasogastric tube with isotonic solution.

Measure suction output.

■ Name the most common reason for metabolic alkalosis in the adult and in the child.

■ Discuss possible nursing diagnoses in metabolic alkalosis.

■ Discuss how carbon dioxide narcosis can occur if oxygen is given to a patient with respiratory acidosis:

Your patient has just returned to the unit from the recovery room after repair of a hiatal hernia. The orders read:

Morphine sulfate gr 1/6 q 4 h prn for pain.

Oxygen at 5 L prn for dyspnea.

(There are other orders, but consider only these at this time.)

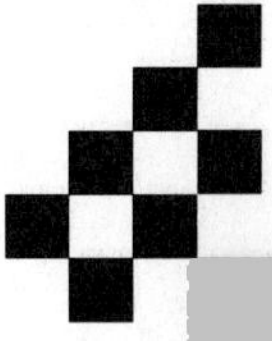

LEG VII-B

How does a hiatal hernia affect respirations? Why? List at least two precautions you would take before giving the morphine and/or oxygen and state why.

Why might you overlook the possible signs of respiratory acidosis for this patient if oxygen is being administered? Relate the procedure of turn, cough, and deep breathe to the acid-base imbalance of respiratory acidosis.

■ Which imbalance does each of the following conditions cause and why? What symptoms are present with each imbalance? The chart has been started for you.

Condition	**Imbalance**	**Symptoms of Imbalance**
Uncontrolled diabetes (diabetic acidosis)	metabolic acidosis	
Severe diarrhea	metabolic alkalosis	
Ulcer patient taking antacid medications		
Vomiting, gastric suction		

What type of replacement IV fluids will each of the above conditions require? Look ahead to Objective 10.

Comments on Assessing Patients

Laboratory reports are of great value in diagnosis. However, normals vary for different individuals because of age, body weight, and surface area. These are "normal limits" expressed as a range. Therefore, the primary test is how the patient looks, feels, and acts. The lab findings may then become confirmatory. This situation places a large burden on the nurse, who must be constantly observant of each patient. Does output equal intake? Does personality change? How? Why? Are respirations rapid, slow, deep, shallow? Does the patient complain of weakness, tremors, tingling? How is the muscle tone: normal, flaccid, tetanic? What is the characteristic of the pulse? Is the blood pressure stable? All of those questions will guide you in evaluating your patient's fluid and electrolyte balance. The earlier you notice symptoms and REPORT them, the earlier treatment can start. In some instances your own nursing action will be all that is necessary. Lucky patient!

2. List and describe as if you were charting the symptoms you see in the following illustration; identify the probable cause (some imbalance) and at least one nursing action you would take. Mark the areas on the figure that indicate problems.

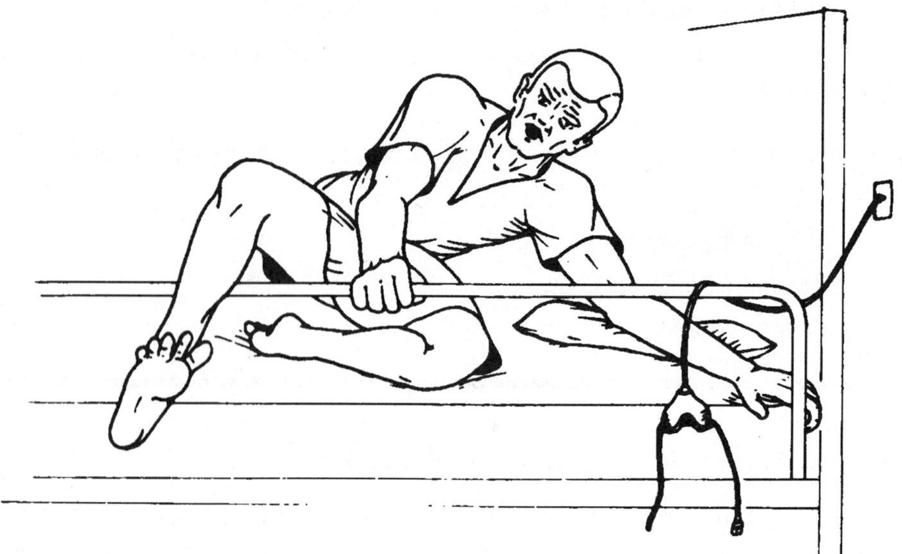

3. **Practice** in campus lab.

■ Check out a box of Laboratory Report Forms. In a small group try to figure out the significance of the reports. Identify acid-base imbalances. State probable signs and symptoms of each patient with a lab report. State what you would look for or do to prevent complications. Speculate as to the cause of the patients' problems.

4. **Plan** for a clinical experience.

▲ Observe breathing exercises given to patients. Evaluate the efforts the patient is making. Talk with patients about the exercises they use at home. Talk with respiratory therapists about how to observe for acid-base imbalances.

▲ Look at patient charts on your patient unit. Evaluate the charting. Find abnormal laboratory findings indicating fluid and electrolyte imbalances. Visit those patients. Compare what symptoms you see with those described on the chart.

▲ Observe and care for patients with acid-base imbalances.

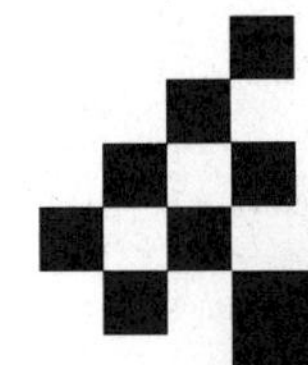

■ C. Extra Added Attractions!

1. **Fill in** the following blanks for acid-base imbalance. Cover the answers.

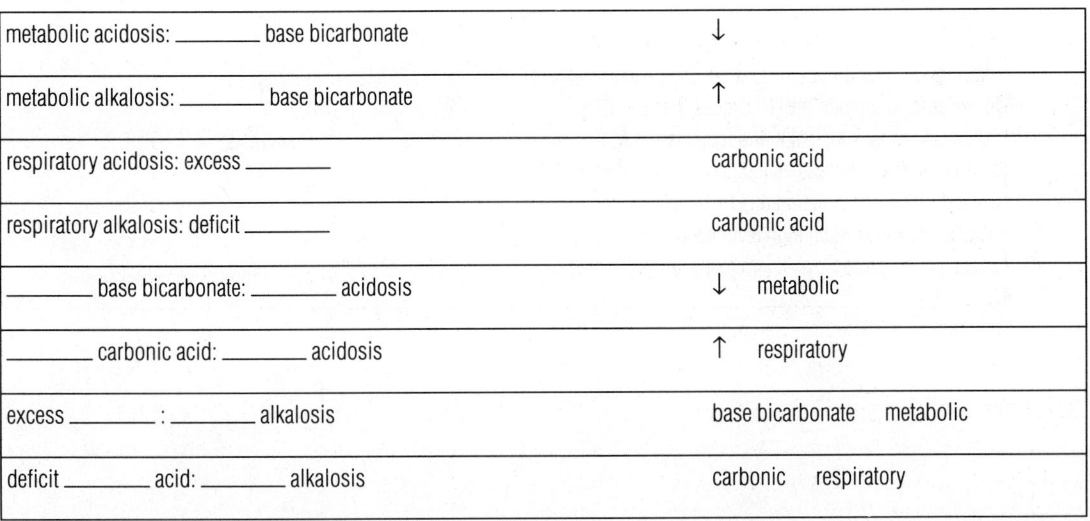

metabolic acidosis: _______ base bicarbonate	↓
metabolic alkalosis: _______ base bicarbonate	↑
respiratory acidosis: excess _______	carbonic acid
respiratory alkalosis: deficit _______	carbonic acid
_______ base bicarbonate: _______ acidosis	↓ metabolic
_______ carbonic acid: _______ acidosis	↑ respiratory
excess _______ : _______ alkalosis	base bicarbonate metabolic
deficit _______ acid: _______ alkalosis	carbonic respiratory

Add an appropriate disease and/or condition to the following spaces:

_______ : _______ metabolic _______________	vomiting, ↑ base bicarbonate, alkalosis
_______ : _______ respiratory _______________	pneumonia, ↑ carbonic acid, acidosis
_______ : _______ metabolic _______________	diabetes, ↓ base bicarbonate, acidosis
_______ : _______ respiratory _______________	fever, ↓ carbonic acid, alkalosis

2. **Explain** the function of the lungs in regulating fluids and electrolytes:

■ Acid-base disturbances are regulated by the action of base bicarbonate and carbonic acid on the medulla.

Fill in the blanks below. Cover the answers.

Excess of H+ (ketosis) due to starvation causes _______ acidosis, _______ in base bicarbonate. To compensate, the medulla sends messages to the lungs to exhale _______. How is this response observed? _______.	metabolic, ↓ carbon dioxide deep rapid respirations
If there is a loss of H+ (vomiting), metabolic _______ occurs with an increase in _______. The lungs, in order to compensate, must now _______ carbon dioxide. How can you tell this action is occurring? _______	alkalosis base bicarb retain slow, shallow respirations

■ The lungs help compensate for metabolic acidosis and alkalosis if they are healthy and receive adequate messages from the brain. If there is a defect in lung function another type of acid-base imbalance can occur!

Fill in the blanks. Cover the answers.

Inadequate elimination of carbon dioxide causes an excess of carbonic acid that is respiratory _______. This can be caused by any blocking of bronchi in lung disease. To compensate for the _______ of carbonic acid in _______ acidosis, the lungs must increase their effort to exhale _______, and the symptoms you can observe, if you observe carefully, are dyspnea out of proportion to effort involved and *hyperpnea* when the patient is at rest. In extreme conditions the H+ excess in respiratory _______ causes loss of K and may lead to ventricular arrest and death. Excessive elimination of carbon dioxide caused by hyperventilation due to anxiety or the body's effort to combat high fever causes a _______ in carbonic acid and respiratory _______.	acidosis excess respiratory carbon dioxide acidosis decrease, alkalosis

LEG VII-B

Parenteral Solutions

Objectives

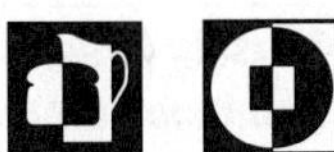

10. List one example of a parenteral solution used in your hospital in each of the following classifications: hydrating, alkalinizing, acidifying, and balanced multiple electrolyte (polyionic). State one nursing observation that should be made when giving each. (Your instructor will provide a list of solutions.)

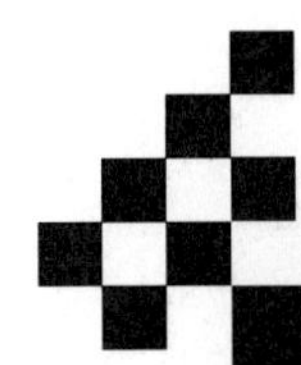

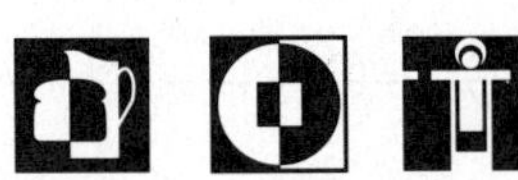

11. Demonstrate how you would use a microdrip set to administer a specified amount of parenteral solution in a given number of hours, and state two observations you would make during the period of administration related to overhydration.

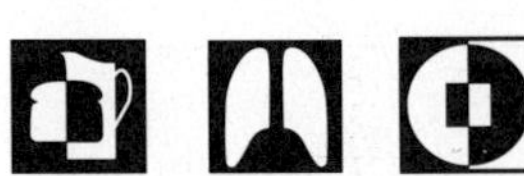

12. Demonstrate safely preparing and adding a bottle of IV fluids to an existing IV infusion, including placing a time tape on the bottle, accurately adjusting the rate of flow, and charting on the records.

13. Demonstrate giving daily care to a venipuncture infusion site and state the rationale for all your actions.

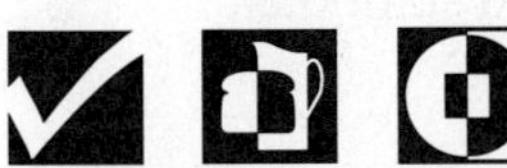

14. List the assessments you would make when your patient's IV stops running and state the appropriate nursing actions you would take.

■ A. What's It All About?

1. Think about what it means when your patient is receiving an IV. Most patients do have IV solutions at some time during their hospital stay. Can you think why? What is the purpose? Or do you just think "fluids, watch for infiltration." There is much more to it. From now on you must know what is in the bottle and the purpose for giving it. Then you will know what signs and symptoms to look for and will be able to evaluate patients before and afterward.

2. Review LEG IV-C, Parenteral Fluid Administration.

3. Read medical-surgical, pharmacology, nutrition, and pediatrics references on *parenteral, intravenous therapy.*

4. View audiovisuals and read articles and books from a list given you by your instructor or read the following:

Metheny, N. M. "Why Worry about IV Fluids?" *AJN,* June 1990, pp. 50–56.

5. Preview:

LEG X-B Legal Responsibilities with IVs
Starting IV Infusions

6. Write your answers to the following questions before attending a group discussion:

(a) Fill in this chart.

Classification (Definition)	**Name of IV Solutions (Common in Your Area)**	**Tonicity**	**Nursing Assessments and Precautions**
Hydrating			
Alkalinizing			
Acidifying			
Polyionic (balanced multiple electrolyte)			

(b) List the names of some oral electrolyte solutions used in your hospital.

(c) How is the daily maintenance requirement of parenteral solutions calculated for pediatric patients? For adults?
Where is the preferred vein for administering IV fluids in adults? In children?
What factors determine the rate at which an IV fluid can be administered?

(d) What solutions would expand the extracellular space (ECS)?
What solutions would move into the cells from the ECS?
What is meant by replacement versus maintenance fluids?
What is the difference between isotonic and balanced solutions?
What is the significance of tonicity (osmotic pressure)?

(e) How many calories are in a bottle of 5% D/NS?
If a patient gets three bottles a day (3000 cc), what purpose do these calories serve?
What is the significance of starvation ketosis?

(f) Why give IV fluids with lactate? When and why would each of the following be used?

D-5-W

D-5-NS

D-5-0.45 saline

(g) If your patient has a fever or an infection, is the need for calories greater or less?
Explain.

(h) When patients are receiving KCl IV, what is the most significant assessment for the nurse to make?

7. Attend a group discussion on "The Nurse's Role in Hospital Malnutrition." Use a dietitian as a resource person. Discuss what can be done to prevent this condition. Be sure that you list specific steps to take and discuss ways to make those steps possible.

Consider the nurse's obligation to the patient who can take oral fluids but who is on IV fluids.

How can you become more insistent, imaginative, persuasive, and successful in promoting normal methods of fluid intake as early as possible?

■ B. Putting It into Action!

1. Practice in campus lab.

- ■ Check out practice materials for "Superimposing IVs." Role play adding a new bottle to an existing infusion so that no air gets into the tubing. Add a time tape and chart the procedure.
- ■ Practice calculating and regulating the flow rate when a microdrip chamber is used. What would you do if the drip chamber is too full to count the drops?
- ■ Practice checking the IV infusion site and changing the dressing.
- ■ List all the actions you could take when an IV stops running. What would you do first? Last?

2. Attend a group discussion on "More on Fluids and Electrolytes—Parenteral Solutions."

- ■ Review and compare your answers with the answers to A.6.

Problems for Solving

What mechanical factors, that you can check, influence the flow of intravenous fluids? How can you increase or decrease the rate of flow without adjusting the flowmeter?

Why is it important that an IV flow rate be slower for a patient who is 81 years old than for a patient who is 41? Why is it more important for a child 3–8 years old than for a young adult?

■ Discuss how you would give fluids to Luis, described below. What observations would be made when giving fluids? How would he be restrained?
What fluid and electrolyte imbalance can occur and why? What signs and symptoms are present?

3/25 Luis—3-yr-old admitted to peds from ED at 11:00 P.M. c̄ dx of dehydration 2° to vomiting.
TPR 101-146-36, R deep, rapid c̄ aromatic smell on breath.
Ht.—39 1/2 , Wt.—30 1/2 lb.
Parents state: Vomiting qh this P.M. Vomiting for past 2 d. No diarrhea.
Immunizations are up-to-date. No exposure to communicable disease.
Speaks Spanish only.
Assessment: Pale, warm, lethargic, occasional crying s̄ tears, lips slightly dry.
Throat not inflamed, skin turgor good

3/25 Admitted.
Dr. orders: Lab work: Bicarb, SGOT, glucose, BUN, S electrolytes, S ammonia now.
NPO except ice chips.
VS q4h.
500 cc D-5-0.45 NS 90 cc/h for 8 h, then 70 cc/h.
Add KCl 2 mEq each 100 cc.
Ampicillin 300 mg IV q4h.
Repeat S electrolytes in A.M.

3/26 1000 D-5-0.2 NS c̄ KCl 2 mEq/100 cc IV at 70 cc/h.
1400 Sips 7-Up prn.

Notes Made by Nurses while Caring for Luis

3/25	2300	Looks scared, crying. Mother left. Translator here to talk with child. Blood work done. IV started R forearm c̄ 20g angio. Voided 150 cc. Skin warm, dry; moist mucous membranes. Water refused.
	0400	TPR 98-110-20.
3/26	0600	No stools, urine. Slept all night. Awake now. Mother here. TPR 97^8-120-20. Blood drawn.
	0700	Color O.K. No fluids til 3 P.M., then sips 7-Up.
	1000	IV rate decreased. Slept 10–12. Ampicillin 8, 12.
	1100	Up to BR, voided 300 cc. Bathed. TPR 98-114-20.
	1600	Awake, assessment—same except more playful. TPR 98-112-20. Voided 350 cc. Sips 7-Up. TPR 98-112-20. Ampicillin at 4.

LEG VII-B

3. Plan for a clinical experience.

▲ Observe patients receiving IV therapy. Read their charts. What symptoms are recorded? How do they tolerate the therapy? What observations do you make? Talk with patients. How do they feel about IV therapy? How is their IV intake recorded?

▲ Observe or give care to a venous infusion site, following your hospital's procedure.

▲ Change or observe a nurse changing IV solutions. Be sure you can accurately record the fluid received, new solutions started, and keep hourly records on the time tape on the bottle.

▲ Observe infusion monitors or pumps and learn how to operate them. Do they measure drops or cubic centimeters?

Gastric and Intestinal Tubes and Feedings

O b j e c t i v e s

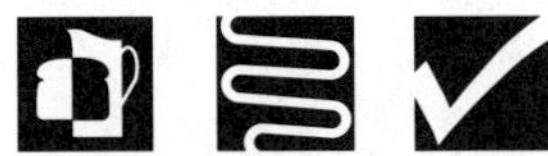

15. Describe or demonstrate the purpose of gastrointestinal intubation, the appearance of the tube, the procedure for insertion, preparation of the patient before intubation, and follow-up nursing care, including observations, use of intermittent suction, and removal of the tube.

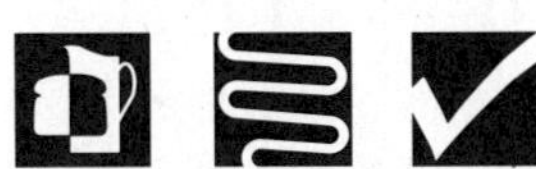

16. Given patients or pictures of patients with gastrointestinal tubes with lumen labeled according to purpose (e.g., suction, balloon), describe how each lumen can be handled (e.g., can it be irrigated?).

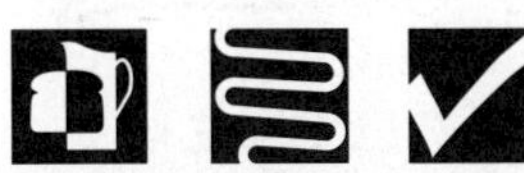

17. Demonstrate giving an enteral feeding via a gastrostomy or jejunostomy tube after writing out a list of the steps you will take to ensure the safety and comfort of the patient before, during, and after the feeding.

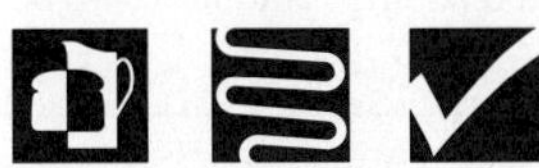

18. Demonstrate inserting a nasogastric tube, taking specific steps to provide for the patient's comfort and checking the location by two different means.

Note: Objective 18 was an Extra Added Objective in Volume I, LEG IV-C.

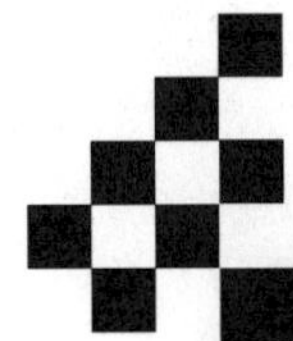

■ A. What's It All About?

1. Think about what a gastric or an intestinal tube means to a person. Usually a serious problem, either internal bleeding or an obstruction. It is uncomfortable to the patient and repulsive and frightening to the family. You can do much to alleviate these feelings by your attitude, presence, and skill. Learn these nursing measures well and remember you are caring for the patient, not just the tube!

2. Review:

LEG I-C Special Mouth Care
LEG IV-C Giving Tube Feedings
Insertion of a Nasogastric Tube

3. Read in medical-surgical, fundamentals, pediatrics, and geriatrics nursing references about *intestinal tubes, gastric tubes, enteral feedings.*

4. View audiovisuals and read articles and books from a list given you by your instructor.

5. Preview: LEG X-B Using Blakemore Tube for Patient with Cirrhosis.

6. Look at the illustrations below. Write what you can do with each of the lumina labeled on the figures below.

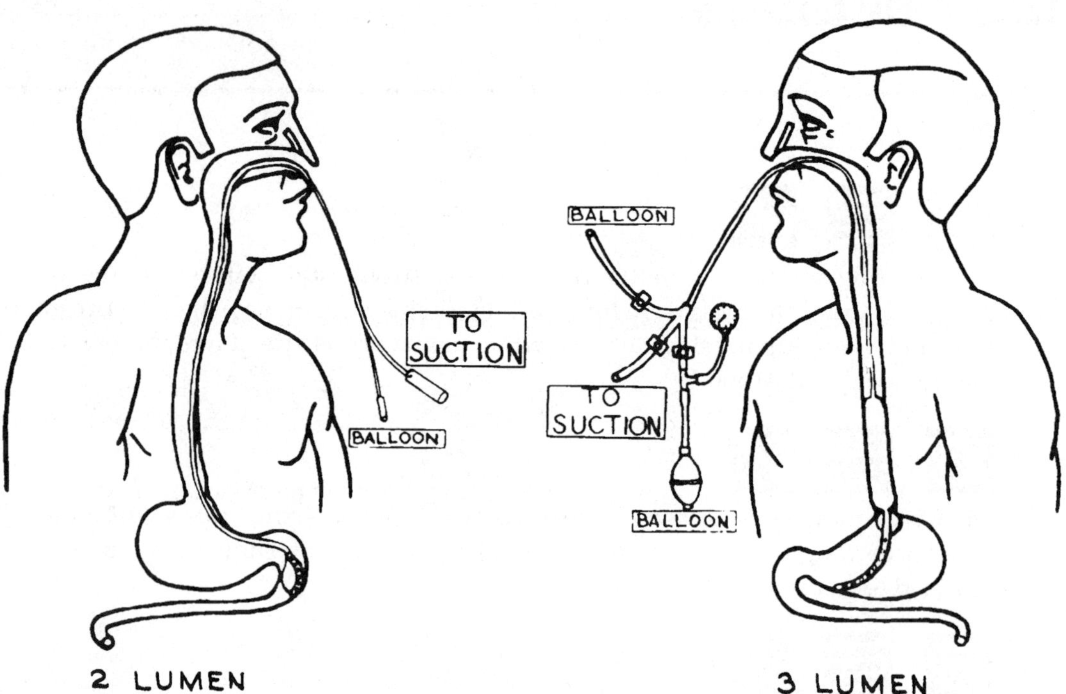

Note: Sengstaken-Blakemore tubes may be used rarely in your area. However, they are stocked in emergency rooms and ICUs and are still important for gastric and esophageal bleeding. Therefore, we believe you should know what they are and how to use them.

Comments on Taping NG Tubes

You will see a variety of "taped noses." To better understand the need for careful positioning and taping of nasogastric tubes, wear one around for a while. Cut off a piece of plastic tubing 3 to 5 inches long; insert it into your own nostril and tape it in place. Wear it for 15 minutes, half an hour, an hour. How did it feel? What did you see as you looked down your nose?

Look at the following illustrations for ideas on anchoring the tubing for best function of the tube and most comfort for the patient.

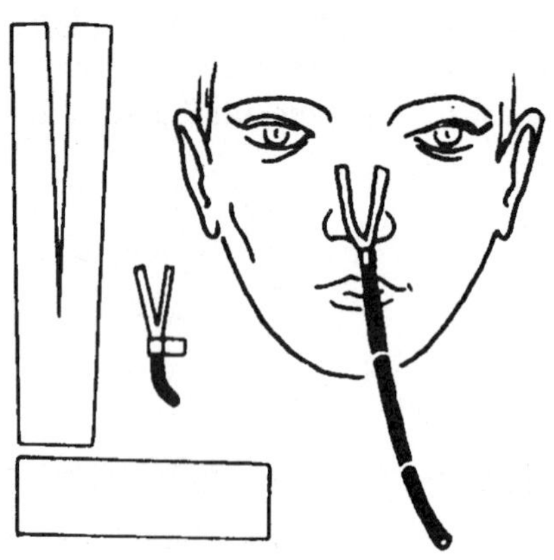

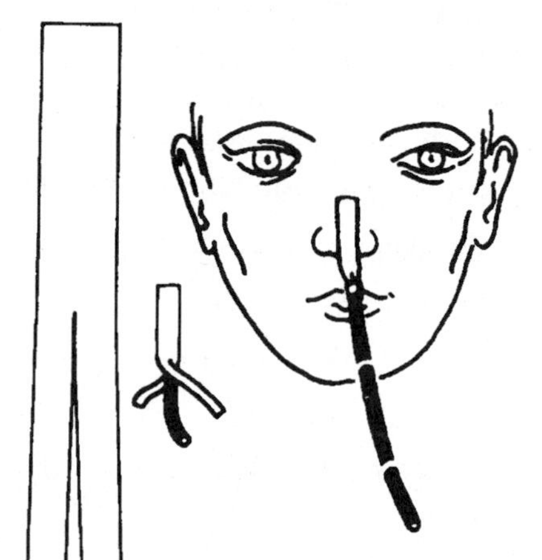

Try these methods. Try some of your own. Above all take time to apply the least amount of the best kind of tape (i.e., paper or plastic) in the correct position! It takes practice.

■ B. Putting It into Action!

1. Write the steps you would take to carry out the following medical treatments:

Intubate for intestinal decompression.
Give jejunostomy tube feeding.
Irrigate Salem Sump tube.
Clamp NG tube for 2h, then open for 1h.

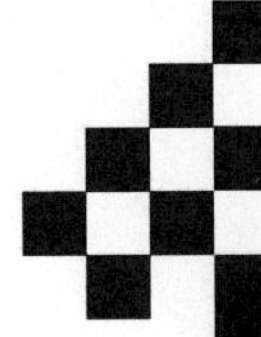

Where do you find out what equipment the physician will need? Does the unit procedure book give you as much information as you need? How do you prepare to assist the physician? What do you need to do to prepare your patient?

When do you apply tape to the nostril to hold the tube in position for the nasogastric tube? For the gastrointestinal tube? Why?

Why does the formula for a gastrostomy tube feeding differ from that for a jejunostomy tube feeding? How?

LEG VII-B

2. Write a nursing care plan for the three patients described below. You are to give routine morning care and irrigate the tubes. For practice, try to figure out what type of drainage tube each patient has in place and what electrolytes are lost via the drainage. In actual practice you would know the name of the tube (for instance, Cantor, Blakemore).

Mrs. Jane Jackson is assigned to your care. She is 34 years old and is hospitalized for observation. She is awake as you enter her room, and you note that the tube coming from her nose has a metal adapter and two lumina.

Mr. Marshall Miller, age 48, has been hospitalized for conservative care of bleeding in the upper gastrointestinal tract. You notice that his tube has three lumina.

George Gevens, age 7, has a tube connected to continuous suction because of peritonitis due to ruptured appendix.

Which opening is which and for what? How can you tell? When in doubt which would you irrigate? *Be sure before irrigating!* If you don't know, *ask!*

3. Attend a small group discussion on "Nasogastric Intubation and Delaying Tactics." Bring with you to the discussion:

Your definition of the term *delaying tactics.*

Five examples, preferably your own, of delaying tactics.

- Discuss how to overcome the need for using delaying tactics.
- Role play using delaying tactics as you prepare to insert or assist with insertion of a nasogastric tube (one nurse, one patient).

How does the patient react to the delay? More or less anxiously? What does the delay do for you, the nurse? Role play an overly quick approach to the nursing action. What effect does this have on the anxiety of the patient and the nurse?

■ List *all* the things that can go wrong as you insert a nasogastric tube (use a chalkboard or add a sheet to this LEG): *Example:* Tube gets "stuck" in the nostril. Across from the "happenings" write the possible causes and what can be done to correct or change the problem. As you think about this procedure, what are *you* really afraid of? When you cannot think of any more possible hazards, stop and look at the list. You have now crossed all the "bridges" before actually approaching a patient. Nothing more can happen (if your list is complete).

■ Role play insertion of a nasogastric tube on "Mrs. Chase" or another model. What problems arise? How does slanting the tube or rotating it help as you begin insertion? Look into the nostril. Do you see a deviated septum? If so, what will you do? What will you do if, after you get the tube into the stomach, you test it and nothing comes back? What could have happened?

■ How will the procedure differ with a child? With an infant?

■ Evaluate your nursing care plans in B.2 above. Revise your plans if you cannot defend them.

■ Now you should be ready to insert a nasogastric tube. You have solved all your problems, and you know how to handle a "happening."

4. **Compare** the following types of enteral feedings.

	Nasogastric	**Jejunostomy**	**Gastrostomy**
Location of tube			
Assessments to make before feeding			
Actions needed to give feeding			
Follow-up assessments and actions			

5. **Plan** for clinical experiences.

▲ Go to several patient units. Find out how to get information about the various decompression tubes. Look in the procedure book.

▲ Give an enteral feeding after writing out the steps you will take and discussing it with your instructor.

▲ Insert or assist in inserting a nasogastric tube, gastric and intestinal tubes.

▲ Observe patients with a variety of gastric or intestinal tubes, some connected to suction, some used for gavage. Look for intestinal decompression tubes with more than one lumen.

▲ Talk with patients about their reactions to intubation, feelings with suction; feelings of thirst; mouth care.

▲ Observe removal of decompression tubes. Is this a fast or slow process? Why?

▲ Give special nose and mouth care to patients with nasogastric tubes. Observe the condition of their skin and nares around the tube and tape. How can you make this procedure more comfortable? Irrigate and/or check tubes for patency. Describe the drainage. Read the output records during the periods of time the tubes have been in place. Which of the patients' electrolytes needed to be replaced? How was it done?

Have I Learned?

The following questions are for you to answer in order to find out if you have met the Objectives. All of the Objectives in LEG VII-B are covered in this series of questions. Pick a quiet time and answer them. Answers are found at the end of this selftest.

No space has been left for answering the questions related to the "doing" Objectives. Use a separate sheet of paper for those answers and then use the answers in clinical or campus lab for your own evaluation.

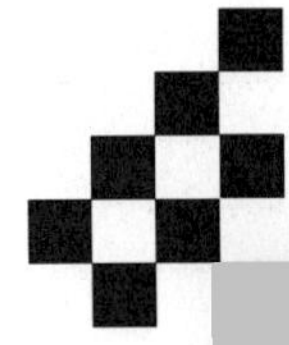

LEG VII-B

Objective **Question**

1 **1.** Write a brief statement that describes how each of the following helps maintain the fluid and electrolyte balance within our bodies.

semipermeable membranes

plasma proteins

kidneys

gastrointestinal tract

nervous system

hormones

electrolytes

2 **2.** During the flu season, three members of the Jones family developed the flu with symptoms of vomiting and diarrhea for 3 days. After 2 days it was necessary to hospitalize both the 11-month-old Jones baby and the grandmother for dehydration. The father was ill, but did not develop a severe dehydration. Why did two become dehydrated and not the third?

3 **3.** You are caring for patients with dehydration related to one of the following causes. State a desired outcome and two nursing actions for each.

fluid volume deficit related to diarrhea

fluid volume deficit related to inadequate fluid intake secondary to depression

potential complication: hypovolemia secondary to hemorrhage

fluid volume deficit related to nausea and vomiting

3 **4.** Identify one problem for each person described below and use the nursing process to solve the problem.

A young woman who is a secretary for a busy young vice president of a corporation has frequent watery stools.

An infant has had diarrhea for 2 days.

4 **5.** Take your Fluid and Electrolyte Assessment Checklist to the clinical area and use it to observe one patient with a potential or existing fluid and/or electrolyte imbalance. Study the chart, and at the end of your experience list three independent nursing actions that would assist this patient to regain a normal fluid and electrolyte balance.

Ask another student to observe the same patient and complete the above. Then compare your observations and ideas.

5 **6.** Your clinical assignment is to care for a patient with ulcerative colitis who has been admitted with frequent loose stools and skin breakdown. The evening before your lab, you review this health problem and discover that the diarrhea could cause the following three fluid and electrolyte imbalances. Write down two observations you will be looking for related to each imbalance as you care for the patient tomorrow.

increased sodium

decreased potassium

decreased magnesium

5 **7.** Describe one patient with Na loss. Include the cause and at least three symptoms.

6 **8.** State two nursing actions specific for alleviating the symptoms of nausea, vomiting, and diarrhea related to the following. Describe why vomiting or diarrhea probably occurred.

drug allergy

intestinal obstruction

vertigo

postoperative course

7 **9.** Describe how lung function, vomiting, and diarrhea can cause respiratory and metabolic acidosis or alkalosis.

8 **10.** Which body system is primarily involved in allowing respiratory acid-base imbalance to occur?
Which system fails when a metabolic imbalance occurs?
List three ways that an imbalance is regulated by the body.

9 **11.** Describe two patient situations that might cause metabolic alkalosis.

9 **12.** List two observations that you would be looking for when caring for the patients you described in Question 11.

10 **13.** Name one parenteral solution in each of the following categories and describe one nursing precaution or observation you would make when giving it.

(a) hydrating

(b) alkalinizing

(c) acidifying

(d) polyionic (balanced)

11 **14.** Explain to another student how you would use a microdrip set. Assume that you are to give 5% D/0.2 NS to a young child. The doctor orders 500 cc to be given in a 6 hr period.

What would the flow rate be? The child should receive _______ cc/h.

List two observations you would make to prevent overhydrating the child.

11, 12, 13 **15.** Role play or demonstrate any of the following. Write down the steps you plan to take. Ask another student to use your list to evaluate you. Be prepared to state your rationale for your actions.

(a) use a microdrip and set the drip rate.

(b) add IV fluids to an existing IV infusion.

(c) change the dressing at a venipuncture infusion site.

14 **16.** List six assessments that would be related to failure of an IV infusion to run and state what actions you would take to solve the problem.

15, 17, 18 **17.** Be prepared to demonstrate any of the following. Bring a list of the steps you will take and be prepared to answer questions regarding assessments, safety, and comfort of the patient and purpose of the procedure.

- **(a)** Insert a nasogastric tube.
- **(b)** Remove a nasogastric tube.
- **(c)** Assist with insertion of a Miller-Abbott tube.
- **(d)** Assist with removal of a Miller-Abbott tube.
- **(e)** Give a gastrostomy tube feeding.
- **(f)** Give a jejunostomy tube feeding.

16 **18.** Describe what each of the labels on the intestinal tubes in the following figure indicates and the purpose of each lumen.

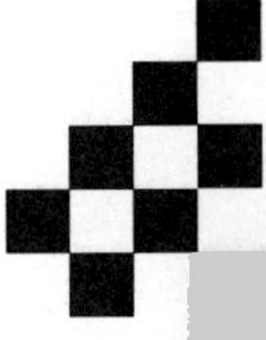

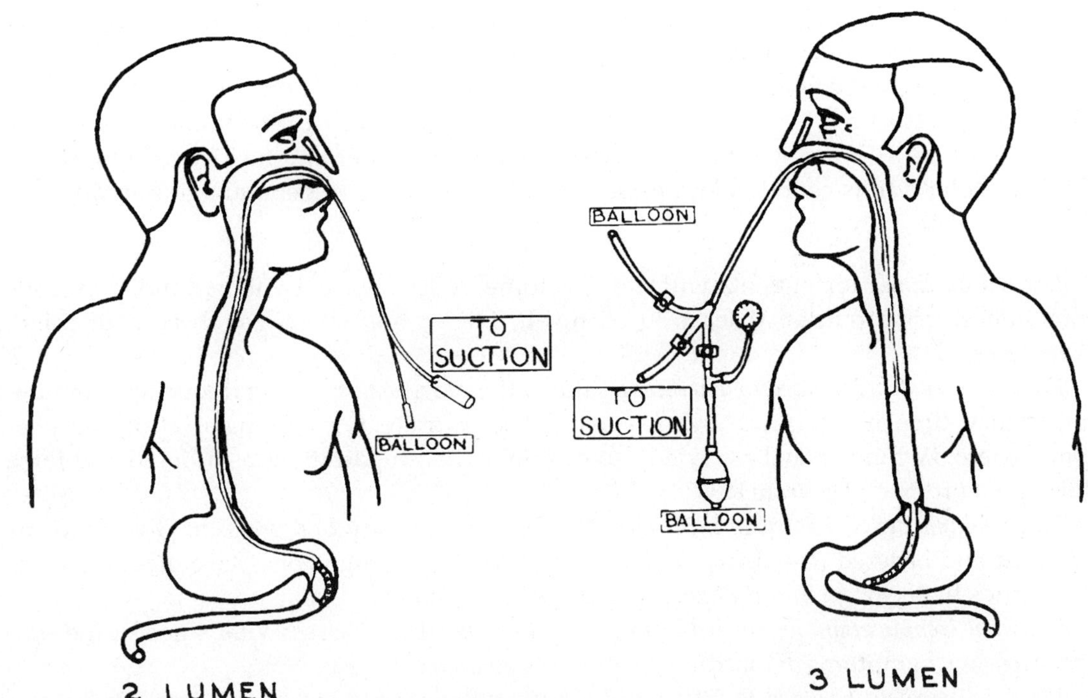

LEG VII-B

■ Answers to Have I Learned?

LEG VII-B

1. *Semipermeable membranes* allow water and selected electrolytes to move between the ECF and ICF.

Plasma proteins hold volume within the vascular space.

Kidneys regulate extracellular volume, electrolyte levels, and pH by conserving or excreting water and electrolytes.

Gastrointestinal tract reabsorbs most fluid. Fluid and electrolytes are replenished by diet.

Nervous system regulates the kidneys and the hormones.

Hormones are released and circulate through bloodstream to target organs. Aldosterone causes sodium retention and thus water retention and potassium loss. ADH causes the body to conserve water.

Electrolytes regulate the osmolarity and volume of body fluids.

2. The infant has a higher percentage of body weight composed of fluid and yet has a smaller reservoir for fluid. His metabolic rate is higher; his kidneys are immature and require a greater amount of water intake and output.

The grandmother has a reduced sensation of thirst and thus a reduced intake of fluid. Her kidneys also need a greater output of urine because they cannot concentrate urine as efficiently as in earlier years. She may be a mouth breather and be losing fluid in that fashion. Older adults cannot adapt easily or rapidly because of general aging in all body systems.

3. *Desired outcomes* for patients with fluid volume deficit: normal volume; moist mucous membranes; urine output at least 30 cc/h; BP, HR in normal range; absence of thirst.
Nursing actions:

Fluid volume deficit related to diarrhea: Evaluate the diarrhea by noting frequency, amount, consistency, time of occurrence and associated discomfort (e.g., cramping). If symptoms become severe, IV fluids may be needed. Give antidiarrheic medications as ordered and force fluids po if ordered. Accurate I&O.

Fluid volume deficit related to inadequate fluid intake secondary to depression: Give fluids as tolerated and ordered (small frequent amounts). Watch for signs of electrolyte imbalance. Push fluids by trying to find patient preferences.

Potential complication: hypovolemia secondary to hemorrhage: Assess vital signs, urine output, dressing, symptoms of bleeding. Give fluids as ordered.

Fluid volume deficit related to nausea and vomiting: Report symptoms observed. Prepare to give IV fluids as ordered. Watch for signs of other imbalances.

4. Compare your answers in a GES.

Secretary: Embarrassment or fear of embarrassment related to urgency and frequency of bowel movements.

Infant: Dehydration and excoriation. Signs to look for: dry diapers (no urine), sunken eyes, sluggish movements. Check your list with at least one other student. Compare how you used each of the steps of the nursing process to help solve the problem.

5. Did you ask the patient questions about subjective symptoms? Did you take the patient's vital signs or compare a recent one with earlier ones? Did you find any lab results that indicated an imbalance? Any nursing notes that described assessments? Your nursing actions may have included the following:

Monitor IV fluids frequently and carefully so the flow rate does not vary.

Record the I&O accurately—alert visitors to this need.

Make frequent written assessments of the patient.

Give special attention to dry areas or where edema may be present.

Check for a safe environment—rails, lights, furniture.

6. *Increased sodium:* thirst, dry sticky mucous membranes, irritability, restlessness, excitement, decreased urinary output, increased temperature and pulse, and S $Na^{+} > 145$ mEq/l.
Decreased potassium: anorexia, soft muscles, abdominal distention, irregular pulse, S K^{+}, 3.5. mEq/L.
Decreased magnesium: tremor, disorientation, neuromuscular irritability, irregular pulse, and paresthesias.

7. You may have a variety of answers for this one. Postoperative patient with continuous suction, allowed sips of water, and has symptoms of apprehension, anuria, and abdominal cramps. This is an example of a Na↓ probably due to too much oral water, which allows Na to be excreted in excess amounts.

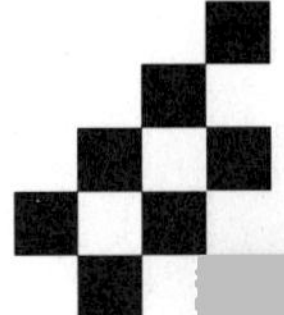

8. *Drug allergy:* Stop the medication until the physician is notified. Restrict fluids, provide rest for the patient, and then try a carbonated drink if allowed.
Intestinal obstruction: Fecal material may be contents of vomitus due to reverse peristalsis. Check vital signs and bowel sounds; look for abdominal distention, passing flatus. Report immediately; usually a surgical emergency.
Vertigo: Avoid quick motion when changing position. Limit physical activity after eating; limit visual work. Give antiemetics or sedatives as indicated. Vertigo triggers nausea mechanism.
Postoperative course: Inform the patient that this is only temporary and a fairly common result of anesthesia; drugs as ordered; restrict fluids (oral); IV may be ordered or sips of carbonated drinks.

9. *Lung function:* Hyperventilation, deep rapid breathing results in blowing off of carbon dioxide; results in depletion of carbonic acid, and plasma pH is elevated. Can occur with hysteria, fever, anxiety—*respiratory alkalosis. Respiratory acidosis* results from hypoventilation or respiratory embarrassment due to impairment in exhalation of carbon dioxide. Any respiratory depressant (e.g., lung disease or morphine) can cause an elevated plasma bicarbonate to compensate for elevated ECF carbonic acid.
Vomiting: Causes loss of chloride secretions of gastric juices, which causes an elevated plasma bicarbonate and *metabolic alkalosis.* Usually potassium deficit occurs that complicates the situation and prevents correction of the imbalance unless the potassium deficit is corrected first. *Metabolic acidosis* occurs with a deficit in the base bicarbonate in plasma due to decreased food intake, diabetes mellitus, or generalized infection. Ketogenic diet or renal failure can also cause this. If vomiting should occur with metabolic acidosis, it may help the acidosis compensation.
Diarrhea: Occurs with metabolic acidosis and complicates the situation.

10. Pulmonary system, Renal system

(a) Chemical buffers and ion exchange dilute the H^{+} in the ECF.

(b) The lungs compensate.

(c) The kidneys compensate.

11. Use of potent diuretics.

Antacid use at home to ease gastric ulcer pains.

Gastric suction.

Prolonged vomiting.

12. Muscles are hypertonic.

Shallow breathing.

Tingling.

13. **(a)** 5% glucose in normal saline—watch for symptoms of overhydration, dyspnea, cyanosis, puffy eyes, moist lung sounds.

(b) 1/6 molar sodium lactate—watch for symptoms of alkalosis (overcompensation).

(c) Ammonium chloride in water—watch for acidosis.

(d) D/5/LR—check urinary output.

14. Flow rate is 84 cc/h. Microdrip at 60 gtt/ml should drip at 84 gtt/min. Observe for cough that is moist, dyspnea, cyanosis, engorged neck veins, puffy eyelids.

15. Attend a GES. Demonstrate skill as requested. Compare what your observer saw you do with your skills list.

16. Your assessments might include: drip chamber is empty; bottle is empty; tubing is kinked; air vent is closed; tubing is full of air or blood; bottle is hanging too low.

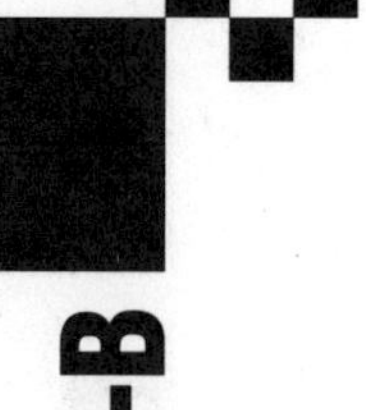

Your solutions will vary but can include repositioning the patient's arm, applying pressure to vein beyond the end of the catheter (needle), and observing for change in drip rate. If the dripping stops, the catheter is still in the vein. If there is air in the tubing, you need to remove it with your instructor's assistance before adding an additional bottle of solution.

17. Attend a GES.

18. *Two-lumen tube:* Balloon is for injection of mercury or air. No suction should be connected to it; no irrigating solutions can be instilled into it. It could be labeled "Hands off" or "Don't touch" just to remind you. The suction-labeled opening can be connected to suction and used for irrigating. This lumen connects with the holes at the tip of the tube, allowing for suctioning and irrigating.

Three-lumen tube: One balloon labeled "Opening" goes to esophageal balloon and is closed by a clamp at prescribed pressure. A manometer is attached to this tube. Other balloon opening is to gastric balloon, which is inflated with air to hold the tube in place. The other opening is labeled "Suction" and is used for suction and irrigation. Irrigation may be required to keep the tube patent. Suctioning is continuous to keep the stomach empty to prevent vomiting and dislodgement of esophageal balloon.

What Will I Learn?

LEG VII-C Cardiac and Hypertensive Problems

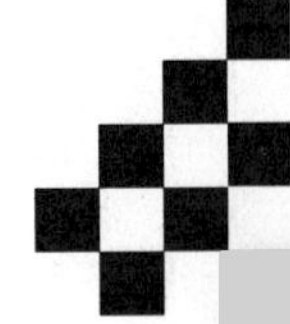

In LEG VI-C you learned about patients with problems of getting oxygen into their lungs and ridding their bodies of carbon dioxide. In following the pathway of the oxygen molecules, you will see that they join the hemoglobin in the red blood cells and travel through the pulmonary vein directly into the heart where they are then quite forcefully expelled into the body's vast network of arteries, arterioles, and capillaries. This is a simple enough process that can be traced on a drawing, yet it is so complex that failure of one of the parts along the way will throw the rest of the body into "emergency measures." It may be the **Regulatory** measures (for example, rapid pulse rate, pooling of fluid in ankles, chest pain, cyanosis) that tell the patient or doctor and nurse that something has gone wrong and that the rest of the system is compensating (regulatory function) to carry the load until the defect can be corrected. These are the signs and symptoms, along with diagnostic tests, that will tell the doctor if the oxygen is getting through, how much permanent damage has occurred to the body, and how long it will be until the system will return to normal operation. It is a frightening prospect to have something go wrong with such a vital **Body System.**

Patients with heart disease offer you the opportunity to perfect general nursing skills, to become familiar with common signs and symptoms, and to recognize and accept attitudes of patients with chronic disease. You have time now to "put it all together"—all you have learned up to this point in Levels One through Six to give total patient care.

Your goal in this LEG will be to prepare yourself to accept these patients as they are and help them cope with their **crises.** Some will face severe changes in their self-image. A few will face the greatest loss of all—their impending death and with it the loss of their feelings of immortality.

Rarely will you see a patient in the acute phase of heart disease if your hospital has a coronary care unit (CCU). This LEG will introduce you to nursing care of patients with cardiovascular problems and offer you the opportunity to study without the pressure of life-saving techniques used in CCU.

What's Ahead in Later LEGs

LEG XI-C Care for Patients in the Acute Phase of Cardiac Illness

LEG XII-C Nursing Care of Patients Requiring Cardiovascular Surgery

Overview of Learning Experiences in LEG VII-C

Objectives	Campus Lab/ Self-Practice	Group Discussions/Lectures	Clinical Lab Focuses
Alterations in Cardiac Function **1.** Lifestyles leading to alterations in cardiac function **2,3.** Pathophysiology, causes, and symptoms of heart problems **4.** Effects of stress		**B3.** Physiologic changes in heart disease	**B4.** Review charts of and look for adults and children with cardiac problems Look for recorded symptoms of heart problems or risk factors.
Diagnostic Tests and Nursing Assessment **5,6** Diagnostic tests **7.** Physical assessment **8.** Apical-radial pulse	**B3.** Apical-radial pulse Physical assessment Cardiac monitors	**B2.** When to start CPR	**B4.** Study and observe diagnostic tests of cardiac patients Attend a code; observe team Do physical assessment, count radial pulse Observe cardiac monitoring
Planning Nursing Care **9,10.** Rationales for medical orders and nursing goals **11.** Pharmacology **12.** Discharge planning for the hypertensive patient **13.** Community resources		**A11.** Talk with dietitian **B1.** Teaching the patient with increased blood pressure GES Objectives 12, 14	**B7.** Examine diets; talk with patients Care for a patient with signs of heart failure Write a NCP Change occupied bed from top to bottom Weigh patients with edema Talk with patients with hypertension; assess learning needs; write teaching plan and discharge plan Observe heparin injections being given Talk with a pharmacist about drug interactions Visit AHA office

LEG VII-C

■ Overview of Learning Experiences in LEG VII-C (cont.)

Objectives	Campus Lab/ Self-Practice	Group Discussions/Lectures	Clinical Lab Focuses
Basic Needs after a Myocardial Infarction **14.** Meeting the basic needs of a convalescing MI patient **15.** Approaches to uncooperative behavior **16,17.** Assessing tolerance to activity	**B1.** Getting a post-MI patient out of bed	**B4.** Needs of the patient convalescing from an MI	**B5.** Care for patient post-MI; write a NCP Give cardiac medications Visit cardiac rehabilitation department Look at lab work
Acute Care Requirements Related to Fluid Excess **18.** Problems related to fluid excess **19.** Planning nursing care for patients with acute CHF	**B2.** Practice drawing up emergency medications Teaching a patient to take own pulse	**B1.** Caring for patients with potential fluid excess GES Objective 19	**B3.** Care for patients with CHF; observe for fluid excess Examine emergency medications Observe and assist with rotating tourniquets Review charting Review Clinical Performance Expectations

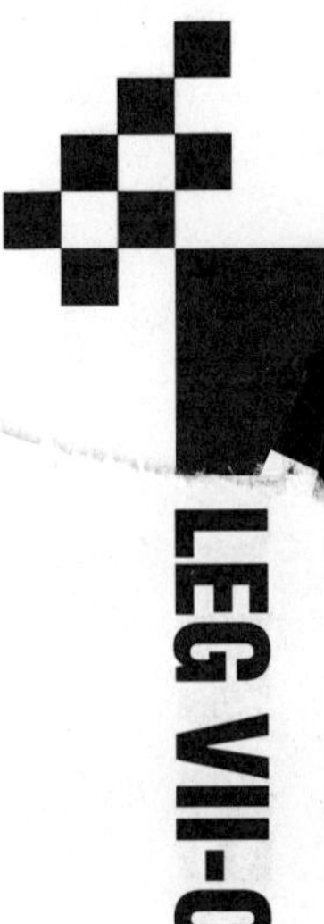

LEG VII-C

New Terms

aerobic
afterload
arrhythmia
digitalization
embolism
hypertension
  borderline
  controlled
  essential
  primary
  secondary
infarction
ischemia
necrosis
preload
prophylactic
pulse pressure
pulsus alternans
telemetry
thrombosis

Abbreviations

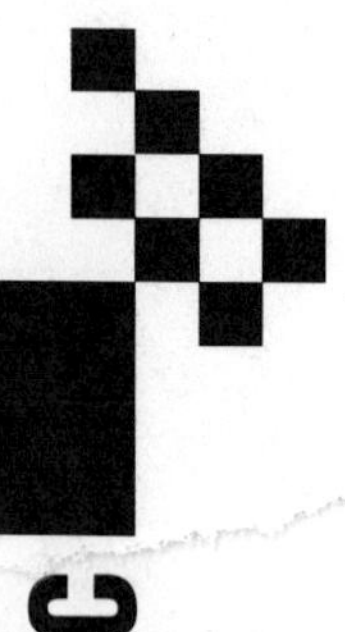

ASHD
CAD
CCU
CHF
CO
HIHD
HTN
JVD
MET
MI
MRI
PND
PT
PTCA
PVD

LEG VII-C

Alterations in Cardiac Function

Objectives

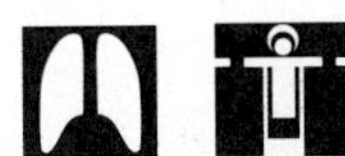

1. Describe three lifestyles that can lead to alterations in cardiac function.

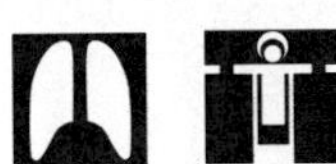

2. Explain the physiologic changes leading to and occurring in left heart failure, right heart failure, angina pectoris, and myocardial infarction, and list the signs and symptoms for each disturbance.

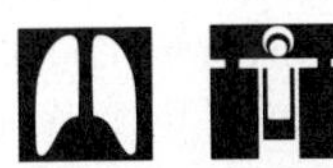

3. List a possible cause and the symptoms of chronic heart problems including: hypertension, congenital heart defects, and rheumatic heart disease.

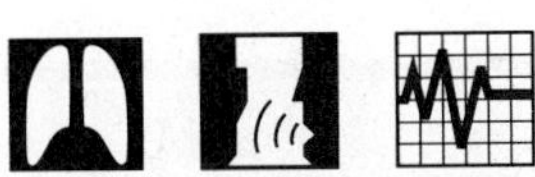

4. Given a list of statements about the effects of stress on the circulatory system, select those that are correct and describe two ways to reverse those effects.

LEG VII-C

A. What's It All About?

1. **Think about** heart disease, the number one killer in the United States. What do you know about the structure and function of the heart and blood vessels? How does this body system work with other body systems to keep a person well? What signs and symptoms can you recognize to direct your nursing care of the patient with cardiovascular problems to provide comfort, support, and encouragement?

Knowing the anatomy and physiology of the heart and circulatory system as it relates to heart disease (not peripheral vascular disease) is your responsibility as you study this LEG. You may have had a human anatomy and physiology course several months or years ago, or you may be taking the course now and be either just beginning or about to begin studying the heart and blood vessels. Whatever your situation, you must learn the parts and general functions of each.

2. **Review:**

LEG I-B	Holistic Health Care and Stress
LEG II-A	Assessing and Charting TPRs
	Assessing and Charting Blood Pressure
LEG VI-B	Adaptation to Stress
LEG VI-C	Recognizing Hypoxemia and Hypercapnea

3. Read medical, anatomy and physiology, surgical, and pediatrics references about *anatomy and physiology of the heart and circulatory system, epidemiology, risk factors, pathophysiology and manifestations of chronic heart failure, congestive heart failure, hypertension, heart defects, effects of stress, stress reduction, healthy lifestyles,* and *cardiovascular problems.*

As you read, list the common signs and symptoms for the diseases listed in Objectives 2 and 3.

4. View audiovisuals and read articles and books from a list given you by your instructor or read the following:

Gawlinski, A., and G. Jensen. "The Complications of Cardiovascular Aging." *AJN,* November 1991, pp. 26–32.

5. Review signs and symptoms of lack of oxygen in the body from LEG VI-C. List two or more signs of hypoxemia in the patients described below:

Mr. Rawlins is 44 years old, hospitalized for the third time in the past 2 years with a "heart attack" better known medically as a myocardial infarction (MI). He was hospitalized this time because he was experiencing severe "crushing" pain in his chest radiating down his left arm. Mr. Rawlins's doctor told him that each succeeding attack leaves further scar tissue on the heart, and prolonged rest and care is indicated. Because of his previous attacks, Mr. Rawlins is extremely apprehensive and discouraged because he foresees another period of 6 to 8 weeks of ospitalization and rest at home. On admission his BP was 80/60; pulse rapid and weak; color ashen; and skin cold and clammy. He was immediately placed in a coronary care unit (CCU).

Mrs. Campbell is a 35-year-old housewife with a history of rheumatic heart disease at the age of 15. She noticed that recently she tired easily in doing her housework, that she was short of breath in going up and down stairs, and that she was increasingly irritable with her husband and children. She also noticed that at the end of the day there was some swelling of her feet and ankles.

She had been told after her bout with rheumatic heart disease that she might have to restrict her activities, and she had experienced all these things previously, so that she did not consult her doctor even though these symptoms were lasting much longer than before. One night after an especially hard day of housework she awoke unable to catch her breath, gasping and choking. She woke her husband, who called the doctor. The doctor recommended that she go immediately to the hospital.

6. Write answers to the following questions as you read or review the structure and function of the normal heart.

(a) Describe the heart, including type of tissue, size, purpose, and location.

(b) Which of the four heart chambers is usually the largest and most heavily muscled?

(c) Describe what happens to the blood from the time the left ventricle contracts until it returns ready for another contraction. Include in your description the following terms: aorta, right atrium, vena cava, right ventricle, pulmonary artery, pulmonary veins, left atrium, oxygen, nutrients, carbon dioxide, coronary arteries.

(d) How does pulmonary circulation differ from circulation to other parts of the body?

(e) What is stroke volume?

(f) Describe the control system to maintain a regular beat.

(g) How can you tell what is the minimum amount of pressure exerted by the blood against the walls of the arteries?

(h) How can you gauge the elasticity of the blood vessel walls?

(i) When is pulse pressure increased? When is it decreased?

(j) How can the heart be adversely affected by our lifestyles? Describe your lifestyle including your pattern of activity and rest, exercise, diet, level of stress, and whether you smoke. (Don't forget to include your own genetic factor.) What risk factors for heart disease exist? Can they be modified?

(k) Why does disease in a blood vessel or heart valve affect the rest of the body? Explain the physiologic changes that occur with coronary artery disease (angina or myocardial infarction) and rheumatic heart disease. How can these changes lead to heart failure?

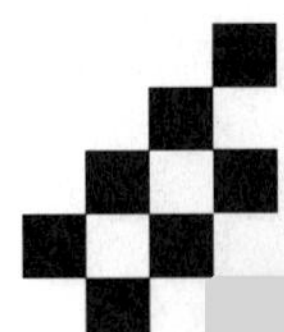

(l) List symptoms of infants that could indicate congenital heart defects. How do these symptoms differ from symptoms of adults in heart failure?

(m) Why do patients with COPD develop heart failure? Which side of the heart is affected? What symptoms appear?

(n) List five of the most common congenital heart defects. Indicate whether each is a cyanotic or an acyanotic defect.

Be prepared to discuss the answers to the questions above in relation to nursing care; for example, location of the heart and taking apical pulse, heartbeat and drugs, function of the heart and blood vessels, and your nursing observations for later Objectives.

7. Write the effects of long-term stress on each of the following:

(a) heart rate

(b) cholesterol deposits on blood vessel lining

(c) blood clotting time

(d) coronary blood vessel size

(e) release of epinephrine

(f) arterial blood pressure

(g) blood viscosity

Which of the above effects are related to the following diseases?

angina pectoris
myocardial infarction (MI)
congestive heart failure (CHF)

List all the stress reduction methods you know about. Share your list in your group discussion.

■ B. Putting It into Action!

1. Obtain a copy of "Heart Drawings" from your local heart association and insert here. Draw in the changes that occur with each of the following conditions: MI, angina pectoris, CHF (left and right sides), rheumatic fever, tetralogy of Fallot.

2. Explain to another person the difference between an MI, angina, and CHF. Have the person ask questions and ask for clarification until it is quite clearly understood by both of you. Having an explanation challenged will stimulate you to seek more information on a subject that you don't really understand and that you have simply memorized from a book.

3. Attend a small group discussion on "Physiologic Changes in Heart Disease."

■ Compare MI, angina, and CHF. Look at the changes in the heart and blood vessels.

■ Explain compensatory mechanisms that permit adaptation.

Frank-Starling mechanism
catecholamine release
cardiac hypertrophy
renal adaptation

■ Discuss changes in the cardiovascular system of the elderly patient. How would your assessment and intervention differ if adapted for age?

■ Describe the pain experience and how pain is relieved.
How does cardiac pain differ from pulmonary chest pain or musculoskeletal pain?

■ Explain the relationship of obesity and hypertension to heart disease.

■ Discuss how lifestyles contribute to or prevent heart disease. What is meant by Type A behavior? What part does smoking play in peripheral vascular disease (PVD) and heart disease? What are the acceptable systolic and diastolic levels of blood pressure for different age groups?

■ What does it mean if the brachial systolic pressures in the arms are different? Is it different when lying down than when standing? Why?

■ Discuss the answers to the questions in A.5 and A.6.

■ Role play and discuss the following situations:

Note: The student assuming the patient's role in the first situation should take a few moments to try to feel and imagine what the patient's fears and questions might be as well as his or her blocks to learning and changing.

Nurse explaining to a 55-year-old obese man with a BP of 180/126 about the relationship between heart disease, obesity, and hypertension.

Woman telling her neighbor about the dietitian she heard speaking at her women's club about the "Whys and Hows of Reducing Cholesterol in the Diet."

Husband explaining to his wife how and why she should reduce the stress and anxiety related to her job.

4. Plan for a clinical experience.

▲ Review charts of adults and children who have been diagnosed as having cardiac problems. Look for recorded symptoms of heart problems or risk factors.

▲ Look for adult patients with diagnoses such as arteriosclerosis, atherosclerosis, coronary artery disease, coronary occlusion, cor pulmonale, hypertension, angina pectoris, MI, and CHF.

▲ Look for children with diagnoses such as patent ductus arteriosis, and tetralogy of Fallot.

Diagnostic Tests and Nursing Assessment

O b j e c t i v e s

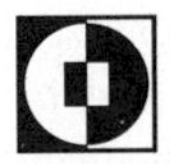 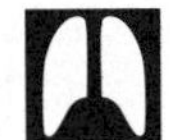

5. Given any of the following lab reports (including their normal values), state its purpose and whether the result is normal or abnormal for a patient having experienced a myocardial infarction: serum triglycerides, WBC, sedimentation rate, prothrombin time, clotting time, partial thromboplastin time (PTT), enzymes (CPK, LDH, SGOT).

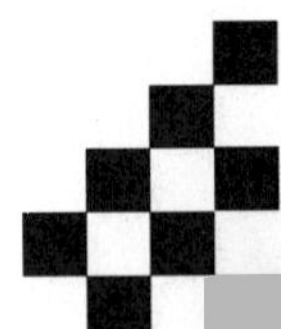

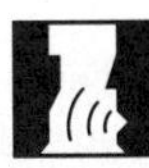 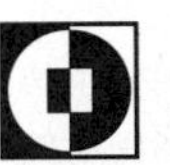 

6. Given a list of descriptions, select the ones that best describe an electrocardiogram and an echocardiogram to a patient.

 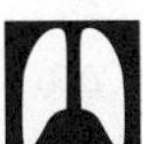

7. Demonstrate making a systematic physical assessment of a patient with impaired cardiac output, using the criteria established by your instructor.

 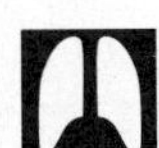

8. Demonstrate accurately counting an apical-radial pulse with another student for 1 minute.

LEG VII-C

A. What's It All About?

1. Think about the physiologic changes you studied with the last Objectives. The physiologic status of cardiac patients changes continually and must be assessed by an alert, knowledgeable nurse. You can use your new skills in listening to lung sounds from LEG VI-C. The diagnostic tests give the physician much important information, but your observations may be even more important in evaluating a patient's progress or detecting deterioration.

2. Review:

LEG II-A Nursing Process—Assessment: Observation and Physical Assessment
LEG II-B Physical Assessment of Maternity Patient

3. Read about *diagnostic tests, apical-radial pulse,* and *physical assessment of the cardiac patient,* in medical-surgical and skills textbooks, and review *CPR techniques* in a CPR handbook.

4. View audiovisuals and read articles and books from a list given you by your instructor or read from the following:

Konick-McMahan, J. "Jugular Vein Distension: Trouble in the Heart's Right Side." *Nursing89,* February, pp. 100–102.
"What to Teach a Patient about Holter Monitoring." *RN,* May 1991, p. 77.

5. Preview LEG XII-C Cardiac Diagnostic Procedures and Physical Assessment.

Comments on Use of Clinical Time

Laboratory test results have increasingly important implications for nursing care. Nurses must be able to read them accurately and take action as necessary. Many physician's orders are based on the lab result that is telephoned to the nurses' station. By the time you complete the fourth LEGs Volume, you should be able to anticipate the signs and symptoms of a patient with a particular lab result. Not every patient has typical signs and symptoms, but at least you will be alert to what you should be looking for. Start now.

There are many lab tests in LEG VII-C, Objective 5. You will need to spend from 30 minutes to an hour each week studying patient charts, observing patients, and relating your findings to the lab reports of diagnostic tests, medications, and treatments. This time is not wasted. A suggested use of clinical time to allow for the varied kinds of experience you will need follows:

If you are scheduled for 8 hours of clinical lab time a week, you will have 4–5 hours of actual patient care and still will be able to spend 2 hours in pre- and postconference and 1–2 hours for chart study and special observations such as those in the laboratory, physical therapy, and x-ray.

There is time—if it is planned and if you are ready to use it well.

6. Read lab reports on patient charts and note whether each is normal or abnormal for a patient 24 hours or more after an MI. There may be numerous lab reports that can be confusing when looking for a specific report (e.g., WBC or SGOT) in a patient's chart. To decrease this confusion, each type of report form is labeled and color-coded (e.g., chemistry may have a black border and hematology may have a red border). Look at your local hospital forms.

■ B. Putting It into Action!

1. Select from the following list of phrases those that could *correctly* and *clearly* describe an EKG to a patient. Use these phrases plus some of your own to explain to a lay person who has never had an EKG what it is and how it is obtained. Ask this person to imagine having one done that day and to ask you questions about it.

A visual record of electric currents in the heart.
A photograph of your pulse.
A tracing of your heart's activity.
A way of recording on paper what your heart muscle is doing.
A picture of the electrical activity of your heart.

How does an EKG differ from a cardiac monitor?

What do enzymes tell you about patient illness and progress?

How does an echocardiogram differ from an electrocardiogram? Imagine you are explaining them to a 10-year-old child. What fears might or might not be expressed? How can you encourage a child to ask questions and reveal concerns?

What is a stress test? When is it given and where? What precautions are taken to protect the patient?

2. Attend a small group discussion on "When to Start CPR."

■ Describe how external heart massage and mouth-to-mouth resuscitation would be given to each of the following unconscious people:

Six-month-old Gary found covered with a pillow in his crib.

Mr. Nokord, a 54-year-old laryngectomee found floating on the top of a swimming pool.

Jack Worker, who is bleeding slightly from a leg wound after a car accident.

Mary, 6-year-old who fell out of a tree while playing.

Mark, a teen-ager with a fractured jaw that is wired together who just received a penicillin injection.

How would you determine that a cardiac arrest had occurred? How can you determine accurately that the patient is getting an air exchange during mouth-to-mouth resuscitation? How would the procedure change if you were using a plastic airway with a mouthpiece for the patient and the rescuer?

■ Obtain a copy of the cardiopulmonary resuscitation procedure used in your hospital, including a list of duties of hospital personnel, and insert it into this LEG. Using this procedure and taking the parts of the following people, role play finding a patient, who was alert the last time you visited him, now lying apparently unconscious in bed with the head of the bed elevated, taking deep gasping breaths. You feel for a radial pulse and can find none. You look at his eyes and find his pupils dilated.

Role players: Patient, nursing student who discovers the patient, the head nurse, aide, doctor, ward clerk, switchboard operator, EKG technician, respiratory therapist.

Discussion questions after the role playing: How do you know if cardiac compression is effective? Would the compression differ for each patient mentioned above? Would you get an EKG tracing before or after starting inflation of the lungs? Why? What do the A-B-C letters stand for in resuscitation? Who is legally allowed to do cardiopulmonary resuscitation in your state?

3. Practice in campus lab.

■ Practice taking an apical-radial pulse with two other students. You will need a stethoscope. Which of the following apical-radial pulses is correct? Why?

$$\frac{\text{A-84}}{\text{R-76}} \text{ or } \frac{\text{A-76}}{\text{R-84}}$$

How many watches do you need to take an apical-radial pulse? When would you need to check the apical-radial pulse? What does a deficit tell you?

■ If you were about to give a patient digoxin and counted the radial rate and found it to be 58, which of the following would you do next and why?

Not give the medication and chart the pulse rate.

Count the patient's apical-radial pulse rate.

Count the patient's apical rate.

Give the medication and chart the pulse rate.

Check to see what the pulse rate has been before.

Tickle the patient to wake him up.

Get the patient out of bed for exercise.

■ Practice setting up a cardiac monitor and applying the electrodes according to the guidelines of your local agency.
What assessments and daily care are required when a patient is being monitored?

■ List the information you will want to obtain during a physical assessment of a patient with impaired cardiac function. Include: what information you want to obtain from an interview, what observations you will make, and how you will use the techniques of assessment (i.e., observation, percussion, palpation, and auscultation). How will this assessment differ from the one you make of a patient with impaired respiratory function, and how will it be similar?

■ Practice making a physical assessment of a cardiac patient after viewing a demonstration by your instructor or watching an audiovisual.
Does your physical assessment include:

General observations: color, degree of distress, diaphoresis

VS: Temperature for low-grade fever

Pulse: rate, rhythm

Respirations: rate, character

Blood pressure in both arms

Heart sounds: S1, S2, and abnormal sounds

Lung sounds: rales, wheezes

Extremities: edema

I&O, weight

Did you include reading the chart to compare your findings with previous assessments? What would they tell you?

4. **Plan** for a clinical experience.

▲ Study the diagnostic tests done for patients with impaired cardiac function. Anticipate the symptoms that would occur because of the information obtained from the tests, then examine the chart for evidence of the symptoms. Visit the patients and ask them to share with you some health history and current problems.

▲ Attend a code in your hospital. Observe the responsibilities of each member of the emergency team.

▲ Count apical-radial rates. Practice on infants and adults. Report any irregularity.

▲ Observe or assist with the physical assessment of a patient with impaired cardiac function.

▲ Observe or assist with setting up or attaching a patient to a continous cardiac monitor.

▲ Observe diagnostic tests: EKG, echocardiogram, esophageal echocardiogram, stress test, and cardiac catheterization.

Planning Nursing Care

O b j e c t i v e s

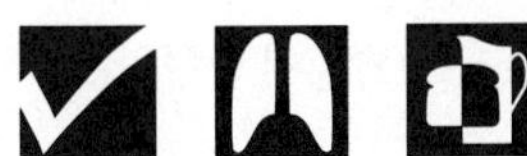

9. State the purpose for each of the following treatment orders for patients with impaired cardiac output (CHF): measure intake and output, daily weight, apical-radial pulse, semi-Fowler's position, low-sodium and low-cholesterol diets, oxygen, bed rest, vital signs, paracentesis. Then write a nursing care plan for a real or hypothetical patient.

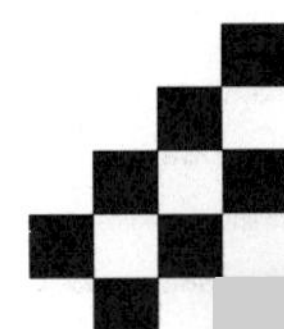

 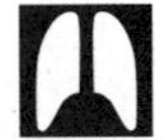

10. Compare the goals of nursing care for patients with angina pectoris and patients convalescing from a myocardial infarction.

11. Given a list of nursing actions, select those you would take when giving each of the following classifications of drugs: anticoagulants, antiarrhythmics, diuretics, cardiac glycosides, antianginal, narcotics, tranquilizers, stool softeners, ACE inhibitors, adrenergic blockers, calcium antagonists, vasodilators, antihypertensives, and antihypotensives.

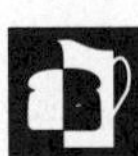  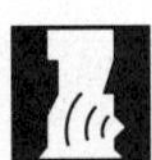  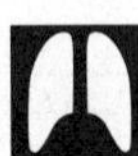

12. Prepare a discharge plan for a hypertensive patient that includes information related to medications, nutrition, drug therapy, exercise, and rest to achieve an optimum level of wellness.

13. List three community resources that support the cardiac patient at home.

■ A. What's It All About?

1. Think about your daily routines and how they are disrupted by an illness such as the flu or some other minor problem that requires you to have more rest and to take medication. Do you ever forget to take the medication? Are you too busy to rest? Why can't you take the idea of rest to heart and stop all your activities and just "get well"? "It's so good for you." "You'll feel better that way." Pat phrases are meaningless to both a busy person who is not confined to bed and a person who is too sick to get out of bed. It takes more than a pat phrase to get your patient to "do what is best." Your skills and energy will be severely tested.

How would you feel if you were told that you could not salt your food from now on? What if you were also told that butter and most meats are taboo because of their "high amount of the wrong kinds of fat"? You feel well, and the dietary controls probably don't appeal to you. Now, consider the patient with heart problems plus dietary controls. These patients need help to cope.

2. Review:

LEG II-A Nursing Process—Assessment: Observation and Physical Assessment
Assessing and Charting TPRs
Assessing and Charting Blood Pressure
LEG II-C Assessment: Interviewing and History Taking
Measuring and Recording Intake and Output
LEG IV-C Nursing Process: Planning and Implementation
Weighing on a Balanced Scale
LEG VI-C Assessing and Preventing Respiratory Problems

3. Read in medical-surgical, pharmacology, nutrition, and skills textbooks about *nursing care teaching, medications,* and *treatment for impaired cardiac function and peripheral vascular disease.*

4. View audiovisuals and read articles and books from a list given you by your instructor or read from the following:

Feury, D., and D. T. Nash. "Hypertension: The Nurse's Role." *RN,* November 1990, pp. 54–60.

Hill, M. N., and S. L. Cunningham. "The Latest Words for High Blood Pressure." *AJN,* April 1989, pp. 504–510.

Rodman, M. J. "Hypertension: First-Line Drug Therapy." *RN,* January 1991, pp. 32–40.

Rodman, M. J. "Hypertension: Step-Care Management." *RN,* February 1991, pp. 24–31.

Solomon, J. "Managing a Failing Heart." *RN,* August 1991, pp. 46–51. (See insert on compensation.)

Thompson, V. L. "Chest Pain: Your Response to a Classic Warning." *RN,* April 1989, pp. 32–38. (See insert, "Angina: Teaching for Discharge.")

5. Preview:

LEG XI-C Acute Heart Problems
Abnormal Heart Sounds
Arrythmias
Chest Pain
LEG XII-B Anticoagulant Therapy
Cardiac Surgery

6. Complete the following chart or write drug cards.

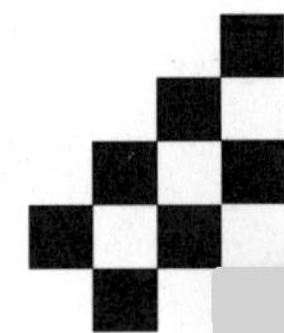

Drug	Class	Action/Use	Side Effects	Nursing Responsibility
digoxin				
quinidine				
Inderal				
Minipress				
Procardia				
Aldomet				
heparin				
nitroglycerin				
Coumadin				
Lasix				
Capoten				
Aldactone				
Apresoline				
Morphine Sulfate (MS)				

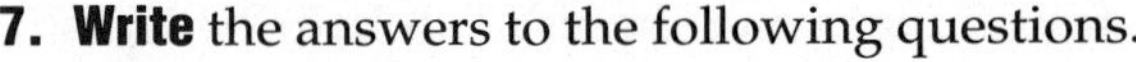

7. Write the answers to the following questions.

(a) What is meant by a "digitalizing" dose? What side effects can occur? What are the symptoms of digitalis toxicity?

What is the difference between digoxin and digitalis with respect to dosage and excretion?

Differentiate between a maintenance dose and a digitalizing dose of digoxin, and teach an elderly patient about it.

Describe therapeutic and toxic effects of digitalis preparations. What puts a patient at risk for toxicity? What are the nursing implications?

(b) Make a list of each class of diuretics: K+ sparing, thiazide, carbonic anhydrase inhibitors, other. What are the nursing implications when giving each type of diuretic?

(c) What is the step-care approach to the treatment of hypertension?

(d) How does the level of serum potassium in the body affect the heart rate? How can potassium be given in the diet?
List three foods containing potassium.
What observations would you make related to loss of potassium and to increased potassium?

(e) Identify the therapeutic range of prothrombin time and clotting time. What is the expected change from normal? When is it unsafe to give heparin or Coumadin? When is heparin used therapeutically? When prophylactically? What is the difference in dose? What are the nursing implications for a patient on heparin or Coumadin? What is the antidote for each?

(f) How is nitroglycerine paste applied? What teaching needs are present for a patient receiving a long-acting vasodilator?

(g) How do the following affect the heart rate?

Isuprel
atropine
vagus nerve
potassium
calcium

(h) What is a beta-adrenergic blocker? Which drugs fit in this category? What does it mean if they are nonselective? Name those drugs. Why would beta-1 adrenergic drugs be better for cardiac patients than beta-2 drugs?

(i) How do calcium channel blockers work? What are they used for? What nursing actions are indicated?

LEG VII-C

8. Visit your local heart association office and browse through their booklets. Find out what is available for your patients and how to obtain educational materials. Can patients call and ask for information? Can nurses arrange to have a supply of specific booklets available on the patient unit?

List three to five booklets you have found that could be used to help patients at home. Describe briefly how you could use each (for example: pamphlet, "Save Food $ and Help Your Heart"). Go over one idea in the booklet each time you have contact with the patient and review the first idea (listening to how and if it was tried) before going on to a discussion of another suggestion.

9. Keep a dietary record of your intake for 24 hours. Underline every food that is high in sodium, and circle each food that is high in saturated fat. What modifications do you need to make in your diet to prevent hypertension and coronary artery disease? *List them.*

Write down a personal dietary goal for this week. Keep it small so that you won't get discouraged, and then next week evaluate your progress and write a new goal.

10. Write a menu for moderate sodium-restricted and fat-controlled meals for 1 day.

Go to the supermarket and shop for the meal. Check prices and salt and fat content on labels. Check content of dairy products, margarines, salad dressings, peanut butter, cooking oils for the presence of unsaturated, saturated, and hydrogenated fat. Read the labels on canned soups and vegetables for sodium content. Check the special foods section, too. Bring your menu and prices to the group discussion with the dietitian, along with your questions. (This experience should give you a feeling for how confused patients can be when given a diet prescription without adequate teaching.)

11. Talk with your hospital dietitian about fat-controlled and sodium-restricted diets. Come prepared with questions to ask, which may include the following:

What types of diets are prescribed in your hospital to reduce elevated serum lipids? (Be sure you know what serum lipids are and how they are formed.)

What percentage of your total calories each day could be obtained from fat if you were on a fat-controlled diet? Compare this percentage with that allowed on a diabetic diet. What similarities are present?

How many milligrams of sodium do most Americans consume daily?

How many do they need?

■ B. Putting It into Action!

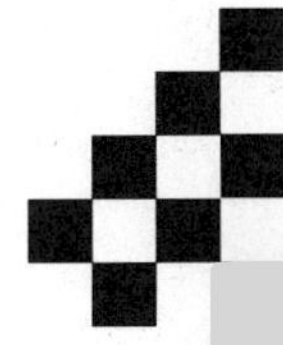

1. Attend a group discussion on "Teaching the Patient with Increased Blood Pressure."

■ To prepare for this session select a patient from your clinical area or use a case study given to you by your instructor. Work with another student to design a teaching plan that will prepare the patient for discharge. Present your plan to the group and be prepared to answer questions. Here are some items to include in your presentation: symptoms that are present, definition and effect of hypertension on the body, how to measure blood pressure, medications and how they work in the body, present or potential side effects, diet, exercise and stress, how age affects the ability to learn and change lifestyle.

■ Investigate the cost of the patient's medications for 1 month.

■ What effect can antihypertensives have on sexual activity?

■ What kind of visual or practice experiences can you think of to help your elderly patient learn about storing medications properly, checking the expiration date, possible interactions with other drugs?

■ How would you discuss the signs and symptoms of toxicity or overdose without frightening the patient? It is important for a patient to recognize what may be a fluid and electrolyte imbalance that can be corrected with diet and fluids. How can you help your patient learn to recognize an imbalance?

LEG VII-C

2. Select from the following rationales which explain each of the patient's medical orders. If a suitable rationale is not included, write it in. The patients' admission diagnoses and symptoms are described under A.5 on p. 214.

Medical Orders	**Rationales**
MR. RAWLINS	(a) slows and strengthens the heart rate and decreases O_2 need of heart muscle
_____ Complete bed rest	
_____ Immediate family only to visit	(b) reduces anxiety and associated increased blood pressure and heart rate
_____ Demerol prn	(c) will detect shock or heart irregularities
_____ EKG	(d) reduces the risk of emboli formation
_____ Sed rate	(e) used to regulate the dosage of anticoagulants
_____ CBC	
_____ SGOT	(f) decreases abdominal distention that interferes with respiration
_____ Prothrombin time	(g) prevents straining at stool that increases arterial blood pressure, which might cause rupture of weakened heart muscle
_____ Heparin	

_____ Vital signs q2h for 3 days, q4h 1 week, then qid	(h) reduces return of venous blood to the heart and decreases pulmonary congestion
_____ Bland low-calorie diet	(i) determines exercise tolerance and recovery of heart muscle
_____ Gradual increase in activities and use of bedside commode	(j) helps reduce pulmonary congestion by causing pooling of blood in the periphery
_____ Coumadin	(k) prevents skin breakdown, venous stasis, weakness, and joint stiffness
_____ Feed	(l) relieves hypoxia, which can lead to cardiac arrhythmias
_____ Oxygen 4L/m prn	(m) increases oxygen supply and relieves dyspnea and anxiety, so decreases work of heart
_____ Restoril hs prn	(n) reduces stress and anxiety
_____ Doxinate	(o) reduces straining, which increases intrathoracic pressure and decreases venous return
MRS. CAMPBELL	(p) provides information on fluid overload
_____ Complete bed rest	(q) may indicate tissue necrosis and inflammation
_____ Oxygen by mask	(r) a decrease in activity will decrease O_2 need and heart work so promotes recovery of heart muscle
_____ Low-sodium diet	(s) maintenance of some activity and self-care improves psychologic recovery
_____ BP, apical-radial pulse, R q4h	(t) may increase or decrease anxiety and needs to be monitored by the nurse
_____ Digitalize	(u) pain and anxiety cause more pain and anxiety and increase oxygen need
_____ I&O	(v) assists in assessing if area of infarction has enlarged
_____ Weigh daily	(w) excess fluid interferes with diffusion of oxygen into cells.
_____ Morphine q4h prn	
_____ Semi-Fowler's position	
_____ Lasix	
_____ Ativan	

3. List the independent nursing actions you would want to take with each patient and select a rationale for each. Use a separate sheet of paper.

4. Select which of the nursing actions in the right column might have caused the situations occurring on days 4, 6, and 7 described in the left column.

Situation	Nursing Actions
_____ Mrs. Campbell was ordered to be weighed daily while still on bed rest. The bed scale was used, and this is a record of her weights for 3 days: Day 1: 160 lb Day 2: 156 lb Day 3: 153 lb	(a) weighs patient at any time of day (b) weighs patient before breakfast daily (c) balances scale before weighing a group of patients
_____ Which of her medications would account for this weight loss? Review medical orders under B.2.	(d) balances scale before weighing each patient
_____ On day 4 she weighed 157 lb. Which of the actions on the right might have caused an error in weighing?	(e) records weight on piece of paper as soon as completes weighing patient (f) sometimes forgets to record weight immediately and writes it from memory
_____ What symptoms would be observable if the patient were beginning to retain fluid again?	(g) keeps a list of all patients to be weighed and brings it up to date daily
_____ On day 5 Mrs. Campbell weighed 150 lbs. On day 6 there was no weight recorded. Which of the actions on the right might have caused this omission?	(h) looks through patient file daily for patients to be weighed (i) delegates responsibility to nursing assistant who has been evaluated as satisfactory in ability to weigh patients
_____ On day 7 the patient was getting out of bed, and the nurse brought the scale into the room. When she returned, she found the patient weighing herself. Her weight was 150 lbs. Is this weight accurate? Why?	(j) delegates responsibility to nursing aide, who has no idea of why patients are being weighed or need for accuracy

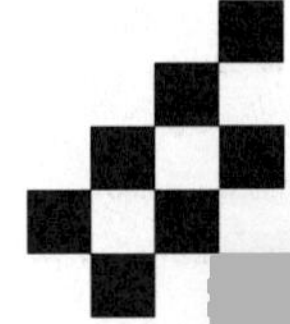

LEG VII-C

5. Write why each of the following nursing diagnostic statements might be seen in the patient with impaired heart function. State how you would know a problem exists, and list one important assessment and one intervention.

alteration in cardiac output
alteration in tissue perfusion
potential complication: arrhythmia
alteration in family processes
sensory perceptual alteration
potential injury: drug complications

6. List at least eight important points to use when assessing teaching needs of a patient on digoxin, nitroglycerin, or an anticoagulant.

Work in three groups to create a teaching plan for one of the drugs listed above.

7. Plan for a clinical experience.

▲ Care for patients with signs of heart failure. Write a nursing care plan before caring for the patient if possible. Include a rationale for each medical order and nursing intervention. Include an assessment of risk factors and identify predictable complications. Reevaluate it after caring for the patient and make changes as necessary. Present it in postconference.

▲ Demonstrate changing an occupied bed from top to bottom. Why do you think this might be necessary?

▲ Weigh patients with edema.

▲ Talk with patients with hypertension. Assess their learning needs and begin a teaching plan. Write a discharge plan that includes assistance to modify lifestyle and considers the patient and family needs and community resources available.

▲ Observe heparin being given and review the lab work. Find out what the antidotes for heparin and Coumadin are.

▲ Talk with the pharmacist about drug interactions, especially those occurring when patients are on cardiac glycosides and diuretics. Discuss antihypertensive therapy.

▲ Visit your local American Heart Association (AHA) office and other community resources to learn what services are available to your patients. Share your findings in a postconference.

▲ Observe and/or assist with a paracentesis. Note and summarize in postconference the nursing responsibility.

▲ Examine the sodium-restricted and fat-controlled diets being served. Talk with the patients about taste and satisfaction. Assess their level of understanding regarding their diet. If they need to remain on the diet after discharge, when should their teaching program begin?

Basic Needs after a Myocardial Infarction

Objectives

 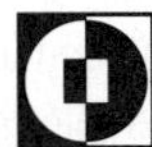

14. Describe how basic human needs are met for and by a patient convalescing from a myocardial infarction.

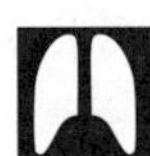 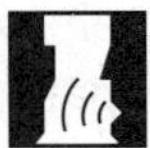

15. Given a patient situation in which the patient is being uncooperative, describe your reaction to the behavior and list two helpful approaches you could take to determine the reason for the patient's behavior.

  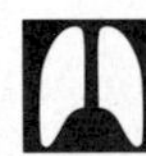

16. List and sequence the activities for an MI patient to allow for a gradual progression to a normal but modified lifestyle.

  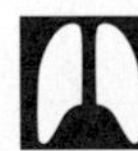

17. Identify signs that might occur during or after activity that indicate exertion is too great.

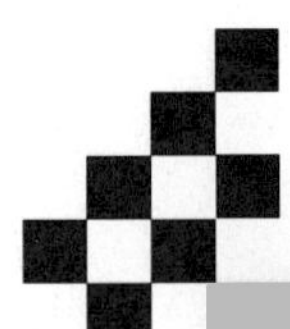

A. What's It All About?

1. Think about nursing care. What aspect is most important? The acute, critical, life-and-death stage? It seems so on television. But what happens to the patient whose life is saved? We have an obligation to help meet this patient's needs through the period of convalescence as he learns to modify his lifestyle and resume former activities. Why shouldn't the patient be anxious and hostile and think "Why me?" Nurses must place a high value on continuing supportive care to help the patient adapt.

2. Review:

LEG I-B	Holistic Health Care and Stress
LEG IV-A	Therapeutic Communication Skills
LEG VI-A	Depression
	Psychosocial Assessment
	Assisting People to Express Grief
	Helping Adapt to Loss
	Healthy Response to Crisis
LEG VI-B	Adaptation to Stress

3. Read about *stress reduction, relaxation techniques, helplessness, lifestyle changes, coping, physical and psychologic needs of patient during convalescence and at home, cardiac rehabilitation,* and *sexuality* in medical-surgical, anatomy and physiology, and psychiatric nursing references.

4. View audiovisuals and read articles and books from a list given you by your instructor or read the following:

Gleeson, B. "After an MI—How to Teach a Patient in Denial." *Nursing91,* May, pp. 48–56.

Note: Journal articles are the most current written materials. Textbooks may run a year or more behind the most current techniques and treatments involved in patient care. Use them selectively as references. Be alert to new ideas. Attend lectures. Television series and news journals frequently have good information. As you come across new material, make notes in the readings section; cross out the old information and add the new.

LEG VII-C

5. Describe the types of expected behavior of the patient during each stage of adaptation after an MI. For each stage, describe the nursing actions that are most helpful. This kind of question is to stimulate you to anticipate problems and, therefore, prepare to care for patients convalescing from an MI. Share your ideas and information. Add to this section after you have observed many patients.

6. Write answers to the following questions.

- **(a)** What is cardiac rehabilitation?
- **(b)** What is collateral circulation, and why is it important?
- **(c)** Describe an abnormal response to exercise.
- **(d)** What symptoms would indicate cardiac stress after sexual intercourse?
- **(e)** What is life like at home during the first year after an MI?

B. Putting It into Action!

1. Practice in campus lab.

- Role play getting the following patient out of bed. Have another nursing student or a family member play the patient.

> Mr. Glee has been on bed rest after a severe MI. His vital signs have been stable, and the doctor has ordered progressive ambulation. He has been allowed to sit on the side of the bed for 10–15 min and has tolerated this with no ill effects, so today he is to walk a few steps and sit in a chair for 15 min.

How can you learn what the patient's feelings are about getting up? What might they be? Why would you want to know?
How do you feel about getting him up? Afraid, confident, nervous?
How do you communicate your feelings to a patient? By your face, your voice, your hands? Think it through! If you expect to feel nervous, is it because you don't know what unexpected event might occur, such as the patient's becoming faint or having chest pain or getting short of breath? Plan ahead. Know exactly what you will do if any of those events does occur! Be prepared and the patient will know you can handle the situation with calm intelligence. If you are calm, the patient's anxiety will decrease, and he will tolerate the activity better. *You are the key person.*

What will be included in your assessment before getting the patient up? After he is sitting on the side of the bed? After he has walked? While he is sitting in the chair? After he has returned to bed? List them here.

1.
2.
3.
4.
5.

Why continue to assess the patient at these intervals? Record your practice on a charting form available in your hospital. Insert it here.
Make up a description of the activity accomplished and your observations of the patient's tolerance to it.

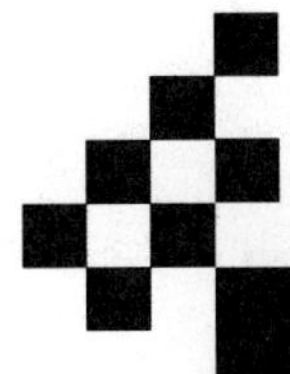

2. List your daily activities. Sequence them in terms of energy cost. Indicate the proportion of the day you spend sitting, walking, bicycling, and so on. How much exercise do you get daily?

3. Arrange these activities in sequence according to the amount of energy (METs) expended.

brushing teeth
sitting at a desk
walking slowly
shopping
showering
taking tub bath
jogging
reaching
straining at stool
lifting up arms
walking briskly
scrubbing floor on hands and knees
scrubbing floor with mop
riding bike
playing tennis
playing golf
stooping
pushing up in bed

4. Attend a small group discussion on "Needs of the Patient Convalescing from an MI."

■ List the basic needs on a chalkboard or overhead projector. Identify those that would be problems for the patient during the first week and second week of convalescence. List the problems across from the need. Write out as many nursing goals and interventions as you can think of as a group.

■ How does your list fit with the following general goals for MI patients?

Allow patient to resume a satisfactory and productive life.
Decrease the risk of any more heart problems.

Use the nursing diagnosis statement "adjustment, impaired." Identify the risk factors, if present, and behavior seen. What are important nursing interventions?

■ What nursing interventions and discharge planning would be helpful for the spouse of Mr. Glee, p. 230?

5. Plan for a clinical experience.

▲ Care for patient after an MI. Begin a nursing care plan before giving any care. Complete it when your care is finished. Describe the patient's behavior and compare it with your preconceived idea. Try to identify which stage of adaptation the patient is in. Include learning needs.

▲ Give medications to patients with heart disease. Read charts of patients with heart disease.

LEG VII-C

▲ Look at the lab work, treatment plans, reactions to care. Visit the patients and make observations related to their diseases.

▲ Visit the cardiac rehabilitation department if available in your community. Discuss their program with the nurses. Find out what information is taught and what teaching methods are most effective. Inquire about the educational preparation needed by the nurses in order to work in that unit.

Acute Care Requirements Related to Fluid Excess

O b j e c t i v e s

  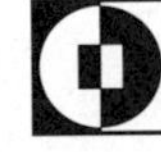

18. Given situations of patients who have symptoms of fluid excess, state at least one possible cause (e.g., body system problem, medication or medical therapy, or a combination of these) and the related nursing interventions.

 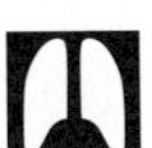 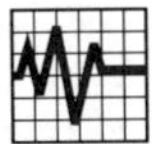

19. Given a description of a patient being admitted to the hospital with acute CHF and a list of medical orders, describe the nursing care for the first 8 hours; state your rationale and include an evaluation that indicates the treatment plan is effective. Write a nursing care plan.

LEG VII-C

A. What's It All About?

1. Think about heart failure, a very frightening experience. Patients in heart failure can be critically ill one minute and then respond well to treatment. This is a chronic progressive disease. Many patients have learned to live well with controlled therapy. *Listen* to your patients. They can help you learn to help other patients with failing hearts. Your careful assessment and evaluation can prevent catastrophe!

2. Review LEG VII-B, Fluid and Electrolyte Balance during Illness.

3. Read about *heart failure, fluid overload,* and *emergency drugs* in medical-surgical, pediatrics, and pharmacology references.

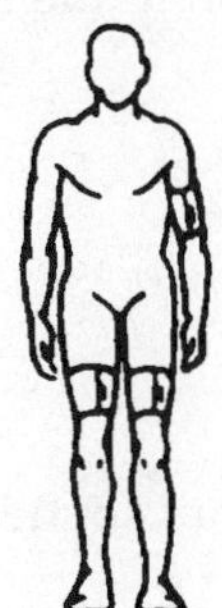

1. Time 9:10 a.m.

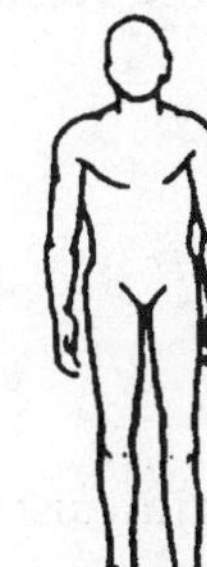

2. Time ______

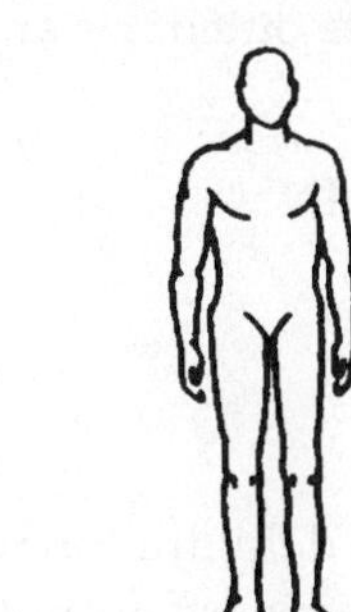

3. Time ______

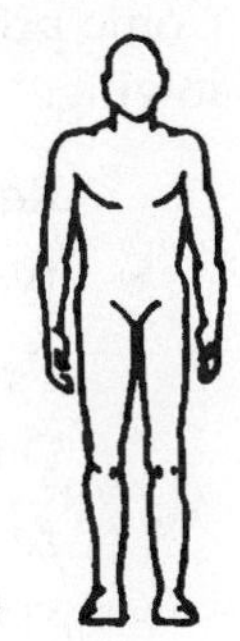

4. Time ______

4. Draw tourniquets on the patient diagrams, indicating how and when they are rotated. Physician's order reads: "Rotate tourniquets q 15 min."

Why are rotating tourniquets used?

Why might patients with fluid excess have a need for rotating tourniquets? How do the tourniquets help them? Bring your answers to the group discussion.

5. Shade in blue on the figure below the areas where signs of ECF excess could occur. List three nursing actions you would take to help the patient.

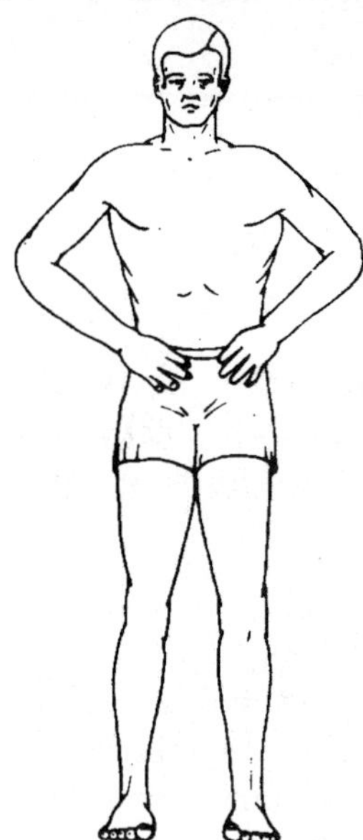

List as many symptoms of fluid excess as you can think of. Describe the pathophysiology that causes excess fluid.

LEG VII-C

■ B. Putting It into Action!

1. Attend a small group discussion on "Caring for Patients with Potential Fluid Excess."

■ To prepare for this group, bring your nursing care plan for a patient with CHF from Objective 9 or complete a case study assigned by your instructor.
Bring some reference books with you to the meeting.

■ Decide on two or three of the patients in the plans and discuss the nursing care for the first 8 hours after admission. What signs and symptoms were present? How did these change with treatment? Does the change tell you the treatment was effective? Come prepared to discuss outcomes and nursing interventions in relation to the following:

Record I&O carefully

Weigh daily

Rest

Diuretics

Assess for signs of dehydration with rapid diuresis: stable BP; fullness of neck veins; hematocrit; urinary output; skin turgor

Check boney prominences; meticulous skin care

Low-salt diet

Signs that the treatment is effective:

Decrease in pitting edema

Weight loss

Good urinary output

Absence of neck vein distention

Decrease in pulmonary congestion

Decrease in circulation time and venous pressure

■ Describe the difference in signs and symptoms and nursing interventions for right heart failure and left heart failure.

Right Heart Failure		Left Heart Failure	
Signs and Symptoms	**Interventions**	**Signs and Symptoms**	**Interventions**

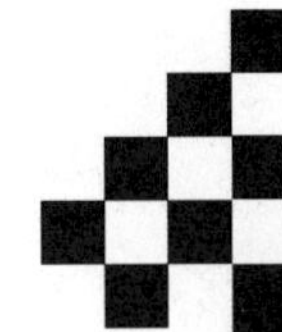

LEG VII-C

2. Practice in campus lab.

■ Practice drawing up emergency medications. Use a 50-cc syringe and needle and a 30-cc ampule and vial. Fill the ampule with water and practice drawing up the solution. You will find it takes several tries to develop a technique to draw it up quickly without spilling it or getting air in your syringe.

Occasionally, this amount of medication must be given in an emergency situation. Be prepared. Develop this skill now!

■ Role play teaching Mr. Glee (p. 230) to take his pulse. Did you make a plan first? Did it include assessing the patient's current knowledge and explaining the significance of the rate?

3. Plan for a clinical experience.

▲ Care for patients with CHF. Assess for fluid excess. Observe their symptoms and behavior now. Read about their problems on admission and ask the patients to describe how they felt before coming into the hospital. Write down the medications they received and be able to explain the rationale for medical and nursing treatment.

▲ Examine the emergency medications on the patient unit. Which drugs might be given for hypotension, cardiac arrest, heart block, pulmonary edema? What equipment would be needed to administer them?

▲ Observe and assist with application and use of rotating tourniquets.

▲ Chart your observations and nursing care. Then look at the charting critically. Does it include all the steps of the nursing process? Is it organized, clear, and concise? Are there any double entries?

▲ Review the **Clinical Expectations** for Level Seven on the Why page.

Have I Learned?

The following questions are for you to answer in order to find out if you have met the Objectives. All the Objectives in LEG VII-C are covered in this series of questions. Pick a quiet time and answer them. Answers are found at the end of this selftest.

No space has been left for answering the questions related to the "doing" Objectives. Use a separate sheet of paper for those answers, and then use the answers in clinical or campus lab for your own evaluation.

Objective **Question**

1 **1.** List and briefly describe three lifestyles that can increase the risk of developing heart disease.

2 **2.** Which of the following best describes what occurs to the heart with angina?

(a) The left side of the heart has weakened and is unable to move the blood out easily.

(b) There is a blockage in the coronary artery and oxygen can no longer reach the heart muscle and tissue dies.

(c) The blood vessels become sclerosed and offer abnormal resistance to the blood flow.

(d) There is a temporary reduction in the amount of oxygen in the myocardium, and pain occurs.

3 **3.** Name one probable cause and at least two symptoms of the following diseases:

Hypertension

Congenital Heart Defects

4 **4.** Write whether these statements are true or false.

(a) Stress decreases the viscosity of the blood.

(b) Stress increases the cholesterol levels in the blood.

(c) Stress increases the heart rate.

4 **5.** Describe two ways to reduce the effects of stress on our bodies.

(a)

(b)

5 **6.** Write the purpose of each lab test for a patient with an MI and state whether the result is normal or above normal and whether it is expected for this patient.

SGOT (8–40 units) 180

PTT (control 15) 25

6 **7.** Mr. Goforth is scheduled to have an EKG. He has never had one before and asks you what will happen during the test. Your best reply will be:

(a) "The machine makes a picture of the electrical activity of your heart."

(b) "You are connected to a machine with wires, and the electrical current is recorded on a graph."

(c) "The technician will place small straps on your wrists and ankles, and you will be asked to just lie quietly. The straps are connected to the cardiograph machine, and it records on a graph. The graph tells exactly what your heart is doing at that moment. You will feel nothing."

(d) "An instrument is moved over your chest. The high-frequency sound waves are recorded on graph paper. You just lie quietly."

7, 8 **8.** Describe counting an apical-radial pulse and making a systematic physical assessment. Ask another student to evaluate you, according to criteria provided by your instructor. Imagine that your patient has a cardiac problem.

9 **9.** While giving you a diet history, your patient tells you that she likes to have the following foods for breakfast: tomato juice, fried egg, bacon, bagel, lox (smoked salmon), cream cheese, cucumbers, radishes, tomatoes, coffee with cream and sugar. Which of these foods will need to be omitted if she is on a sodium-restricted diet?

9 **10.** Write the purpose for each of the following orders for patients with CHF:

Diuretic

Intake and output

Weigh daily

Apical-radial pulse

Semi-Fowler's position

Oxygen

Bed rest

Vital signs

Paracentesis

10 **11.** Compare goals and rationales for nursing care for patients with angina pectoris and patients convalescing from myocardial infarction.

11 **12.** Place the letter of the correct action(s) in front of each drug classification.

_____ anticoagulant

_____ antiarrhythmic

_____ antianginal

_____ antihypertensive

_____ diuretic

_____ cardiac glycoside

(a) check dosage daily

(b) check BP and P frequently

(c) watch for hematuria, ecchymosis

(d) don't give aspirin

(e) check prothrombin time

(f) check pulse before giving

(g) instruct patient to dissolve tablet under tongue

(h) give into subcutaneous fat pad and avoid massaging area after injection

(i) allow patient to keep at bedside and take when needed with a doctor's order

(j) watch for dizziness, fainting, headache

(k) have patient sitting or lying when taking drug

(l) instruct patient about increased voiding

12 **13.** Role play teaching a patient with hypertension about self-care after discharge. Bring a sample list of medical orders and educational materials you would want to use.

13 **14.** List three agencies or people in your community who have a service to offer the cardiac patient at home.

14 **15.**

> Mr. Bland is recovering from an MI that occurred 3 days ago. He is on a bland, fat-controlled diet. He is allowed to shave and feed himself but not bathe yet.

List the basic needs and how they can be met for this patient. Under each need state one potential complication or problem that could occur (for example, need for activity: complication might be thrombophlebitis).

15 **16.**

> You are told to give Mr. Breeze a bath this morning, as he is on bed rest after a myocardial infarction. When you enter the room, you find him sitting at the edge of the bed smoking. You know he is not supposed to smoke and not to sit up yet, either. He gives you a look as if to say, "I dare you to stop me."

What two actions could you take to find out why he is disobeying the doctor's order and to help him follow the prescribed treatment plan?

16 **17.** Describe a patient with a myocardial infarction both before and after the MI. (Use a nursing history or data base form.) List the patient's activities (before and during the hospital stay), and then sequence those activities that will allow the patient to gradually progress in terms of energy cost to resuming a normal but modified life pattern.

17 **18.**

> After a walk to the mailbox one evening, Mr. Roberts noticed that he was slightly short of breath but did not feel tired. His pulse rate was above 100 for about 15 min. The following day he felt too tired to repeat the trip.

Which of these symptoms indicates the walk was too strenuous?

18 **19.** State one possible cause and one nursing action for each of the following patients' fluid excess problem.

> Mr. Puffen has chronic heart disease and is admitted to the unit with poor color and dyspnea.

> Mrs. Reno has been complaining of voiding only scanty amounts of urine for 2 days, even though she is thirsty and drinks "plenty of water." Her face is puffy, and her ankles have pitting edema.

19 **20.** Write a nursing care plan for a patient with CHF during the first 8 hours after admission.

Answers to Have I Learned?

LEG VII-C

1. Lack of regular exercise, diet high in sodium and saturated fats, smoking, high stress level.

2. **(d)**.

3. *Hypertension*

Cause: The cause of primary hypertension is unknown. Theories of causes include: heredity, salt and water metabolism, kidney function disturbances, emotional stress, obesity.

Symptoms: Sustained elevation of diastolic pressure, headache, dizziness, fatigue, nervousness.

Congenital Heart Defects

Cause: Rubella in expectant mother during first trimester.
Irradiation or drugs such as thalidomide.
Maternal malnutrition and heredity.

Symptoms: Acyanotic: loud harsh murmurs, frequent respiratory infections, normal growth and development.
Cyanotic: CHF in infancy, dyspnea, easy fatigability, slow growth and development, frequent respiratory infections.

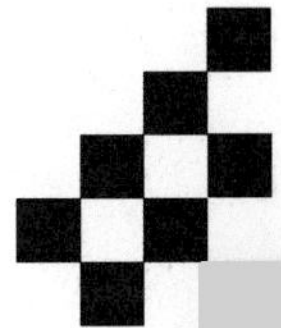

4. **(a)** false, **(b)** true, **(c)** true.

5. Relaxation techniques, exercise, biofeedback, acupressure, meditation, develop new coping behaviors.

6. *SGOT:* To detect tissue damage such as necrosis of heart muscle. It is expected to be elevated if an MI has occurred.

Prothrombin time: Indicates how quickly the blood will clot. When the patient is receiving a medication to change the amount of prothrombin in the blood, blood is compared with another person's (control sample) who is not receiving such a medication. The patient's prothrombin time, or the time it takes the blood to clot, should be longer than the control's time but not more than twice as long. If it is more than twice as long, no further medication should be given without physician's verification.

7. **(c)** is the best answer because it tells the patient specifically what will happen and how it will feel as well as the purpose of the procedure.

8. Write down each of your observations as you complete your assessment. Then compare your observations with your list from your clinical lab experience. Did you include everything, or were some things overlooked? You must develop a pattern of assessment because you won't be able to have lists in your pocket as you work.

One person counts the radial pulse for 1 minute while a second person counts the apical rate, using a stethoscope, for the same minute. The two rates are recorded as A/R. Your observing student should see you and another person do this.

9. Bacon and lox would be omitted. A *sodium-restricted diet* allows a moderate amount of salt in cooking, but no salt is to be added at the table. Avoid salty foods.

10. *Diuretic:* Remove excess water and sodium from body.
Intake and output: Assess fluid balance.
Weigh daily: Assess fluid balance.
Apical-radial pulse: Detect difference between heart rate and pulse.
Semi-Fowler's position: Improve breathing.
Oxygen: Increase supply and decrease work of the heart.

Bed rest: Decrease work of the heart and relieve signs and symptoms of decompensation.
Vital signs: Detect changes in the circulatory system.
Paracentesis: Remove fluid from abdominal cavity.

11. *Relief of pain:* Required by both. Angina treated with medication (e.g., nitroglycerin) to dilate coronary blood vessels. MI treated with narcotic (e.g., morphine) and oxygen.

Rest: Required by both. Angina requires a short period of rest until pain subsides. MI requires extended bed rest to decrease body's need for oxygen while heart muscle is healing.

Diet: Both may require fat-controlled diet to reduce the formation of atherosclerosis. MI may require sodium-restricted or low-calorie diet to reduce fluid, weight, and prevent distention.

Exercise: Encouraged for both as tolerated to promote collateral circulation. An exercise program is carefully prescribed by the physician.

12. *Anticoagulant:* **(a)**, **(c)**, **(d)**, **(e)**, **(h)**.
Antiarrhythmic: **(f)**.
Antianginal: **(b)**, **(e)**, **(g)**, **(i)**, **(j)**, **(k)**.
Antihypertensive: **(b)**, **(j)**.
Diuretic: **(b)**, **(j)**, **(l)**.
Cardiac glycoside: **(f)**, **(i)**.

LEG VII-C

13. Attend a GES. Take turns teaching about medications, nutrition, exercise, and rest. Include simulated family members.

14. Your answer might include the American Heart Association, Visiting Nurse Association, homemakers.

15. Attend a GES to evaluate your plan.

16. **(a)** Make an observation of what you see (e.g., "I see you are sitting up and smoking although Dr._______ wishes you to lie quietly in bed and avoid cigarettes.") This gives the patient an opportunity to explain why he is doing it.

(b) Empathize with the patient (e.g., "It must be hard to lie in bed all day and not smoke when you feel well"). This tells the patient that you can accept his feelings even though his behavior disobeys the doctor's orders. Use the bath time to review the reasons why he should not smoke.

17. Your descriptions will vary (use a real person). Every activity is measured in METs for the energy expended (e.g., self-care activities are mostly in the range of 2.5 calories; slow walking is 3, showering is 4, and brisk walking is 5). This sequence would be followed while in the hospital. The energy requirements on the job should be examined (e.g., Is it a brisk-walking or sitting job? Does it require lifting or running?).

Exercise tolerance needs to be built up gradually until it meets the job requirements, or perhaps modified (e.g., perhaps the patient should not take work home, should avoid long driving trips, should schedule a quiet restful lunch time).

Your answer should also include a description of the patient's normal recreational interest and the energy costs. Bike riding and swimming are strenuous; golf is not. The patient needs to understand that preparation for these activities is important, but if the patient is not prepared, then they can be harmful. A maintenance exercise program will also be designed for the patient once an optimum level of activity is achieved.

18. Symptoms present are: slightly short of breath; elevated pulse for longer than 5 minutes; tired the following day.

19. *Mr. Puffen's* heart disease and poor circulation probably contributed to his fluid excess. Your best effort upon admission is to elevate the head of the bed and stay with him until he is well settled and feeling your interest and concern. Give medication or oxygen as ordered.

Mrs. Reno probably has a history of chronic kidney disease, and the oliguria is a symptom of an acute phase. That her body is retaining fluid indicates a need for medication and physician's care. In the meantime, give her complete bed rest. Elevate the legs slightly to help venous circulation. Report signs of potassium excess and metabolic acidosis. Low-potassium and low-protein diet will help, plus added calories.

20. Attend a GES to compare and discuss your plan.

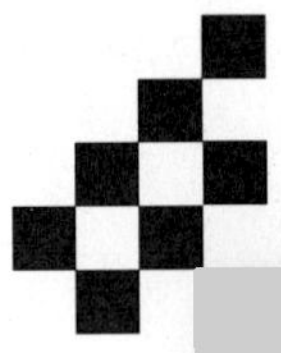

LEG VII-C

Why Should I Study?

You are more than halfway through Volume II and should have acquired a working knowledge of how the body functions in time of stress and crisis as it strives to maintain a balance of its fluids, gases, and electrolytes when a dysfunction occurs. You, as a responsible nursing student, can recognize how a patient is coping with a dysfunction and how you can organize your nursing actions to further facilitate the body's ability to overcome its problems and to help your patient help him- or herself.

In Level Eight you will learn how the body functions, during childbirth and the puerperium, and how you can help the mother to experience this normal body function in her own best way. You will experience ways to help a new mother be successful as she learns to mother her new infant, and you will learn how to give physical care to both mothers and babies. The gastrointestinal body system will also be explored, and you will find out how you can apply the ups and downs of food and fluid to actual patient situations. You must apply all of your working knowledge as you increase your ability to give intelligent, skillful care to your patients.

To meet the **Clinical Performance Expectations** for Level Eight, you should be able to:

1. Search out information in the health agency on your own initiative.
2. Seek any additional information you need to know about your patients and take steps to find this information, whether it involves asking questions or reading further in the chart (e.g., lab reports).
3. Know your own limits of knowledge and skill (based on self- and instructor-evaluation) and ask for assistance when an experience requires you to exceed those limits (for example, you can give intramuscular injections safely, but you request supervision when giving your first subcutaneous heparin injection).
4. Use *each* patient contact to obtain the most information possible and give the best care you can (e.g., make numerous observations when in a patient's room to give a medication and listen to what the patient is saying so that you can respond therapeutically).
5. Report and record information in sufficient detail for clarity.
6. Modify nursing care plans on the basis of evaluation of outcomes.
7. Explain the relationship between the nursing diagnosis, the patient's condition, and the treatment plan.

You will make better use of your time as you find yourself attempting to assume greater responsibility for patient care. Strive to increase your efficiency by careful and complete planning of increasingly complex clinical experiences. Look at your own performance critically and continue to identify your strengths and weaknesses. Are you still weak in the same areas as you were in Level Six? What have you done, specifically, to improve them? Now is the time to identify your problem areas and to actively begin to solve those problems. Talk with your instructor to find out what experiences are available to give you additional practice. Don't procrastinate! Be honest with yourself. Seek help and help yourself. Your behavior can be strengthened.

What Will I Learn?
LEG VIII-A Labor and Delivery

The process of labor and delivery is a normal physiologic event. You have already studied antepartum, and in this LEG you will focus on intrapartum, or labor and delivery. You will learn the normal progression of labor and delivery and the related nursing care. These experiences and the classroom content will also prepare you for future study and application of your knowledge to the complications of labor and delivery in LEG XI-A.

You will learn how to help the mother in labor by teaching her breathing exercises, how to save her strength until the time, during the second stage of labor, when she needs it most. You will learn to observe for signs of the progress of labor. You will learn which signs require additional and different nursing interventions to prevent complications.

You may have the opportunity to see many or few deliveries. Make the most of each opportunity. Be ready! Be prepared in your coursework so that you know what to expect, how to find out what you need to know, and how to proceed in this very specialized part of the hospital.

You will learn what is involved in each of the stages of labor. The first three stages of labor have very standard definitions. The fourth stage of labor is defined differently according to the source. Our definition of the fourth stage of labor will be from the time of the delivery of the placenta to the second hour after delivery, when the immediate postpartum checks have been completed. During this time, the mother begins her involution process and the fetus begins adjustment to extrauterine life.

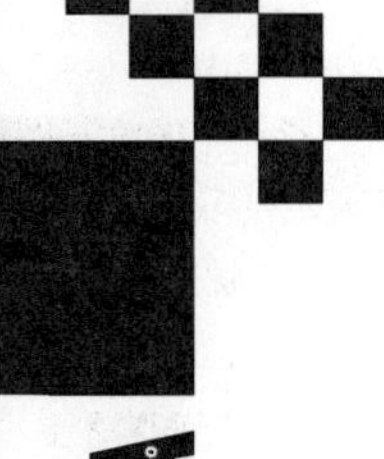

What's Ahead in Later LEGs

The complications of labor and delivery will be studied in LEG XI-A, Volume III. Look ahead to see how this LEG fits into the total subject, especially if you have patients with complications.

■ Overview of Learning Experiences in LEG VIII-A

Objectives	Campus Lab/ Self-Practice	Group Discussions/Lectures	Clinical Lab Focuses
Growth and Development of the Fetus **1.** Fetal development		**B1.** Fetal development	**B8.** Check for position and size of fetus
Admission and Assessment of a Patient in Labor **2.** Admission and assessment of a patient in labor **3.** Nursing interventions to decrease fear, pain, discomfort **4.** Observing attitudes about pregnancy and childbirth **5,6.** Stages of labor **7.** Assessments and interventions in Stages I and II	**B3.** Breathing patterns	**A4.** Normal labor and nursing care of the patient in labor **B1.** Labor **B9.** Assessing a patient in labor	**B11.** Observe and assist with admission Sit with mother during labor Observe patient in three stages Give care to patient in labor Talk to mothers 2–3 days postpartum Teach or coach three patients to change breathing patterns Attend a class on psychoprophylactic methods
Monitoring a Patient in Labor **8–10.** Monitoring (assessing) FHR **11.** Assessing cervical dilatation **12.** Assessing uterine contractions **13.** Nursing care during labor	**A5.** Study electronic monitoring graphs	**B5.** Nursing care of the patient admitted in labor	**B6.** Assess FHR in prenatal clinic and listen to FHR before, during, and after contractions Observe and time uterine contractions Apply a transducer and a tocotransducer Read graphs from electronic monitoring
Anesthesia and Analgesia **14,15.** Types of anesthesia and analgesia **16.** Nurse's role in giving analgesia **17.** Drugs used during labor		**A6.** Obstetrical analgesia and anesthesia **B1.** Analgesia and anesthesia	**B3.** Observe patients receiving anesthesia and analgesia Follow three patients from early stages of labor Observe a cesarean section

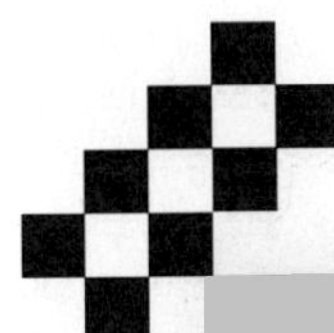
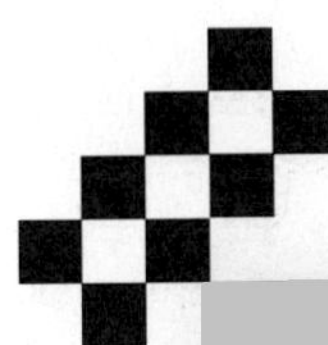

■ Overview of Learning Experiences in LEG VIII-A (cont.)

Labor and Delivery

Objectives	Campus Lab/ Self-Practice	Group Discussions/Lectures	Clinical Lab Focuses
Second and Third Stages of Labor **18.** Physiologic and psychologic changes in the second stage of labor **19.** Teaching and assisting with breathing patterns **20.** Mechanisms of labor **21.** Nursing care in Stages I and II **22.** Third stage of labor		**A5.** Mechanisms of labor **B1.** Giving support to patient in labor GES Objective 19	**B3.** Observe second stage of labor Observe transfer of mother to delivery room Observe changes in breathing and pushing during second stage Assist with delivery Observe LDR and LDRP arrangements
Signs of Placental Separation **23.** Observing for placental separation		**A5.** The third stage of labor	**B1.** Observe for signs of placental separation
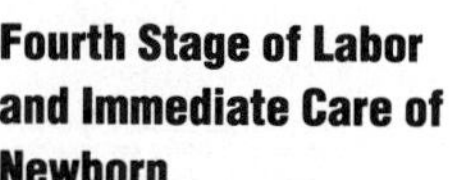 **Fourth Stage of Labor and Immediate Care of Newborn** **24.** Nursing care during the fourth stage of labor **25.** Assessing the fundus **26.** Immediate care and assessment of the newborn	**B2.** Assessing the fundus Postpartum check	**B1.** Effect of medications on mother and baby and assessment and care of the newborn GES Objective 25	**B4.** Observe infants immediately after birth Observe mothers during fourth stage Assist with care of new mother and infant immediately after delivery Observe how baby's nose and mouth are suctioned

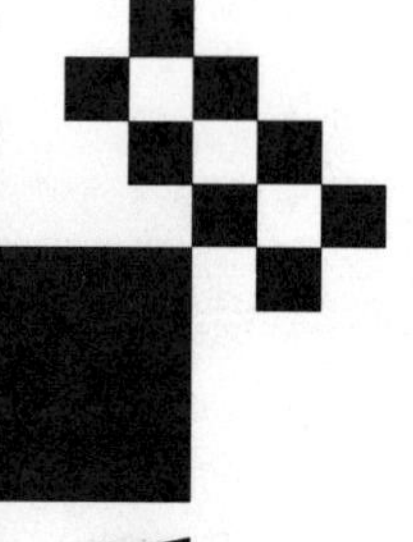

New Terms

Apgar
biophysical profile
caput
caudal
contraction
- acme
- decrement
- increment

contractions
- duration
- frequency
- interval

crowning
deceleration
- early
- late
- variable

descent
dilatation
Dubowitz assessment
duration
effacement
effleurage
engagement
episiotomy
fetal heart rate (FHR)
fetal lie
fetal narcosis
interval
labor
- Stage 1
  - Phase I
  - Phase II
  - transition
- Stage II
- Stage III
- Stage IV

laryngospasm
lightening
maternal hypotension
mechanisms of labor
meconium
neglect
overprotection
oxytocin
perfectionism
presentation
presenting part
physiologic bradycardia
placenta
- expressed
- manual
- retained

rejection
show
station
tetanic contraction
ultrasound
uterine contraction
vertex

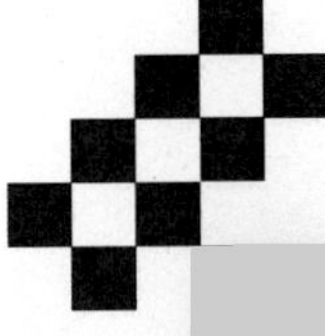

Abbreviations

DTR
FHR
LDR
LDRP
NIAL
PIH
VBAC

LEG VIII-A

Growth and Development of the Fetus

O b j e c t i v e

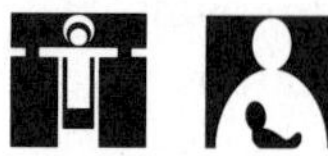

1. Describe fetal development during the first, second, and third trimesters, either in detail for each lunar month or by summarizing development occurring during each trimester (three months), including length, weight, and one or two developmental characteristics (appearance and/or movement) of the fetus.

Note: Objective 1 was an Extra Added Objective in LEG II-B.

A. What's It All About?

LEG VIII-A

1. Think about the tiny cell that becomes a human being in approximately 9 months, automatically, without being reminded when to grow, move, eat, sleep, and so on. Fetal development is in precise stages, each stage essential to the next. As each lunar month passes, there are fewer dangers to the fetus. Fetal development is not only interesting or fascinating; it is good to know so you can help the mother to understand and to cope with her own physical changes. Modern technology has allowed fetal surveillance to provide information and assessment regarding the well-being of the fetus throughout the pregnancy.

2. View audiovisuals and read articles and books from a list given to you by your instructor.

3. Read about the physiology of the *placenta, fetal circulation, amnion, chorion, fetal development, obstetrical positions and presentations,* and the *assessment of fetal well-being.*

Review LEG II-B for the physiology of ovulation, menstruation and conception, and development of the embryo. You are responsible for this content and will need to use it as you study and practice in labor and delivery.

4. Answer the following questions as you read:

(a) How would you describe a mature placenta in size and appearance?

(b) List some growth and development characteristics of the fetus from zygote through gestation:

first month embryo (4 weeks):

second month (8 weeks):

third month (12 weeks):

fourth month (16 weeks):

fifth month (20 weeks):

sixth month (24 weeks):

seventh month (36 weeks):

eighth month (40 weeks):

5. **Differentiate** between the weeks described as follows:

- **(a)** the period of the ovum
- **(b)** the period of the embryo
- **(c)** the period of the fetus

6. **Summarize** the fetal growth and development for each trimester.

7. **Discuss** the use of ultrasound as a tool to assess fetal well-being. Describe specifically the components of the fetal biophysical profile.

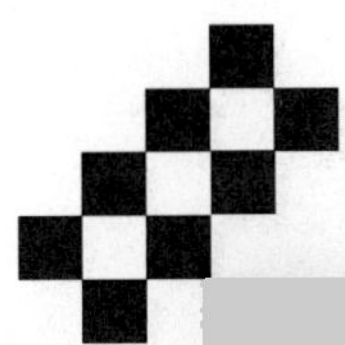

■ B. Putting It into Action!

1. **Attend** a group discussion on "Fetal Development."
Bring your list of characteristics from A.4 or A.6 for this discussion.

■ Consider the following:

What are some physiologic changes you might expect to observe (subjective or objective) in the mother for each stage of fetal development? Compare your answers with the physiologic changes given in a maternity reference.

What are the nursing implications?

Explain to another how the placenta develops. Choose words that would help a new mother understand how the placenta develops and how it functions.

What hormones are produced by the placenta?

Explain the fact that there is no direct communication between the maternal bloodstream and that of the fetus even though the placenta has many functions. Identify and elaborate on the functions of the placenta.

Why is the fetus vulnerable to certain dangers during the first trimester? Discuss the placental barrier. Discuss the teratogenic effect of drugs, x-rays, rubella, viruses, diseases, smoking, and environmental dangers.

■ Discuss the developmental tasks for each trimester of pregnancy. List these on a board as each is mentioned. Note the pattern as pregnancy progresses. Why is it important that each developmental task be completed before the new mother goes into labor? (Much of this will be review from antepartal care in Volume I.)

2. **Look** at a drawing in one of the maternity texts illustrating fetal circulation. Study this so that you could identify the following structures even if there were no labels on the drawing. (Cover the labels). Identify the umbilical vein, umbilical arteries, hypogastric arteries, aorta,

pulmonary artery, ductus venosus, ductus arteriosus, foramen ovale, superior vena cava, inferior vena cava.

Which of these structures are found only in fetal circulation?

Where in fetal circulation is the highest percentage of oxygen? Of carbon dioxide?

Look ahead to LEG XII-C to read about congenital heart defects and their repair.

3. **Describe** the three germ layers formed during the development of the embryo.

4. **Describe** what the initials mean for common positions and presentations: LOA, ROA, ROT, LOP, ROP, LSP, and LMA. Which are most desirable? How might each of them affect the mother and baby?

5. **Identify** the fetal presentation that occurs most frequently. Of the most common presentations, identify several groups within that category and describe the relationship of the fetus's head to its body.

6. **Compare** and contrast the types of breech presentations with the shoulder and brow presentations.

7. **Review** Leopold's maneuvers as you practiced in LEG II-B. What features of the fetal lie in the cephalic, breech, and shoulder presentations are discovered with Leopold's maneuvers?

8. **Plan** for a clinical experience.

▲ Observe in an obstetrical office or clinic or in labor and delivery. Check for the position and size of the fetus. Do this as many times as possible.

▲ Accompany an expectant mother during an assessment with ultrasound. Why was ultrasound used? What are possible findings in her particular case?

Admission and Assessment of a Patient in Labor

Objectives

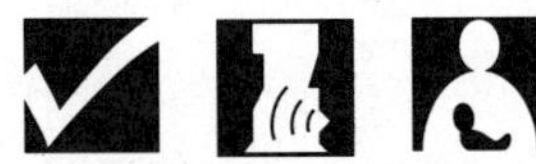

2. Demonstrate or role play admitting a patient in labor using an intrapartal assessment form or tool.

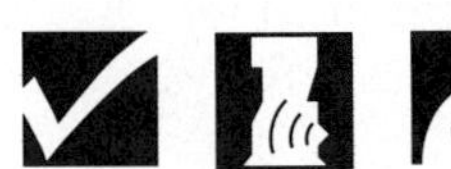

3. Demonstrate or role play assisting a patient during labor; apply nursing actions that would minimize fear, pain, and discomfort; include several Lamaze or psychoprophylactic techniques that may be used with relaxation.

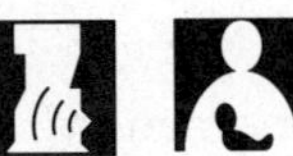

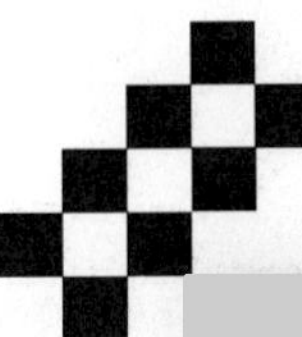

4. Given statements about pregnancy and childbirth, identify which ones display an accepting attitude and which ones display fear or rejection.

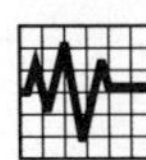

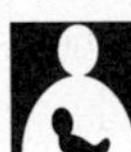

5. Describe orally or in writing two major events that occur during each of the four stages of labor.

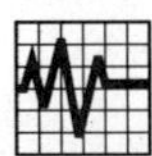
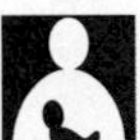

6. State the purposes, the average length of time for each stage of labor, including the phases of Stage I, and the muscle groups involved for a primigravida and a multigravida.

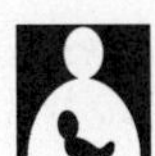

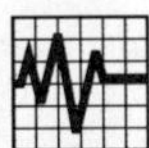

7. Identify the standard of care and frequency of nursing assessments of the mother and fetus during Stage I (Phase I, II, and transition) and Stage II of labor.

■ A. What's It All About?

1. Think about the meaning of the word *labor*. What does it mean to you as a student, a working person, a mother-to-be, a 17-year-old primigravida who is shy and quiet, a 36-year-old multigravida, talkative and self-assured?

What is involved in labor outside of the delivery room (e.g., preparation, job to be performed, time required, reward)? Compare this meaning as you think about and study labor and delivery.

Think about food and fluid intake and urinary output in relation to a person doing hard, physical labor (muscle output). Think about that person's vital signs. How is each affected by hard labor? Compare these reactions and needs with those of the mother-to-be and fetus in labor. Why are these observations by the nurse so important?

2. Read a variety of maternity and psychiatric nursing references. Look in the index under *fears during labor, rejection, attitude of the mother, role identity, culture and child bearing,* and the *establishment of nurse-patient relationship.*

Review LEG III-C and LEG V-B. Relate concern, anxiety, and pain of other patients you have observed with the discomfort and pain of labor and delivery.

3. View audiovisuals and read articles and books from a list given you by your instructor.

4. Attend a lecture on "Normal Labor and Nursing Care of the Patient in Labor."

■ B. Putting It into Action!

1. Attend a small group discussion on "Labor."

Include at least two mothers (and fathers) in the group, if possible. Select at least one of the following topics:

■ *Cause and Signs of Labor.* What is known about this phenomenon?

Consider the following:

> Two patients are admitted to the labor unit in early labor. Marit is a shy, quiet, teen-age primigravida of Scandinavian descent who is accompanied by her mother. Dolores is Hispanic, middle-aged, very talkative, and accompanied by her husband, Eduardo.

Discuss these questions related to the situations above.

How do you know what each mother-to-be is thinking? Feeling?

How can you let them know you care and want to help?

What explanations can you give to each for what is going on?

How may the person accompanying the woman in labor affect the labor?

What are the theories regarding the origin of labor?

How does each patient know the significance of the various signs of true labor?

Why is this important?

What if one sign doesn't occur?

What if one sign occurs out of sequence?

How would these questions or concerns differ for each of the patients? Why?

What if:

(a) a patient, pregnant for the third time, stated she had a very "bad" experience the last time she was in labor?

(b) the mother-to-be can't afford this new baby or doesn't want a baby or can't care for one at this time? How would these situations probably affect the mother's attitude toward pregnancy or labor? How can you tell when the signs and symptoms are more than those of normal fears and concerns? What cultural variations are related to perceptions of labor?

■ *Labor and How to Minimize Fear, Pain, and Discomfort.* Role play or discuss some specific nursing actions to minimize fear, pain, and discomfort with another student for the two patients above. Ask for criticism and suggestions from the group members to aid you in becoming more effective in giving supportive care. Discuss the behavioral signs that would alert you to the fact that a mother-to-be has strong feelings of rejection or abnormal fears concerning labor. You may want to diagram these on the board and then discuss your nursing action when these signs are noted.

■ *Admission of a Patient in Labor.* Think about admission of any patient to the hospital, about the purpose of the hospitalization, and how this influences the patient's attitude. How does admitting a patient in pain differ from admitting one who is not in pain? Relate these thoughts to admitting patients in labor—both primigravidas and multigravidas. Remember to always review your patient's medical and obstetrical history.

Does your admission form have a space to note the *time of last meal?* Why is this important? Discuss the importance of noting the *anticipated analgesia/anesthesia* and *blood type, Rh, hemoglobin, hematocrit,* and *pediatrician* for the baby. (Some of this information will be on the prenatal record.) Be sure that you develop the habit of noting these clues for each and every patient.

2. Talk with a mother about her labor. You may even ask your own mother to share her experience with you. How did her labor progress the first time, the second, the fourth? What about the signs of approaching labor? Did they all occur? In what sequence? What was her reaction? How did this reaction change after the first experience? What would your response be if the mother stated, during the course of the conversation:

"I had a dry birth."

"I was in labor three weeks."

"My grandmother told me not to raise my arms or the cord would get knotted."

"I was a forceps baby."

3. Attend a Lamaze class or another class in childbirth preparation with a classmate. Support each other as you rehearse breathing techniques with the other couples in attendance. Reverse roles practicing as coach and mother. In a group discussion, share your experiences with your teacher and classmates. Discuss the class content, breathing techniques, teaching techniques, and visual aids used in the class.

4. Attend another group discussion session lead by your teacher. Identify signs and symptoms of abnormal fears and rejection related to pregnancy and childbirth.

5. Explain what is occurring with each of these symptoms:

lightening

show

ruptured membranes

What nursing observations and care are required with each?

LEG VIII-A

If the membranes ruptured while the patient was hospitalized in labor, what assessment must be done immediately to ascertain the status of the fetus? If the membranes rupture while the patient is at home, what should she do?

6. **Write** your feelings about each stage of labor.

- Which stage or phase of labor concerns *you* most? Why?
- Which is easiest or most difficult for the mother? For the baby? Why?
- What ideas do you have that you want to try in order to give support to a mother-to-be and help the progress of each stage of labor? What is the FHR?

7. **Compare** the following obstetrical terms as they relate to progress during labor:

Dilatation and effacement

Descent, engagement, and station

8. **Examine** the chart on p. 255, Labor and Delivery Information Board. This is a sample of a chalkboard that indicates the patients' progress in labor. Note all the abbreviations. Try to figure out what they mean. You will find your laboratory experiences less confusing if you have some idea of the meanings of these terms and references. Fill in the chalkboard schedule for the patients under "Special Questions You Want to Ask" on p. 256. (Use pencil.)

Which of the questions below could you answer by looking at the chalkboard?

1. How many patients in labor?
2. What stage is each patient in?
3. Is each a multipara or primipara?
4. What is the FHR for each?
5. Whose membranes are ruptured?
6. Who is vulnerable for infection?
7. Which fetuses have reached the level of the ischial spines?
8. How many mothers have had premature babies? Abortions?
9. Which women are in the transition phase of labor?
10. Which patient is not in active labor?
11. Which mother is in labor with a baby with a malpresentation?
12. Which mother has anesthesia that will cover her in labor and delivery?
13. Which mother is in preterm labor?

The following questions may help you plan for your experiences in the labor and delivery rooms. You may want to make a card with information that is applicable to your hospital situation. You may need to research this subject.

When receiving a report from the floor nurse, what specific information do you need about each patient?

What should you do during your hours in lab? Sit with one, two, or more patients? Count FHR? Take BP? Time contractions? Observe a prep? Observe a delivery?

Labor and Delivery Information Board													
Name	EDC wks. gest.	Age	Gravida & Parity	Eff/Dil	Sta.	Pos.	FHR	Mem.	Meds.	Remarks	OB Dr.	Time	Infant wt. Sex Pediatrician
1. Kim	40	21	1-0-0-0-0	C/3	0	LOA	140	I			J.C.	0300	Lund
2. Thompson	41	20	2-1-0-0-1							DEL 0530	N.J.		9-7 F Jones
3. Hawkins	42	32	2-0-0-1-0	20%/2	↑		144	26 hr R		NIAL occasional contractions	K.L.	0500	Hagan
4. Moussa	40	25	5-2-1-1-3	C/5	0	Breech	138	I	Demerol 0530	Paracervical block 0400	J.C.	0730	Thomas
5. Pellegrino	41	27	3-1-1-0-2	50%/1	−2	Vertex	146	0630 R					
6. Lynch	39	21	1-0-0-0-0	C/8	+2	ROP	135	Amniotomy at 0700		at 0500 Epidural block	G.A.	0700	Davis
7.													
8.													
9. Wasake	30	20	1-0-0-0-0				130	0130 R		Rh neg. irregular contractions			

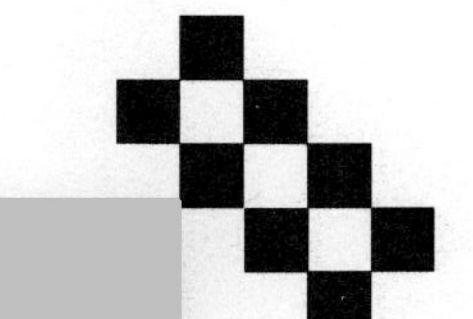

LEG VIII-A

Special Questions You Want to Ask

Who to ask for help? When to ask for help (at a certain point when timing contractions, FHR, etc.)? When to prepare for the physician and what to do? What exactly is your responsibility? Assisting? Observing? Doing? What and where do you chart? What, if any, medications are you to give?

You might want to ask some of those questions to help you prepare for patient care. What more information do you need to take care of the following patients?

> Mrs. Ramos, patient of Dr. Green, has one living child born at term, no prematures or abortions, and is pregnant for the second time. Her membranes ruptured before admission. Her contractions are effective every 3 min; cervix 6 cm with 70 percent effacement and bloody show. The baby is at the level of the ischial spines.
>
> Mrs. Hong, room 8, is having contractions every 5 min with bloody show; membranes have not ruptured, and her cervix is 7 cm and 80 percent. She is Dr. Gray's patient. She has six boys, born at term (one was stillborn), and is still trying for a girl.
>
> One hour later: Mrs. Ramos: contractions every 2–3 min, cervix 7 cm, 90 percent. Mrs. Hong: membranes ruptured. Dr. Gray says, "She is now complete and complete."
>
> Make up your own situations and fill them in until you can do this easily.

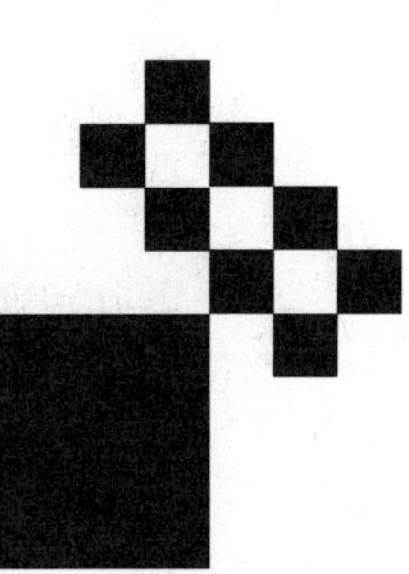

9. Attend a group discussion on "Assessing a Patient in Labor.

Bring your assessment records of your patient from the beginning of her pregnancy, or from the first time you met her while you were studying antepartal care. You should have a complete antepartal data base. If some students have more complete information than others, compare the value of this information. What more would you want to know before your patient is admitted in labor?

Bring a sample of the admission history form that is used in the labor room of your hospital. Be sure that you know the meaning of each term on the form, such as gravida, 4-digit parity, para, EDC.

Discuss the intrapartal assessment form used in your birthing situation. Do you think of this as just paperwork? Or have you discovered that this is a real part of giving nursing care? Discuss the benefits of having this information. If you find assessment records incomplete, what steps can you take to promote better use of these tools?

10. Fill in the chart entitled Nursing Assessment during Labor, with the nursing assessments that are required to meet the standard of care expectations for labor. Under the Uterine Contractions portion of the chart, identify also the normal frequency and character of contractions in Stages I and II of labor.

Nursing Assessment during Labor							
	Specific Vital Signs				Uterine Contractions		
Stages and Phases of Labor	**Mother TPR, BP**	**Frequency**	**FHR**	**Frequency**	**Expected Normal Character of Contractions**	**Expected Normal Frequency of Observations**	**Frequency of Nurse Observations**
Stage I, Phase I							
Stage I, Phase II							
Stage I, transition							
Stage II							

11. Plan for a clinical experience.

▲ Observe and assist with the admission of patients in labor in the early part of first stage and in the last part of first stage, either multigravida or primigravida or both. Record your observations. Bring your record to postconference.

▲ Sit with a mother during labor. Select a patient who is in the first stage of labor and stay with her, giving support and nursing care throughout labor. (It would be ideal to do this several times with patients in each stage.) Assist the mother as necessary. Are you minimizing her discomfort? How can you do more? Ask for assistance from the registered nurse or your teacher.

▲ Observe a patient in each of the first three stages of labor. At the completion of each of these observations record your feelings and observations. Bring this record with you to postconference.

▲ Give care to a patient in labor with at least three specific nursing actions in mind. Your goal is to minimize fear, pain, and discomfort for your patient. How is your own anxiety level? What can you do to lower it? Yes, get more self-confidence by practicing, practicing, practicing! Bring your recorded observations to postconference.

▲ Talk with mothers two to three days postpartum and ask them about their feelings regarding labor and delivery both before and after. What would they like to have their partner or the nurse do next time? What was done that was exceptionally helpful to them? How did this delivery compare with the last one? How does she feel about another?

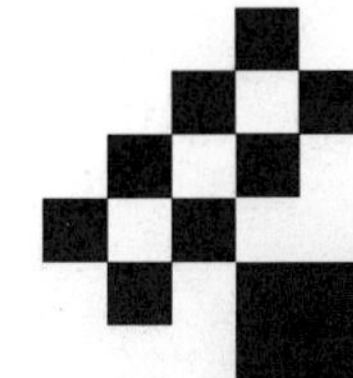

▲ Read charts that have been set aside by your instructor. Look for the stages of labor in each. Note the duration of labor, multipara or primigravida, amount and kind of analgesia and anesthesia given and during which stages. Note the expected date of confinement (EDC), the date of the first prenatal visit, differences in ages of patients, differences in vital signs upon admission and during labor, intake of food and fluids, including history taken at admission, urinary output, and need for catheterization, if any. Look ahead to see the progress of labor. Compare the labor progress of multigravidas and primigravidas. Describe the variations in delivery. How was the postpartum course? What kinds of nurse's notes do you see? Identify differences in charting in labor, delivery, and postpartum versus charting patients' records in medical-surgical nursing. Routine? Special comments? What would you do if you were caring for these patients? How would you record signs and symptoms of fear and rejection?

LEG VIII-A

▲ Teach or coach at least three patients to change their breathing patterns. This should be during the early part of the first stage of labor. Continue to care for and coach these patients as they actually need to change their breathing patterns in order to see how successful your teaching has been. (If you are not able to follow these same patients, try to arrange with a staff member to tell you how successful your patient was in changing her breathing pattern.)

▲ Attend at least one class for psychoprophylactic method for childbirth. Ideally you will be able to attend a class with your "case study" parents. Talk with the instructor of the classes and find out what each class includes, such as orientation, breathing patterns, and so on. How many techniques can you assist with? How do these techniques affect the circular effect of fear, pain, and tension?

Note: You may combine some of these experiences for one clinical session (for example, sitting with a patient and teaching breathing patterns).

▲ Support the coach in labor as he coaches the laboring patient. Identify the techniques being successfully used by the coach and encourage them. Talk with your instructor to assist you in intervening, when the coach needs assistance or redirection to assist the woman in labor.

▲ Observe mothers as they attend their daughters in labor. Attend a class led by your teacher or a prepared childbirth instructor. Discuss ways you can assist the mother of the woman in labor. What feelings and concerns might this mother have as she sees her own daughter in labor?

Monitoring a Patient in Labor

Objectives

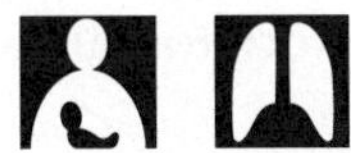

8. Demonstrate accuracy in locating and monitoring the fetal heart rate (FHR).

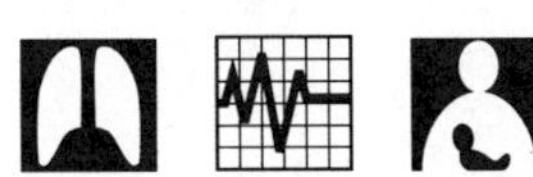

9. Differentiate between early, late, and variable decelerations of the FHR.

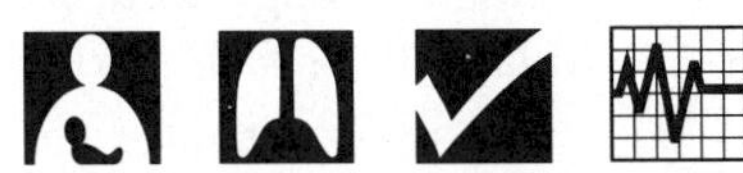

10. Identify the significance or risk to the fetus whose FHR exhibits early, late, or variable decelerations and identify the related nursing interventions.

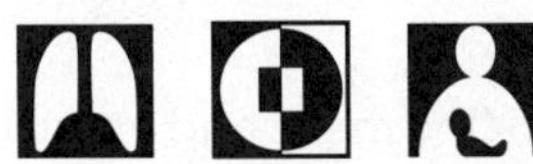

11. Given a series of circles (or diameters of circles) representing stages of cervical dilatation, (a) identify the average size of the cervix at the beginning and end of each stage of labor and (b) discuss the relationship and significance of dilatation, effacement, and station.

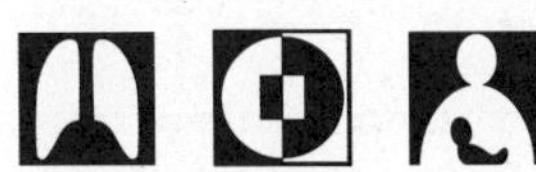

12. Describe in writing and demonstrate timing and recording uterine contractions including duration, intensity, and frequency.

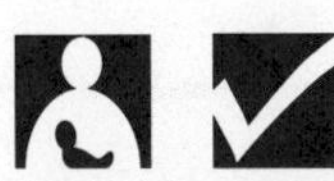

13. Identify the nursing care for the patient experiencing each of the stages and phases of labor.

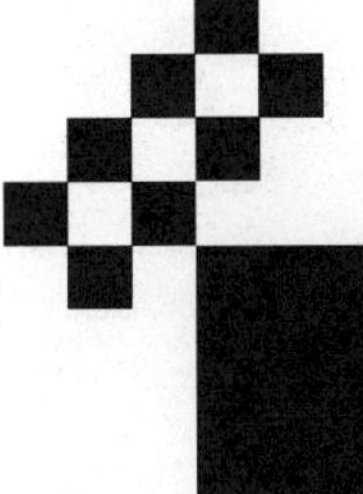

LEG VIII-A

A. What's It All About?

1. Think of the fetal heart rate as a very significant vital sign. The FHR viewed on the fetal monitor strip really is an indication of the brain's control of the fetal heart. Many fetuses tolerate labor very well; others suffer the effects of asphyxia and hypoxia. Frequent assessment of the FHR is essential during labor. Nurses need to know when and how the fetus should be assessed and follow with the correct nursing interventions. Close observations will reveal the status of the fetus during labor.

Seek opportunities to master auscultation of the fetal heart rate. Listen and count the FHR with supervision until you are truly skilled. Report any variation from normal to the physician, staff RN, or your instructor.

Problems for Solving

- How do uterine contractions affect the FHR?
- Where would you expect to hear the FHR if the fetus is in the LOA position? Why?
- Would you listen before, during, or after a contraction? Does it matter? If so, why?

2. Try this! Flex one elbow (raise your forearm) with the other hand on the biceps. Start easy; increase flexion. What do you feel? Is the muscle getting harder? Is it beginning to be uncomfortable? Flex harder and hold that position while watching the clock for 60 seconds. Painful? Why? Now relax your arm. How does it feel? Tired?

Compare this action with uterine contractions of labor (e.g., duration, purpose, force, voluntary, or involuntary). How would you feel if you could not relax and extend your arm of your own free will? Think about it!

3. Review Leopold's maneuvers.

4. Read a variety of references on *FHR* and on *monitoring*. Compare the authors' views. Read your hospital policy book on *routine FHR timing*. Review the nursing literature about *labor, delivery,* and the appropriate *nursing care*. Look in the index under *fetal distress, signs and symptoms,* and *internal and external fetal monitoring*.

5. Obtain a packet of electronic monitoring graphs from your instructor. Identify contraction patterns: duration, frequency, and relaxation periods. Identify the baseline fetal heart rate. Look for indications of early, late, or variable deceleration of FHR. What are the nursing implications of each of the above for the baby? For the mother?

What are the advantages and disadvantages of external (indirect) and internal (direct) monitoring?

6. Explain the use of a Friedman graph during the first stage of labor.

(a) Use specific data that you have about your patient. Plot all the data on a graph and draw some conclusions about the meaning of the curves and implications for nursing care.

(b) Look for the Friedman graph in the charts of all your patients. Compare the events of their labors. How does the shape of the normal Friedman curve vary with different patients?

B. Putting It into Action!

1. Measure the lines below with a metric and an inch ruler. Label each with the number of centimeters and the appropriate average stage of labor. Draw circles around them to simulate a cervix.

Lines Represent Diameters of Dilating Cervix
______________________________ cm
________________________ cm
________________ cm
______________ cm
________ cm
______ cm

Note that 4 in = approximately ________cm
3 in = approximately ________cm
1 in = approximately ________cm
1/2 in = approximately ________cm

2. Fill in the Labor Graph on p. 262 as you observe and care for a patient in labor. Watch for signs of labor progress and fetal descent.

3. Match the following lists for counting FHR:

Patient Condition	**Time Interval for Counting FHR and the Rationale**
_____ 1. After membranes are ruptured	(a) Count FHR q30min because contractions cause stress on fetus
_____ 2. Early period of first stage of labor	(b) Count FHR immediately because the cord may prolapse causing fetal distress
_____ 3. First stage of labor is well established	(c) Count FHR q15min because harder contractions cause more stress
_____ 4. Second stage of labor	(d) Count FHR after each contraction because constant hard contractions increase stress.

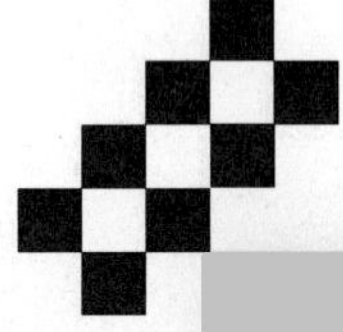

Answers:

1. **(b)**, 2. **(a)**, 3. **(c)**, 4. **(d)**.

Note: Fetal heart rate is the best indicator of the condition of the fetus; careful frequent monitoring of fetal heartbeat is the most important responsibility of the nurse to the infant during labor.

ALWAYS IMMEDIATELY REPORT TO YOUR INSTRUCTOR, THE RN, OR PHYSICIAN A FETAL HEART RATE OUTSIDE THE NORMAL RANGE OF 120 TO 160 BEATS PER MINUTE OR ANY IRREGULARITY OF BEAT!

4. Write a thought paper on assessing fetal heart rate. How do you feel about it? What would you do if you couldn't find it or count it? What facial expression will you have? How long will you try? How do you think the mother-to-be will react to your inability to count the FHR of her baby? What will you do to allay her fears? Discuss this subject with at least one other student or turn your paper in to your instructor for comments.

5. Attend a group discussion on "Nursing Care of the Patient Admitted in Labor."
Identify three nursing diagnoses, the interventions, and the rationale for the care of the following patient at this specific point in time:

> Mrs. Smith is a 19-year-old primigravida admitted to the labor unit in active labor. She has had no prenatal care and no childbirth preparation such as breathing exercises. The friend who drove Mrs. Smith to the hospital had to leave to care for her own children. Mr. Smith is unable to leave work at this time.

LEG VIII-A

LABOR GRAPH

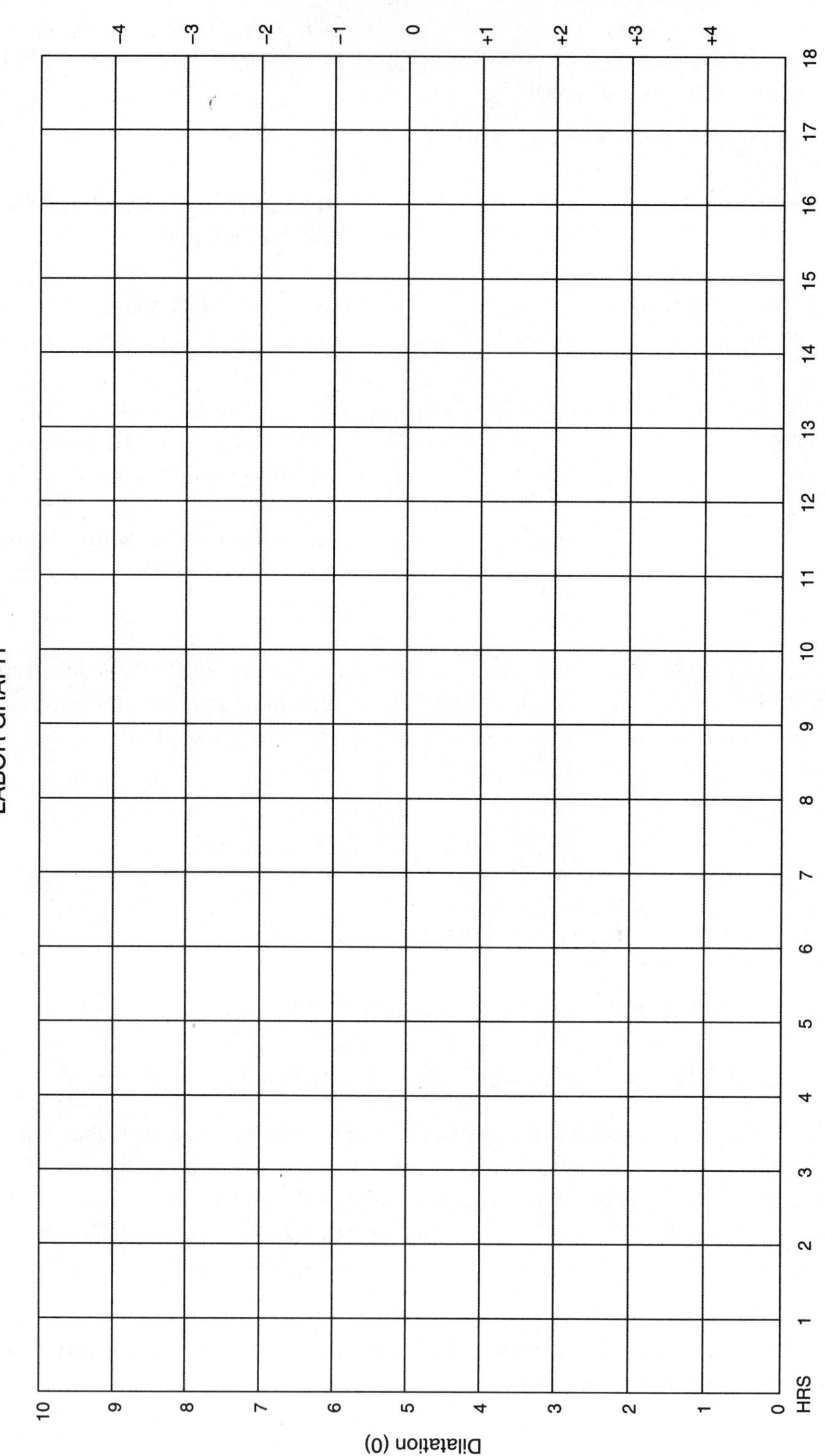

6. **Plan** for a clinical experience.

▲ Listen to and count FHR for 1 minute in prenatal clinic. Check your readings with the RN, a staff member, or your instructor.

▲ Observe and time uterine contractions. Feel the quality of many contractions with your fingertips on the fundus. Be sure you can identify firm, mild, and moderate contractions. Note duration, intensity, and frequency. (This will take at least 15 minutes.) What would a tetanic contraction be like? Validate with your instructor or a staff member until you are sure of what you feel. Palpate for the bladder. If you can recognize the bladder during a contraction on one patient, are you sure that you can find it on every patient? Be sure! How does distention of the bladder affect labor? How frequently should a woman in labor be reminded to urinate?

▲ Use Leopold's maneuvers and apply an ultrasound transducer and a tocotransducer to an expectant mother's abdomen to obtain a clear FHR pattern and to record uterine activity.

▲ Read graphs from electronic monitors. Try to imagine what is going on and what the nurse should do if abnormal readings are noted. Look at the patients' charts and see what was done and what the outcome was for each patient and her baby. What nursing assessments and interventions were performed for these patients?

▲ Work with an RN in labor and delivery. Observe the FHR of the patients assigned. How did the registered nurse handle the variations from the normal FHR? Compare your observations and the explanations with your classmates in a group discussion led by your instructor after this clinical experience.

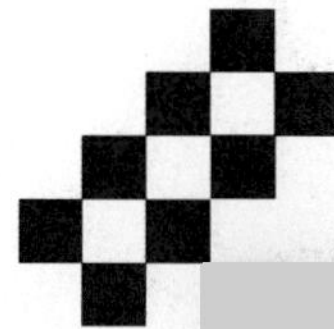

▲ Count FHR for 1 minute on patients in various stages of labor. Check your findings with the RN, staff members, or your instructor.

▲ Observe fetal monitoring. Discuss what you see and hear in postconference. Compare this method with the counting method.

▲ In postconference, discuss the action of the uterine segments during labor and delivery.

▲ Discuss in postconference how the FHR and maternal pulse may be differentiated. In other words, how do you know whether the count of 68 beats per minute heard by auscultation in the lower abdomen reflected the pulsations of the mother or the fetus? Ask your instructor or a maternity staff nurse to help you answer this intriguing question.

Anesthesia and Analgesia

Objectives

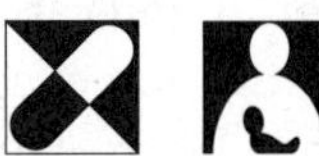

14. Compare and contrast the advantages and disadvantages of the following types of obstetrical anesthesia in relation to their effect on the fetus and the mother: general anesthesia, regional anesthesia including the paracervical block, the pudendal block, the peridural blocks (lumbar epidural and caudal block), and the subarachnoid blocks (spinal, low spinal, and saddle block), and also the local infiltrations.

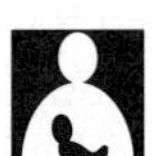  

15. Given one of the types of obstetrical anesthesia from Objective 14, identify in which stage or stages of labor it may be used and describe the nursing assessments indicated following the administration of the anesthesia.

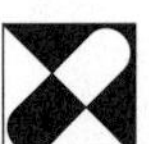  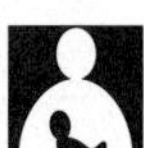

16. Compare and contrast the responsibilities of giving analgesia to a woman at term in labor versus a woman who has pain after a surgical procedure.

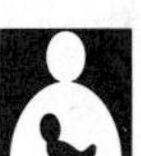 

17. List the drugs and their dosages that are most commonly used in your hospital to achieve analgesia, sedation, and tranquility during labor. Indicate which are least hazardous to the fetus.

■ A. What's It All About?

1. Think about the differences between anesthesia and analgesia. Why is one used rather than the other? How does nursing care for a patient who is under anesthesia differ from that for one with analgesia? Why? What is the major difference between nursing care for patients with general anesthesia and those with local anesthesia? When, during labor, do you think analgesia might be changed to anesthesia? Why?

Review LEG V-B on pain. Explain the subjective aspects of pain and the theories regarding the cause of pain during labor. Why do certain medications work and others not work? Why do certain techniques work for some women and not for others?

2. Read maternity and surgical references and compare patients' reactions to anesthesia and analgesia. Compare the surgical patient's response to anesthesia with that of a maternity patient and her fetus.

3. **View** visual aids related to anesthesia and analgesia.

4. **Consider** the following questions:

Why does a woman in labor have pain?

What causes the discomfort she may have during each stage of labor?

Where does she have pain during each stage?

How do the answers to the above questions influence the choice of anesthesia or analgesia as a patient progresses through labor to delivery?

5. **Consider** the following maternity patients, who have become quite uncomfortable in their labors.

A primigravida in Stage I, Phase II of labor whose fetus is average size and at term.

A grandmultipara at term in Stage I, Phase II of labor.

A primigravida in Stage I, transition phase of labor whose baby at term is estimated to be large, or greater than 8 lb 5 oz.

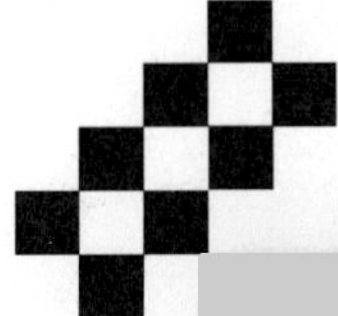

What are the considerations of giving analgesia to each of these patients? Why should it be given or why not?

Would any of these laboring women be candidates for anesthesia at this time? Why or why not?

What nursing assessments should be made on the mother and fetus before giving anesthesia or analgesia?

If the first mother above was given a lumbar epidural block, how would the nurse assess the patient during the administration of the block, the first 15 to 30 minutes after the block and thereafter until delivery?

6. **Attend** a lecture on "Obstetrical Analgesia and Anesthesia" given by your teacher or an obstetrical anesthesiologist.

LEG VIII-A

■ B. Putting It into Action!

1. **Attend** a small group discussion on "Analgesia and Anesthesia." Select one of the following topics:

■ *Patients Receiving Caudal Anesthesia*

Can you explain the caudal anesthesia procedure to your patient? Role play explanation of caudal anesthesia with another student before trying to explain it to a patient. At what point in labor can caudal anesthesia be administered? Does this differ for a multipara and a primigravida? Why? How can you prevent fear in the mother as the sensations change with the onset of effects of this anesthesia? Is this method a one-time injection of medication? Does the medication go into the spinal fluid? If not, where does it go?

■ *Patients Receiving Saddle Block*

Discuss the positioning of patients for a saddle block. What nursing measures should be taken to prevent continual leaking at the puncture site? How would this leakage affect spinal fluid pressure? How would this leakage affect the comfort of the patient? What observations should be made related to bladder function during and after labor? During what stage of labor is the saddle block administered? Why?

■ *Patients Receiving the Following Types of Care:*

Analgesia and local anesthesia

Lumbar epidural

Analgesia only

Natural childbirth

Inhalation analgesia

Discuss how you would approach these patients if you were assigned to care for them during labor and delivery. How will you find out when to ask for help? How will you know when your patient needs more medication for pain? How will you know each of the following: when to help your patient with breathing exercises; if your patient is having good labor contractions or if there are signs of fetal distress? What antagonists are used to reverse the effects of a narcotic?

■ *General anesthesia:*

How does the nurse prepare the patient for general anesthesia?

Compare the risks for the mother and the fetus of general anesthesia versus regional anesthesia.

Give examples of when general anesthesia may need to be the anesthesia of choice. Look ahead to LEG XI-A for complications of pregnancy, labor, and delivery.

How does the general anesthesia childbirth experience compare with the awake and alert expectations of childbirth many mothers anticipate as they contemplate labor and delivery? How may the nurse help the mother to work through disappointment about the childbirth experience if she gave birth under general anesthesia?

What other questions do you want answered? This is your chance to go through all the stages of anxiety before actually observing or assisting in labor and delivery. Plan for your instructor to sit in as a resource person. Role play the situations; make them as realistic as possible.

Note: Each region of the country and many hospitals within regions have different approaches to labor and delivery. The Objectives in this LEG are general, to prepare you to learn the specific differences as you begin to practice nursing in your own hospital (for example, if it is common practice in your area for obstetrical patients to be anesthetized with caudal anesthetic, plan to observe and assist with this procedure and care for the patient following anesthesia). Observe patients with many different combinations of analgesia and anesthesia.

---

2. Complete the chart below.

Anesthesia or Analgesia	Effect on Fetus	Effect on Uterine Contractions	Stage Given	Nursing Actions and Observations
Inhalation	Narcosis			
IV Analgesia, Demerol				Watch for respiratory depression for mother or neonate. Administer small amounts of the diluted drug IV at the beginning of contractions to decrease the drug concentration going to the placenta. Maternal hypotension.
Lumbar epidural		Retards	I or II	
Local anesthesia		None		
Pudendal		Does not slow contractions		
Caudal				

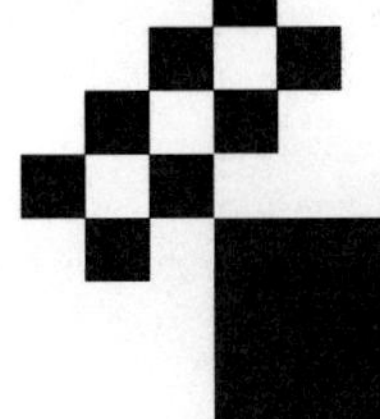

Look at your completed chart. Do the answers make sense? Think about it! The effect produced by the drug indicates when it can be used safely. This rule applies to all drugs. If an anesthetic produces fetal narcosis and/or inhibits uterine contractions, would you expect it to be given early or late in labor? Why? What do respiratory depression and maternal hypotension mean to the nurse as he makes observations and gives nursing care? Remember your goal—*you* are to be the nurse.

Think about this: your patient is medicated appropriately either with analgesia or anesthesia or both. How can you tell that labor is progressing well just by observing that patient? Discuss with your instructor and observe staff members as they observe patients. Question them. Make the most of your time!

3. Plan for a clinical experience to observe patients in labor.

▲ Observe patients receiving analgesia and anesthesia. Note the stage of labor. Note the sounds each patient makes. Compare the consciousness and actions of patients receiving IM and IV analgesia, inhalation or general anesthesia, or any type of regional anesthesia. Which of the women needed the most constant and complete care by the nurse? Why?

▲ Discuss in a group session led by your teacher the interventions and antidotes used when anesthesia or analgesia has a detrimental effect on the fetus and mother.

▲ Follow three patients from early labor through each stage (patients receiving different types of analgesia or anesthesia; at least one patient a multipara). Observe the use and effect of analgesia and anesthesia. Listen to reports on each of the patients. Make notes. Compare reports with the Labor and Delivery Information Board documentation. Ask questions about what you want to know.

▲ Which methods of anesthesia can be used for a cesarean section? Observe a cesarean section. Share with your classmates your observations of the method of anesthesia used and its effects on the mother and newborn infant.

Second and Third Stages of Labor

Objectives

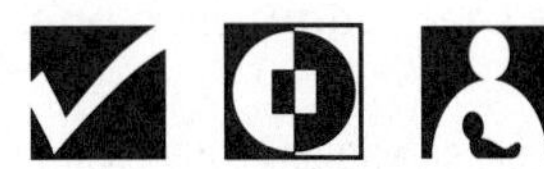

18. Describe, orally or in writing, at least five physiologic or psychologic changes that would indicate labor is progressing.

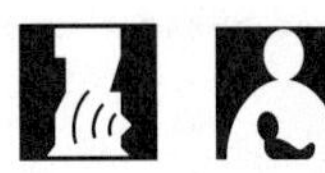

19. Describe in writing or role play with another student teaching a patient effective breathing patterns during the second stage of labor.

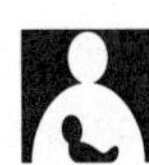

20. Demonstrate the mechanisms of labor for a fetus in the LOA position using a doll or a fetal model and maternal pelvis model.

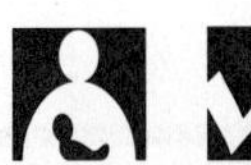
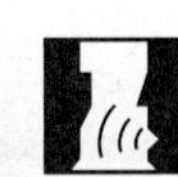
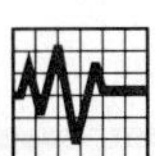

21. Identify the role of the nurse in the second and third stages of labor.

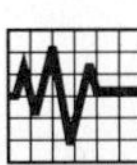
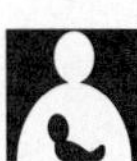

22. Describe the third stage of labor.

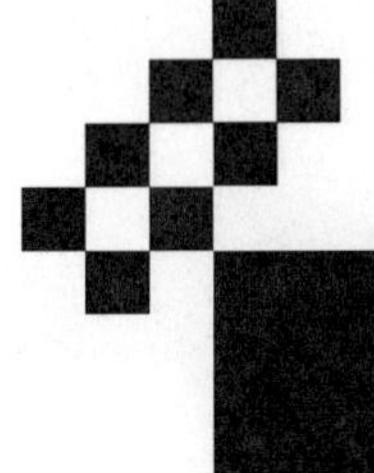

A. What's It All About?

1. Think about the different stages of labor. What happens during the first stage? The second stage? The third stage? When the first stage is complete, a new action is required. What signs and symptoms do you see? Hear? Feel? When can the mother use her own voluntary efforts to assist in the labor process?

Some hospitals still transfer their maternity patients from labor to delivery to recovery and then to postpartum. Economic and convenience factors have influenced change in this process. Many women today labor, deliver, and recover in the original unit to which they were admitted (LDR). Others do the same, but in addition, remain in the room for postpartum (LDRP).

2. Read maternity references on *second stage of labor, third stage of labor, FHR, delivery care, teaching and breathing techniques of second stage.*

3. View audiovisuals, articles, and books selected by your instructor.

4. List some nursing measures to be taken after the rupture of membranes. *What must be done first?* Discuss this with your instructor. What is the rationale behind your interventions?

5. Attend a lecture demonstration on the "Mechanisms of Labor" given by your instructor or another expert in the field.

■ B. Putting It into Action!

1. Attend a small group discussion on "Giving Support to Patient in Labor."

■ Discuss the following situations. Answer the questions that follow each one.

> Sarah Rosenfield, 24 years old, gravida 5, para 3-1-0-3 was checked vaginally one-half hour ago to assess her progress in labor. She was found to be complete and 5 cm. She suddenly clutches your hand and states: "I want to push. Now!"

What nursing assessments must be done now?
How will you communicate with the registered nursing staff or physician?
Can Sarah actually be ready to push? Why or why not?

> Mrs. Beauregard has been pushing for 1 1/2 hours and seems to be showing signs of being very tired. The fetus, according to the fetal monitor, shows early decelerations with contractions and a FHR of 130 baseline. Mrs. Beauregard is a primipara who attended a few early childbirth classes. She is observed by the registered nurse to take a cleansing breath, expel it, then hold the next breath at the beginning of the contraction. Soon she expels her breath and then simply cries out for the duration of the contraction.

What components of the description above indicate that Mrs. Beauregard and her fetus need assistance?
What kind of support does she need and why? Be very specific.
Write a nursing diagnosis based on the description of this moment in her labor.

> Mrs. Mori is in the second stage of her labor and is pushing appropriately and making progress.

How will you manage to assess her, provide as much rest as possible, and alert her to the next contraction—all within the interval between contractions?
What steps would you take to help you become proficient and safe in your nursing care?

■ Role play the following situation. (The purpose of this practice is to anticipate needs and to be prepared!)

> Your patient's physician has just come in and asks you to help her with a vaginal examination of her patient.

What equipment will you need to have handy? Why?
What will you do to assist her?

■ Role play teaching a patient to push. At what stage would this be appropriate? What would you do between contractions to help the patient be comfortable and to rest?

■ Discuss how you would help a patient who has attended prepared childbirth classes when her coach is not there during labor. Be specific about what you would do for each stage because of what is going on and how the patient feels. How would your approach vary if the patient came in the door of the unit in the latent phase versus transition?

2. Write a thought paper about your feelings regarding labor and delivery and turn it in to your instructor for comment.

3. Plan for a clinical experience.

▲ Observe the second stage of labor. Note the transitional symptoms from Stage I to Stage II. Notice the difference in activity and purpose of the mother and the staff during the second stage. What are the major differences?

▲ If your hospital has the traditional maternity arrangement, observe the transfer of the mother to the delivery room. How is the time of transfer decided upon? What does the nurse need to know before the patient is moved to the delivery room? Watch and assist when the patient is helped onto the delivery table. What special precautions are taken when positioning her legs? Why? Does coaching of the patient continue? By whom? Note the reaction of each of the people in the room when the birth is just accomplished.

▲ If your hospital has the LDR or LDRP maternity arrangement, observe when the equipment used in anticipation of an approaching birth is opened and draped. How does this vary from multipara to primigravida? How is the patient positioned throughout labor? How is she positioned for delivery? In what way is the room arranged and stocked to handle the unexpected and expected events of labor and delivery? Share your observations with your classmates in postconference.

▲ Observe the changes in breathing and pushing during the second stage of labor.

▲ Attend postconference. Discuss your reactions to your first childbirth observation experience. If you haven't seen an actual delivery, listen to other students as they discuss their reactions. Notice that at this stage the discussion involves feelings of all kinds: relief, joy, hilarity, exuberance, and even tears. Why? Talk out your feelings and let others state their views. Sometimes students may need clarification of a procedure performed or an unexpected complication of the mother or baby. If you continue to have concerns, talk with your instructor, staff nurses, the physician, or all of them. Then you will be ready for more clinical experiences.

▲ Assist with the delivery of a baby from the beginning of the second stage until the mother is taken to the recovery room. Compare your reactions at this time with those of the first time.

▲ Fill in a Delivery Room Form for at least one patient in labor, preferably several (for example, a multipara, primipara, patients with several types of anesthesia). Your instructor will supply this form. If the form does not provide the opportunity, add the following:

Length of Stage I: hours ____ minutes _____
Length of Stage II: hours ____ minutes _____
Length of Stage III: hours ____ minutes _____

The nurse usually completes this documentation by computing the results from the significant beginning and ending events of each stage.

Signs of Placental Separation

O b j e c t i v e

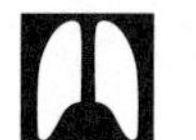  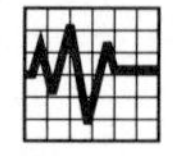 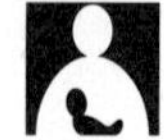

23. State four signs of placental separation.

A. What's It All About?

1. Think about the placenta. What is its main composition? Why? What is the function of the placenta? What would you expect to happen if it should separate prematurely? Think about the signs and symptoms of hemorrhage. If you are charged with the responsibility of guarding against this complication, you must know what you are looking for and how to find it.

2. Read about the *placenta* in references provided by your instructor. Look in the index under *placenta—manual, expressed, retained—Schultz, Duncan.*

3. View audiovisuals on the third stage of labor.

4. Preview LEG X-A, Complications of the Placenta and Hemorrhage.

5. Attend a lecture on "The Third Stage of Labor."

B. Putting It into Action!

1. Plan for a clinical experience.

▲ Observe for signs of placental separation. Be sure that you note the normal symptoms that indicate separation if the delivery is normal. Attend postconference. Discuss this phenomenon. Listen to other students, your instructor, and other resource people as they relate their experiences. Question them about how they observe.

▲ Notice nursing documentation and possible medication administration with the delivery of the placenta. Discuss these and other nursing actions during postconference.

Problems for Solving

What is the difference to the mother whether the delivered placenta is spontaneously expressed or manually removed? What must be done if the placenta is retained? What can occur if a small piece of the placenta is left in the uterus? Which is most desirable and most frequent, a Schultz or a Duncan placenta? Why? You may need to research this topic.

▲ After a delivery, attend a demonstration or explanation of the placental anatomy. Identify the cotyledons. Be sure that all have been expelled. Observe for signs of placental aging, site of insertion of the cord, the amnion, and the chorion. Put on gloves and use a surgical instrument to lift the placenta yourself to see how much this significant structure weighs. You might be surprised!

Fourth Stage of Labor and Immediate Care of Newborn

O b j e c t i v e s

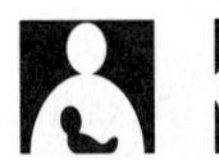 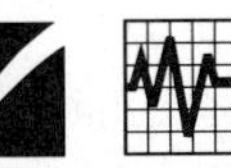 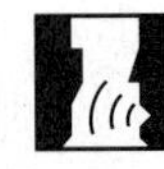

24. Describe orally or in writing the nursing care, including the immediate postpartum checks, during the fourth stage of labor until 2 hours after the delivery.

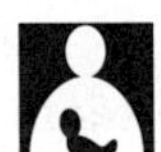 

25. Demonstrate safe, accurate assessment of the fundus, location of the fundus, and proper fundal massage techniques.

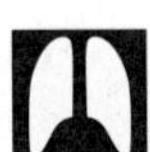  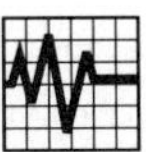

26. Describe, orally or in writing, the immediate care and assessment of the newborn with regard to temperature regulation, Apgar scoring, care of the cord, identification, resuscitation, care of the eyes, and mother-infant bonding.

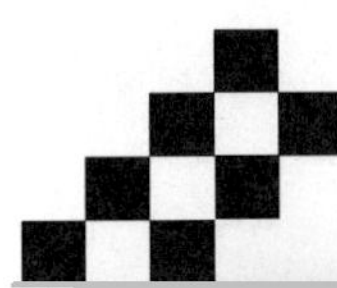

Note: Consider the infant to be an average-size, term infant, vaginal delivery, vertex presentation, birthweight of 3000 grams or more, Apgar score of 7 or higher.

A. What's It All About?

1. Think about the time immediately after delivery. This is a time of tremendous physiologic adjustment for the baby and the mother. Emotionally the mother will be dealing with many feelings. What does this period mean to the mother? To the physician? To the nurse? To the infant? Consider yourself as the nurse. What are your responsibilities?

Remember that the fourth stage of labor has various definitions, but the mother still needs close supervision and a lot of support as she recovers and begins to care for the neonate.

2. View related audiovisuals and read articles and books from a list given to you by your instructor.

3. Answer the following questions:

(a) How does the uterus usually respond after the delivery of the placenta?

(b) Why must the mother be watched carefully after birth even if her baby is normal and delivery was uneventful? How is she assessed?

(c) How does neonatal resuscitation in the delivery room compare with CPR on an adult?

(d) How can bonding be established at delivery if the baby needs nursing intervention and assessment?

■ B. Putting It into Action!

1. Attend a small group discussion on "Effect of Medications on Mother and Baby and Assessment and Care of the Newborn."

■ Review how medication affects the mother and infant during the fourth stage of labor. What patient reactions would you expect from the newborn? From the mother?

> Mrs. Sayer delivered a large baby boy, 8 lb, 2 oz in an unmedicated birth.
>
> Mrs. Jones, delivered a 7 lb, 10 oz girl. She was given IV Demerol during labor. The baby was born 10 minutes after her second dose of medication.

What if Mrs. Sayer's baby boy had an Apgar score of 4? What if Mrs. Jones's baby girl had weighed 4 lb, 5 oz? How would these conditions affect care of both mother and baby?
Try other possibilities and combinations as you discuss and role play situations in the fourth stage of labor.

■ List on a chalkboard the physiologic changes that must occur if the infant is to survive. Think about the differences the infant encounters in extrauterine life compared with intrauterine. What must occur in order for him to survive?

■ Discuss, after you have observed a delivery, caring for a newborn immediately after delivery. Why do you think a knit cap might be placed on a baby's head in the delivery room? What else can be done to conserve a newborn's energy? What is brown fat? Discuss its importance. What are the reasons for taking axillary instead of rectal temperature on newborns?

Discuss in detail how you would go about assessing the condition of a newborn. What guidelines (or forms) are used in the newborn nursery? How can you make yourself consciously aware of assessing a newborn as you give care?

■ Evaluate the following patient situation:

> Baby boy, 6 hours old in crib, on side, dressed and wrapped in blanket. At change of shift, you are giving report to the oncoming nurse as she makes rounds. A 2-inch spot of bright red blood was on the blanket when he was turned over on his back.

What has happened? What would you do? How could this have been avoided?

2. Practice in the campus lab.

■ Rehearse in a simulated scenario the correct techniques to assess and massage the fundus. After a demonstration from your teacher or lab instructor, practice the techniques using models designed for that purpose or make your own. The fundus of a newly delivered woman feels like it is the size of a grapefruit; the next day, the fundus has decreased in size to that of an orange. Place a soft pillow over the grapefruit. Remember to guard the uterus from inversion by placing your left hand in front of the symphysis pubis. The right hand is used to assess fundal height and to massage the uterus. When you do get to the clinical area, you will be amazed to discover that this simulation was very similar to the actual fundus.

■ Practice assessing a classmate in all the components of the immediate postpartum check for two 15-minute intervals.

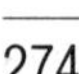

■ Attend a lecture and demonstration given by your instructor on the components of the immediate postpartum check for the mother and the immediate care of the newborn.

■ In a small group discussion, share the approach you would use and explanations you would give when the immediate postpartum check is due in the following situation.

> The patient is surrounded by relatives and well-wishers and she is talking about the baby to someone on a long-distance phone call.

3. Write the rationale for the nursing actions in the chart below for both mothers and infants during the fourth stage of labor.

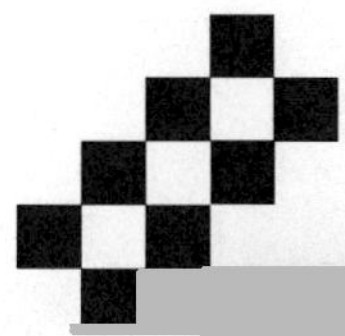

LEG VIII-A

Nursing Actions	Rationales for Mother	Rationales for Infant
Check fundal height		
Massage fundus if fundus is relaxed		
Check fundus with left hand in front of symphysis pubis and right hand on fundus		
Lower legs together from stirrups		
Give backrub, change gown		
Do formal postpartum check q15 min × 4, then q30 min × 2		
Encourage mother to express any emotion		
Note time of birth		
Position infant's head downward		
Gently rub infant's back		
Suction gently		
Conserve heat loss for infant		
Record Apgar score at 1-min and 5-min intervals		
Care for cord, eyes, and identification		
Provide a warm blanket for the mother		

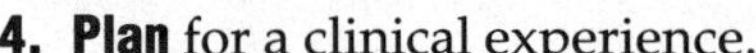

4. Plan for a clinical experience.

▲ Remember to use universal precautions when in contact with the body fluids of the mother and baby and in handling the newly delivered neonate.

▲ Observe infants immediately after birth. Note the Apgar scores and what nursing measures are taken.

▲ Observe mothers during the fourth stage of labor. Note what nursing actions are taken, which are routine department policies, and which are individualized for a particular new mother.

▲ With the approval of your instructor or the staff registered nurse, assist with or care for a new mother and an infant immediately after delivery until transfer.

▲ Observe how the nurse organizes her care for mother and baby within the appropriate time frame.

▲ Observe how the baby is suctioned with the delivery of the head. Is the mouth or the nose suctioned first? Why?

▲ Observe the way the parents are included as the nurse performs the care of the baby.

Have I Learned?

The following questions are for you to answer in order to find out if you have met the Objectives. All of the Objectives in LEG VIII-A are covered in this series of questions. Pick a quiet time and answer them. Answers are found at the end of this selftest.

No space has been left for answering the questions related to the "doing" Objectives. Use a separate sheet of paper for those answers, and then use the answers in clinical or campus lab for your own evaluation.

Objective	Question
1	**1.** Describe in detail or summarize by trimesters the fetal development, including length, weight, and one or two characteristics of the fetus.
2	**2.** Complete an assessment form as you admit a patient in labor. Are you satisfied with your nursing care and record keeping?
3	**3.** List five specific actions to minimize fear, pain, and discomfort during labor.
3	**4.** Describe three psychoprophylactic techniques used for relaxation.
4	**5.** Which of the following statements by a patient in labor would make you think that she had an accepting attitude? Which might indicate fear or rejection?

(a) "This is my first baby, and I'm kind of scared, but maybe it won't be too long."

(b) "How soon do you think I'll have my baby? This pregnancy has seemed so long and uncomfortable, I'll be glad to have it over. Can't you do something to hurry it along?"

(c) "I dream at night that the baby's deformed."

(d) "Hurry with the medicine. I just can't stand the pain any longer. This is so bad, it must be another boy."

(e) "Stay with me, I just can't bear to be alone."

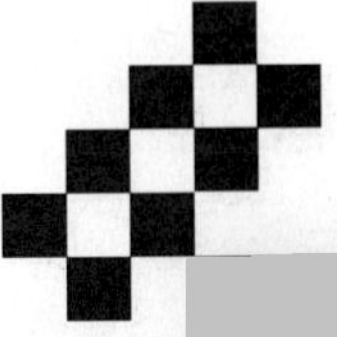

LEG VIII-A

5 **6.** Match the "Events" with the "Times of Occurrence." There may be more than one answer for some events.

Event	Time of Occurrence
____ 1. Complete dilatation of cervix	(a) Stage I beginning
____ 2. Delivery of baby	(b) Stage II beginning
____ 3. Rupture of membranes	(c) Stage III beginning
____ 4. First true contractions	(d) Stage IV beginning
____ 5. Delivery of placenta	(e) Stage I end
____ 6. Discomfort in small of back	(f) Stage II end
____ 7. Begin pushing action	(g) Stage III end

____ 8. Immediate postpartum checks (h) Stage I during

____ 9. Schultz/Duncan mechanism

6 **7.** State the purposes and length of time of each stage of labor and the muscle groups involved (for example, abdominal or uterine).

7 **8.**

> Mrs. McCellan is feeling the urge to push and has just been found on exam to be complete and complete.

What nursing assessments should be done for her according to the standards of care expected at this point in labor?

8 **9.**

> Miss Thompson, SN, was working in the labor unit during her second week in her maternity course. She located the position of Mrs. Ricardo's baby as head down, baby's back on the left side of the mother, and occiput toward the front of the mother's pelvis. When Miss Thompson listened to the FHR for 1 minute, she found it to be beating at what she thought was a rate of 67.

(a) What is the obstetrical position of the baby?

(b) Where should Miss Thompson place the Doppler?

(c) What could Miss Thompson have done to rule out the pulse of 67 as that of the baby? Of the mother?

9 **10.**

> Mrs. Ping's baby's FHR is a mirror image of her uterine contractions. When Mrs. Ping's contractions begin, the FHR begins to decelerate.

What type of a deceleration of the FHR is this?

10 **11.**

> Mr. Kelly is working as the night nurse in labor. His patient Mary Claire Westover's fetal monitor has just revealed she has had several late decelerations to 90 and the FHR has not rapidly returned to baseline.

(a) What is the risk to the baby?

(b) What are some interventions Mr. Kelly could do to assist the fetus?

11 **12.** **(a)** Label the following circles according to the beginning and end of the first stage and the beginning of the second stage of labor.
(b) What is the relationship of significance of dilatation, effacement, and station?

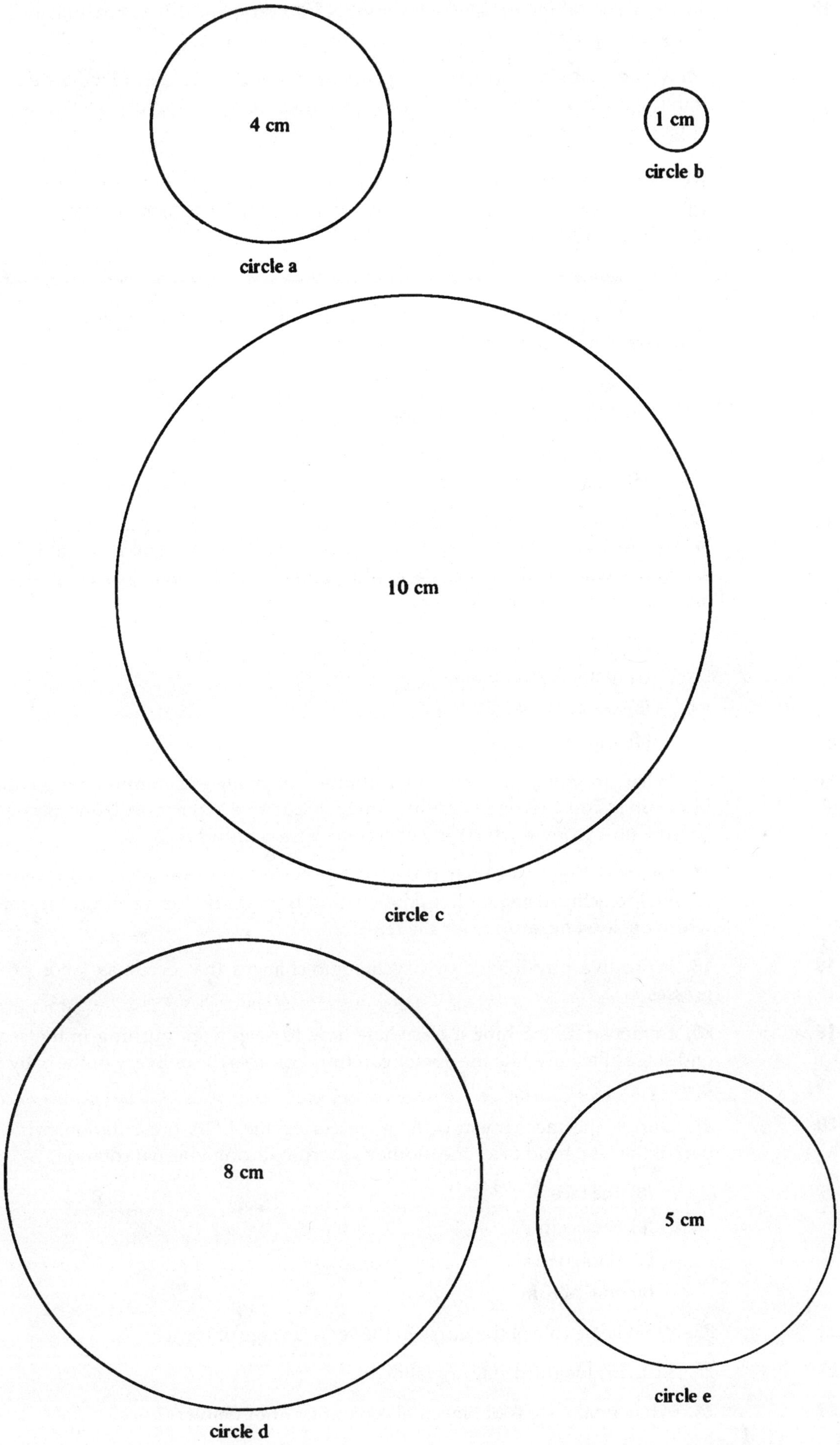

4 cm

circle a

1 cm

circle b

10 cm

circle c

8 cm

circle d

5 cm

circle e

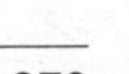

12 **13.** Explain the relationship of duration, intensity, and frequency of contractions to the progress of labor and the effect on the mother.

13 **14.** Write a nursing care plan for a patient in the latent phase of labor. Identify nursing problems she has at the moment. Include also in your plan two problems she may encounter as her labor progresses.

> The patient is a 27-year-old Hispanic woman. English is her second language. Her partner is with her but seems uncomfortable. The couple has not had childbirth education classes. The patient is gravida 3-1-1-0-1.

14 **15.** Which anesthesia used for delivery has the least possible disadvantages that would affect the fetus?

- **(a)** general anesthesia
- **(b)** local perineal infiltration
- **(c)** continuous epidural block
- **(d)** pudendal block

15 **16.** Mrs. Hapip needs something for her pain as she has been in labor for several hours, has made progress to 6 cm, and her baby's estimated weight is 9 lb 8 oz. What regional anesthesia could be selected now that would provide anesthesia for labor and delivery?

- **(a)** saddle block
- **(b)** paracervical block
- **(c)** epidural block
- **(d)** pudendal block

LEG VIII-A

16 **17.** What are some of the responsibilities of analgesia administration the nurse must consider when giving an analgesic to a woman in labor as compared with a woman who is in her second postoperative day?

17 **18.** List the drugs and their dosages that are most commonly used in your hospital to achieve analgesia, sedation, and tranquility during labor. Indicate which are least hazardous for the fetus.

18 **19.** Write five physiologic or psychologic changes that occur as labor progresses.

19 **20.** Demonstrate teaching a classmate how to keep from pushing in the second stage of labor while the doctor carefully controls the delivery of the baby's head.

20 **21.** During the mechanism of labor featuring the LOA presentation, which part of the fetal head faces the mother's sacrum during internal rotation?

- **(a)** the face
- **(b)** the occiput
- **(c)** the left ear
- **(d)** the sacrum

21 **22.** What is the role of the nurse in the second stage of labor?

22 **23.** Describe the third stage of labor.

23 **24.** What are the signs of placental separation after delivery?

24 **25.** What are the primary nursing responsibilities of the immediate postpartum checks after delivery?

25 **26.** Demonstrate the proper assessment and massage of the fundus and lochia using a model and equipment in the campus lab.

26 **27.** Describe how you would assess and care for a newborn including:

resuscitation
temperature regulation
Apgar scoring
care of the cord
care of the eyes
mother-infant bonding
identification

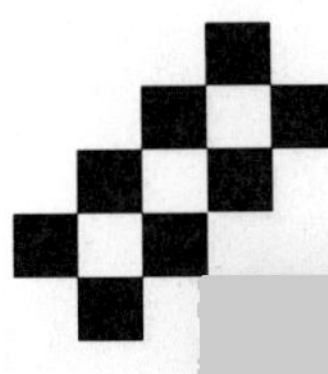

Answers to Have I Learned?

LEG VIII-A

1. *First trimester:* 0 to 8 cm (3 inches); weight up to 30 gm (1 oz); human face, fingers, toes, tail retrogresses; some movement but not yet felt by mother.

Second trimester: Up to 30 cm (12 inches) and 720 gm (1.5 lb); quickening, mother can now feel movement. Opens and closes eyes, regular shallow breathing (not compatible with life); meconium forms in digestive tract; other systems begin to function.

Third trimester: Up to 40–50 cm (15–20 inches) at birth and 3600 gm (7.5 lbs); greatest fetal weight gain and maturation; may suck thumb; develops subcutaneous tissue; goes from poor to good chance of survival at birth.

2. Compare your assessment form with that of another student. Discuss your strengths and weaknesses.

3. Your answer (and nursing actions) should include: interpret the progress of labor and carry out procedures skillfully; sponge bath; oral hygiene; back rub; explanations before a procedure; effective use of touch (e.g., allowing patient to grasp your hand, stroking patient's brow); stay with the patient.

4. Breathing techniques, light chest breathing to help raise the diaphragm away from the uterus.

Effleurage, a light circular motion with the fingertips to massage the abdomen. It is done in rhythm with breathing as a distractive technique.

Concentrating on a focal point.

Cleansing breath, deep breath through the nose and exhaled through the mouth.

Operant conditioning.

5. Accepting: **(a)** and maybe even **(b)**.

Fear or rejection: **(d)** and maybe **(c)** and **(e)**.

One isolated statement is not proof of an attitude. You should be alert to the need for further investigation.

6. 1. **(b)**,**(e)**; 2. **(c)**, **(f)**; 3. **(h)**; 4. **(a)**; 5. **(g)**; 6. **(i)**; 7. **(b)**; 8. **(d)**; 9. **(g)**.

7. *Stage I:* Prepares for Stage II by dilatation and effacement (shortening the cervical canal and enlarging the opening of the cervix). Dilatation and effacement are accomplished by uterine contractions, lasting 8–12 hours.

Stage II: Continues from full preparation of Stage I, 30 to 90 minutes until birth of the baby. Abdominal muscles assist with this phase.

Stage III: Accomplishes the separation of the placenta and expulsion in about 10 minutes after birth of baby. Both uterine and abdominal muscles are involved.

Stage IV: Purpose is to stabilize the mother's condition (e.g., vital signs, control of bleeding, recovery from anesthesia). This stage may last from 6 to 24 hours. Abdominal and uterine muscle groups are involved.

8. Your answer should include some of the following: Examine her to see if she is C/C. Notify physician. Stay with the patient. Check FHR after each contraction, check maternal pulse and BP every 5 minutes. Assist her in breathing correctly, making use of each contraction. Encourage the patient to rest between contractions. The mother should be encouraged to push toward the vagina. Pushing toward the vagina actually relaxes the vagina, but pushing toward the rectum seems to constrict the vagina. The mother should take a cleansing breath, expel it, take another breath, then expel it slightly through pursed lips as she pushes during the contraction. She should repeat this process as long as she has a contraction. Then she should take a cleansing breath and exhale.

9. **(a)** The position is LOA.

(b) The Doppler should be placed in the mother's left lower quadrant. If Miss Thompson was unsure, she could have placed the Doppler in the center of the lower half of the abdomen and then listened to the left or right of center.

(c) Miss Thompson could have palpated the radial pulse of Mrs. Ricardo to see if it was beating at the same rate as the Doppler sounds.

10. Early deceleration.

11. **(a)** Mr. Kelly should be concerned that the baby is experiencing uteroplacental insufficiency.

(b) The mother should be placed on her left side and oxygen should be given by mask. Check maternal vital signs. Treat hypotension if needed. Reposition mother as indicated. Discontinue oxytocin if present. Examine for prolapsed cord. Notify physician. Reassess.

12. **(a)** Circle b (1 cm) for beginning of first stage; circle c (10 cm) for end of first and beginning of second stage.

(b) *Dilatation* is represented by the circles and means the enlargement of the cervical opening to allow the passage of the fetus.
Effacement is the shortening of the cervical canal.
Station is the numerical determination of the degree of descent of the presenting part of the fetus as it relates to the level of the ischial spines.

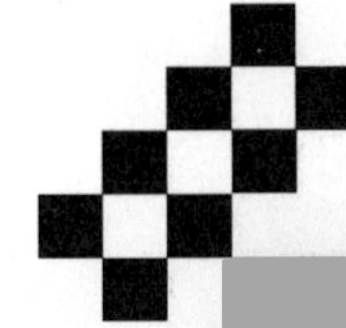

13. Uterine contractions can be likened to blood pressure diastole and systole to allow the heart periods of rest. Frequency, duration, and intensity of contractions must be watched closely. The patient's endurance and eventual success and delivery are dependent on this relationship. Your observations and descriptions will protect her from danger. Intensity is a relative term and takes much experience to judge well. Rule of thumb: mild muscle is somewhat tense; moderate muscle is moderately firm; strong muscle has feel of woody hardness and cannot be indented by pressure of fingers during acme. Note whether muscle relaxes completely between contractions. If any contraction lasts longer than 90 seconds and is not followed by a 2-minute rest interval with complete relaxation, it should be reported immediately because of danger to both mother and infant.

14. Give the nursing care plan to your instructor for evaluation.

15. **(b)**

16. **(c)**

17. Your answer should consider some of the following. The peak of the drug action may occur just as the infant is being born and could affect the infant's adjustment to extrauterine life. Narcotic antagonists need to be available to assist the neonate if necessary. Hypotension as a side effect will affect the baby's oxygen supply via the placenta. The drug needs to be carefully timed according to labor status and projected labor progress. The drug, if given IV, must be given diluted and injected as the contractions begin. This dosage should be given over 3–4 contractions. A woman who is not pregnant does not have the same considerations as the mother in labor. Peak effect and duration of the drug are important for both women, but serious side effects may harm the fetus or slow the labor progress if given at the wrong time.

18. Your answers will vary. Compare with a list provided by your instructor.

19. *Physiologic* | *Psychologic*

Physiologic	*Psychologic*
Dilatation 8–10 cm	Does not want to be left alone Withdrawal, drowsiness Behavioral change
Contractions q 45–60 sec	Depressed, nausea, trembling
Contractions q 2–3 min	Backache, urge to push Highly suggestible, irritable
Dilatation complete	Relief with pushing Totally involved

20. Instruct the mother to pant until she is told to push. When she pushes, help her to push gently not vigorously while the head is being delivered. Assist the mother to follow the physician's instructions at this significant moment. Role play this scenario at a GES for evaluation by your instructor.

21. (a)

22. Your answer should include the following. Support the mother during the second stage; care for her physical and emotional needs; teach her and support her and her partner in proper breathing techniques; monitor vital signs of mother and fetus after each contraction. Assess the equipment needed for delivery and infant resuscitation and inform physician or health care provider of the patient's status. Prepare for delivery in labor room if appropriate or prepare to transfer the patient to the delivery room. Transfer patient by her bed or guerney. Support patient as she prepares for delivery; assist her in positioning. Assist the physician during the delivery; note and record exact time of delivery.

23. The third stage begins after delivery of the baby and ends with delivery of the placenta. Placental separation and expulsion usually occur about 5 minutes after the birth of the baby but may take as long as 15 to 30 minutes to deliver in some cases.

24. Lengthening of the umbilical cord; increased blood from the vagina; the uterus becomes more rounded and firm; the uterus comes forward toward the abdomen.

25. Assess P, R, BP, fundus, lochia, fundal height, perineum, IV fluids, and IV site at a baseline after delivery. Then check vital signs—P, R, BP, fundus, lochia, fundal height, perineum, IV and IV site, pads, every 15 min × 4, then every 30 minutes × 2.

26. Demonstrate proper fundal assessment, fundal massage, and lochia assessment in the campus lab under the supervision of your instructor.

27. *Assess:* Establish airway. If necessary, resuscitate, which may include tactile stimulation, positive pressure ventilation, or oxygen near the face.

Temperature: Dry the infant and place him or her under a radiant heat warmer. Prevent cold stress.

Apgar scoring: Should be done at 1 and 5 min after birth. Repeat again after another 5 minutes if score is less than 7. Evaluate respiratory effort, heart rate, coin reflex, irritability, muscle tone.

Care of the cord: Tie or clamp; assess the cord for 2 arteries and 1 vein.

Care of the eyes: Instill 1 or 2 drops of silver nitrate or ophthalmic antibiotic ointment (if used in your area) in each eye.

Mother-infant bonding: Place the infant on the mother's warm body after he is dry.

Identification: Fill out arm and leg band for baby and matching arm band for mother.

What Will I Learn?

LEG VIII-B Postpartum and Neonatal Care

The delivery has taken place and the new baby has arrived! Now comes a period of adjustment following the long-anticipated birth. The mother will begin immediately the involution process to restore her to her nonpregnant state. This **Regulatory** process is completed rather quickly compared with the many months of gradual changes in her body during pregnancy. Psychologically and physiologically, the mother will be affected as her body adjusts. Bonding of the parents and infant will be enhanced by frequent contacts with the infant as the developing of parenting continues.

The neonate took his first breath at the time of delivery and began his physiologic adjustment to extrauterine life. The first 24 hours after birth are surely significant for the infant as well as for the parents.

Many couples face childbirth and parenting with very little advance preparation. Economic and sociologic changes have affected the family significantly. Frequently, the new parents face this wonderful but sometimes difficult adjustment to parenting in a location far away from their families or a support system. These issues affect the transition to the parental roles.

You will continue to apply your nursing skills from LEG VIII-A and will add many more skills related to the mother, neonate, and families. Assessment skills and teaching skills are used continuously in postpartum and neonatal care. This area of maternity is actually far from routine as there are so many areas of need that can be addressed.

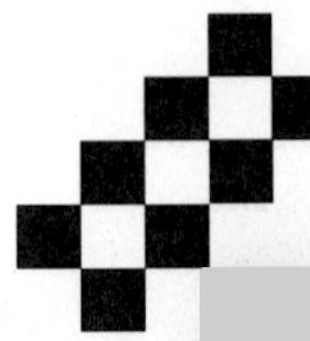

Women spend *much* less time in the hospital nowadays than they used to. Many mothers are discharged with their neonates within 12 to 24 hours after delivery. But the problems, potential problems, and teaching and learning needs are still the same. It is a great challenge to meet the needs of maternity patients and neonates under these time limitations. In the future, more emphasis will have to be placed on assessment, intervention, and follow-up outside the hospital.

What's Ahead in Later LEGs

Complications that may occur in the postpartum and neonatal periods will be studied in LEG XI-A, as will care of the newborn with complications including preterm and postterm infants and infants who are large and small for gestational age. The knowledge of typical postpartum and newborn care will serve you well in LEG XI-A.

■ Overview of Learning Experiences in LEG VIII-B

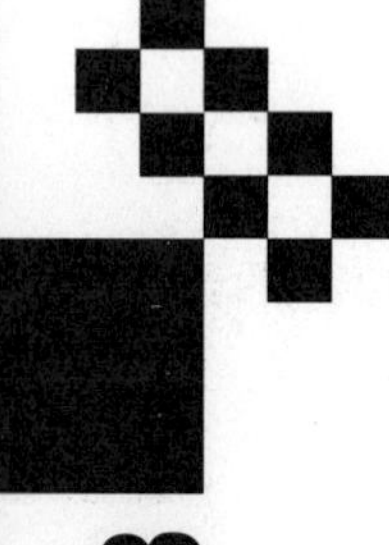

Objectives	Campus Lab/ Self-Practice	Group Discussions/Lectures	Clinical Lab Focuses
Postpartum Assessment and Care **1.** Postpartum physiologic changes **2.** Nursing care plan for a normal postpartum patient **3.** Nursing actions for postpartum problems **4.** Postpartum checks and perineum care	**B4.** Role play postpartum check Assess deep tendon reflexes **B5.** Teaching plan for peri care	**B2.** Normal postpartum physiologic changes GES Objective 4	**B7.** Talk with patient postpartum Care for newborns Care for postpartum patients Do postpartum checks and peri care
Oxytocics in Postpartum **5.** Oxytocics		**A3.** Oxytocics **B1.** Standing orders in postpartum	**B2.** Look at oxytocics being given, observe effect Observe RN performing postpartum checks
Characteristics of the Normal Newborn **6.** Characteristics of a normal newborn		**B1.** Characteristics of a normal newborn	**A3.** Observe through a nursery window **B3.** Observe in newborn nursery Assess newborns Make rounds with a nursery nurse
Breast and Bottle Feeding **7,8.** Breast and bottle feeding **9.** Methods to suppress lactation	**B2.** Teaching about infant feeding and care	**A3.** Breast and bottle feeding **B1.** Assisting mothers to breast feed	**B3.** Find out about bottles used in your hospital **B4.** Observe nurse teach a mother to breast feed Observe mothers/babies breast-feeding; assess condition of breasts Assist with and teach breast and/or bottle feeding
Caring for the Normal Newborn **10.** Use of Apgar scoring **11,12.** Admitting, assessing, and caring for a normal newborn **13.** Teaching newborn care to a mother	**B3.** Assessing a newborn with head-to-toe tool Role play teaching care of a newborn	**A8,9.** Assessing newborns **B1.** Helping mothers with new babies	**B4.** Care for babies in newborn nursery Discharge at least one baby Observe and do procedures in the newborn nursery Observe care of neonate with jaundice Observe and do gestational assessment

■ Overview of Learning Experiences in LEG VIII-B (cont.)

Objectives	Campus Lab/ Self-Practice	Group Discussions/Lectures	Clinical Lab Focuses
Assessing a New Parent's Feelings and Attitudes			
14. Mothering and attainment of maternal role **15,16,18.** Assessing attitudes and emotional needs of the new mother **17.** Assessing for blues and psychoses **19.** Helping a mother have success with her infant **20.** Using positive nursing diagnoses in nursing care planning		**A6.** Postpartum problems **B5.** Postpartum problems	**B6.** Talk with multipara patients Observe, listen, and help mothers Talk with new fathers Read charts Take baby to mother Use assessment tools Research community agencies providing postpartum support
Teenage Pregnancy, Single Mother, Nontraditional Childbearing Couples, and Birth Control			
21. Nursing care for single mothers and nontraditional childbearing couples **22.** Teenage pregnancy **23.** Contraception methods		**A5.** Care of the single mother or Planned Parenthood **B2.** Resumption of sexual intercourse after birth of baby **B3.** Therapeutic communication with a teenage new mother	**B5.** Care for single and/or teenage mothers Identify community resources
Helping a Family Deal with Loss of Health or Life of Infant (EAO)			
24. Helping a family deal with loss of health or life of infant		**A7.** Grief in maternity **B1.** Helping grieving parents	**B2.** Visit the mother of a premature infant Talk with the mother of a stillborn or newborn with a physical anomaly

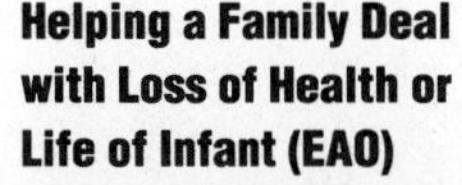

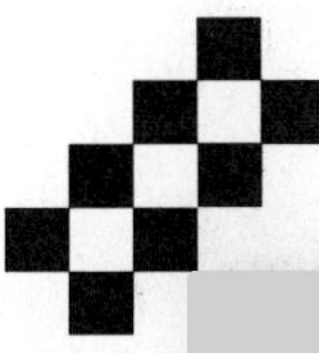

New Terms

acrocyanosis
ambivalence
anomaly
Ballard assessment
Brazelton assessment
caput succedaneum
cephalhematoma
colostrum
diuresis
engorgement
erythema toxicum
fontanel
hematoma
hyperbilirubinemia
icterus neonatorum
involution
kernicterus
lanugo
lochia
  alba
  rubra
  serosa
milia
molding
Mongolian spot
Ortolani's maneuvers
parlodel
physiologic jaundice
pilonidal cleft
postterm
preterm
puerperium
scarf sign
subconjunctival hemorrhage
sutures
term
vernix caseosa

Abbreviations

AGA
EGA
LGA
SGA

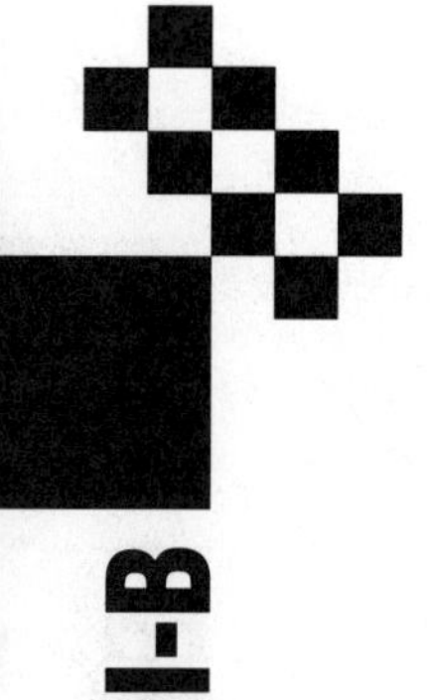

LEG VIII-B

Postpartum Assessment and Care

O b j e c t i v e s

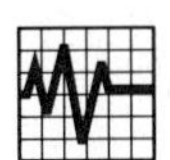 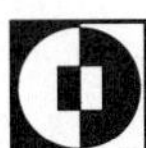 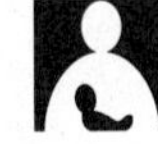

1. Describe the physiologic changes that occur in the following systems postpartum: reproductive, vascular, endocrine, GI, urinary, and in the abdominal musculature.

 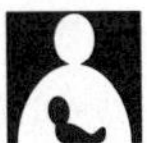

2. Write and implement a nursing care plan including at least one positive nursing diagnosis for a normal postpartum patient including at least one positive nursing diagnosis.

 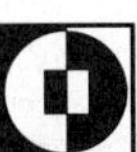 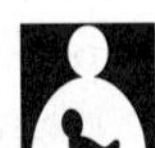

3. Describe, orally or in writing, nursing measures for each of the following conditions: hemorrhoids, engorgement, episiotomy, urinary retention, constipation.

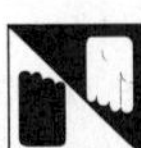  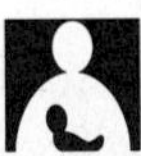

4. Demonstrate carrying out postpartum checks and teaching a new mother to care for herself according to hospital routine to provide clean, dry area for healing to decrease the risk of infection and provide comfort for the patient.

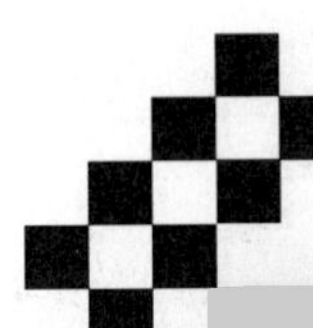

LEG VIII-B

A. What's It All About?

1. Think about the period after childbirth, postpartum, or the puerperium, which lasts from the third stage of labor until the completion of the involution process. What does the new mother feel? Relief? Satisfaction? Anxiety? Anger? Pride in accomplishment? Disappointment? Guilt? Some, none, or all of these? It depends on who the patient is and what has happened to her. This is a period when the new mother's body is undergoing change and her mind is adjusting to new situations. What are the needs of the newly delivered woman as she begins to take up the activities of daily living as a mother? How can you help her, beginning with the first day after delivery until she is discharged?

2. Review the immediate postpartum care described in LEG VIII-A and in your textbook.

3. Read about *postpartum assessment, physiologic changes,* and *maternal role attainment* from a list of books and articles provided by your instructor.

4. View visual aids on the topics listed in A.3.

5. Preview LEG XI-A, Complications of Postpartum.

6. Memorize the following chart. You will find some differences in your readings about the postpartum checks, but generally the steps are the same. The important point here is to establish a routine so that you do not forget any part of it. The first 2 hours after delivery are a very critical period for the new mother, and are referred to as the fourth stage of labor by some authors. It is a time when nursing care and observation are extremely important; the mother is usually completely dependent on the nurse during this period.

Palpate fundus
Slight massage of fundus; observe for bladder distention
Express clots from uterus with massage after the fundus is firm
Measure fundus in relation to umbilicus
Inspect perineum for discoloration and swelling
Inspect and change peri pads
Record BP and P
Offer food and fluid if allowed
Include comfort and safety measures
Chart observations and record pad and chux changes.

■ How often should this check be done the first hour? How often should it be done during the second and third hour if the postpartum course is normal?

What will you tell the mother about what you are doing? How can she help you make the most accurate assessment of her condition?

■ How can the nurse distinguish between bright bleeding and lochia rubra during the early postpartum period?

■ What observations of the episiotomy may be made? How can the nurse detect development of a hematoma during the early postpartum period?

■ When do you include the temperature and respirations in your assessment?

■ When is the mother checked for hemorrhoids?

■ What assessment is done concerning bladder functioning?

■ How is the lochia evaluated in terms of volume, character, and odor?

■ When do you do a regular medical-surgical assessment on your patient?

■ Plan how you would observe, chart, and report if you were asked to do a postpartum assessment for two patients. Assume you have 15 minutes for each. Check your patients in the following areas each shift:

emotional status
breasts
Homans' sign or anterior lateral leg check
fundus
bladder
lochia
episiotomy
bowel function
deep tendon reflexes (DTR)

■ Identify the rationale for perineal care throughout the postpartum period.

■ Compare the observations and principles of asepsis that would be applicable when giving perineal care for a postpartum patient with those that would be applicable when changing a dressing on a surgical patient.

	Observations	Principles of Asepsis
Peri care		
Surgical dressing		

■ B. Putting It into Action!

1. Identify the areas most likely to be a problem during the postpartum period for a new mother.

2. Attend a group discussion on "Normal Postpartum Physiologic Changes."

- ■ Discuss the normal consistency and placement of the uterus immediately after delivery, 12 hours after delivery, and 1–8 days postpartum.
- ■ Discuss how involution occurs.
- ■ What are the changes in vital signs that are normal postpartum adaptations?
- ■ Describe three types of lochia. When does each occur?
- ■ Discuss physiologic changes postpartum. (See Objective 1.)

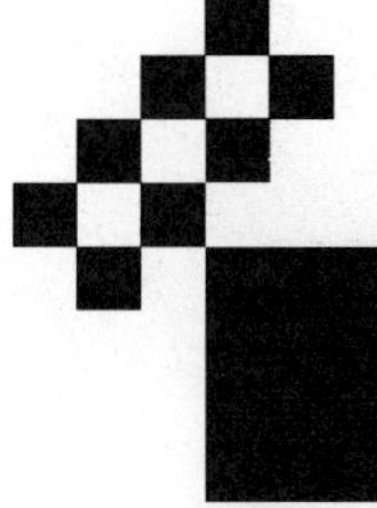

3. Find out the policy for perineal care at your hospital. Observe the procedure as it is given to a patient.

Is the procedure "clean" or "sterile"?

Is equipment disposable or not?

Are cotton balls, cloth, sponges, or tissues used?

Is mild soap or detergent used?

LEG VIII-B

4. Practice in campus lab.

- ■ Role play eliciting deep tendon reflexes (DTR) on your classmate. Memorize the scale of 0 to +4 with normal at +2. Apply this assessment skill to all your patients in antepartum, labor, delivery, and postpartum. Preview in your text and LEG XI-A about pregnancy-induced hypertension (PIH).
- ■ Role play explaining or teaching a new mother about the normal changes in lochia, normal involution of the uterus, and return of menses.
- ■ Role play how to do a postpartum check. Use the list in A.6.

5. Make a teaching plan to teach your patient about perineal care. Include the patient's history and the short-term and long-term goals of teaching this topic. Identify the objectives, teaching techniques or visual aids, and the evaluation process used to accomplish your goals. Submit this teaching plan to your instructor for evaluation.

6. Label the following actions to indicate which should occur during (a) the early postpartum period (1–2 days) and (b) which will occur later, and write your rationale.

____ Ensure several long rest periods
____ Check lochia
____ Push fluids
____ Teach self-care
____ Plan for care of mother and baby at home
____ Give peri care
____ Note breast changes
____ Take vital signs
____ Assist to void
____ Check level of fundus
____ Check perineum
____ Observe for urinary retention
____ Supervise self-care
____ Help mother relive delivery experience

What would you think might exist if, when you palpated the fundus, it was to one side?

7. Plan for a clinical experience.

▲ Talk with patients who have had both vaginal deliveries and cesarean sections. What were their feelings about each? What kinds of nursing care helped them most?

▲ Care for newborn babies delivered vaginally and by cesarean section. Compare their Apgar scores and progress before discharge. Read about each labor and try to understand why the surgery was performed.

▲ Give care to a postpartum patient, including peri care and teaching a mother how to do this herself.

▲ Care for a patient during pregnancy, labor, and postpartum, establishing rapport, making observations, minimizing fear, pain, discomfort, and possible complications. Write a nursing care plan, selecting one period of time on which to focus.

Note: This experience may not be possible for one patient through pregnancy, labor and delivery, and postpartum. If not, care for a different patient during each stage.

▲ Carry out a postpartum check of several patients. Pay special attention to giving maximum care during brief contact with the mother to allow her much-needed rest. Accompany your instructor or the staff RN to the bedside whenever a mother is being checked for the first time.

Oxytocics in Postpartum

O b j e c t i v e

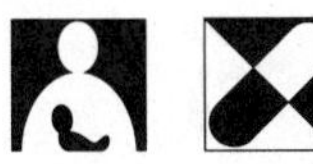

5. Name two oxytocics that may be used after delivery to promote uterine contractions and state the average dose, route of administration, contraindications, and nursing implications.

■ A. What's It All About?

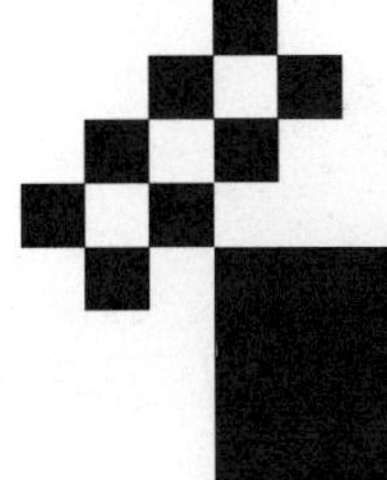

1. Think about medications that affect the uterine muscle. Oxytocins such as Pitocin, ergotrate maleate, and Methergine are frequently listed in the standing orders for women in the fourth stage of labor and in the postpartum period. Pitocin may be used to induce labor under very specific, controlled situations. (Pitocin will be discussed in relation to indication and augmentation of labor in LEG XI-A.) This unit of study refers to the oxytocics used for the purpose of promoting uterine contractions as an action to reverse uterine atony after delivery.

2. Read maternity and pharmacology references. Check the index for *oxytocics.*

3. Attend a lecture on "Oxytocics" in postpartum given by your instructor.

4. Review causes of postpartum bleeding in your textbook and in LEG XI-A.

5. Review assessment of the postpartum patient.

■ B. Putting It into Action!

1. Attend a small group discussion on "Standing Orders in Postpartum."

■ Discuss the following patient situation:

> Mrs. D. has just delivered a 9-lb boy. All is well; Dr. O. orders:
>
> (a) ergotrate maleate 0.2 mg IM q6h × 4 doses or
> (b) Methergine 0.2 mg PO q4h × 6 doses

What is the action/use of (a) and of (b)? What are the advantages and disadvantages of each?

What is your plan of action? Why?

2. Plan for a clinical experience.

▲ Look at the oxytocics in your hospital on the maternity floor. Note which ones are used most frequently and how they are supplied. What kind of containers, what color, and in how large quantities? Why do you think there might be some stocked on the postpartum floor? Check and see. Make flash cards with the name of the medication on one side and some of the other information on the other.

▲ Follow a staff RN as she performs her postpartum assessments. Which patients does she feel are candidates for bleeding? Why are they? Which patients demonstrate a slightly boggy uterus?

▲ Observe the actions and side effects of oxytocics in postpartum. Record them and share with your classmates in a postconference.

LEG VIII-B

Characteristics of the Normal Newborn

O b j e c t i v e

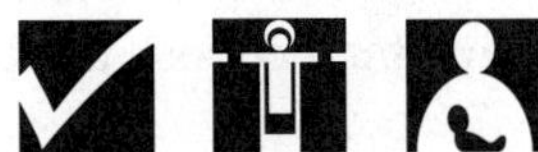

6. Describe, orally or in writing, five physical and behavioral characteristics of a normal newborn, including:

heart and respiratory rates (vital signs)
circulation (differences between fetal and newborn)
periods of reactivity
eight major reflexes
blood values
temperature regulation, heat production, and effects of cold stress

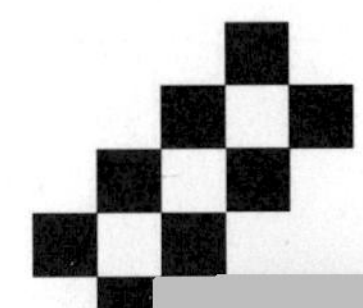

LEG VIII-B

■ A. What's It All About?

1. Think about your first reaction to caring for a newborn. Are you a little anxious about being responsible for a neonate? Are you excited and anxious to hold and cuddle a baby? Perhaps you have never held a baby before and wonder what it would be like. Now you are free to observe and learn the normal behavior of the newborn; later you will be responsible for the nursing care. Enjoy this time and observe as many newborns as possible. When you do care for a newborn, be sure to remember to use gloves and practice universal precautions when indicated.

2. View audiovisuals and read articles and books from a list given to you by your instructor.

3. Talk with a nursery nurse or your instructor. What does she look for in the normal newborn? List the descriptions.

- Go to the nursery (outside the window). What do you see? Write down the similarities and dissimilarities as you observe three babies during morning or evening care.

4. Read one or more references on maternity and pediatric nursing. Look in the index under *neonate, newborn.*

Appraisal (physical assessment) is part of the nursing process. Use this opportunity to review and to build on your knowledge and skills in carrying out the nursing process.

5. Review LEG II-C, Growth and Development of the Infant.

6. Review the colorful visual-aid pamphlet "Variations and Minor Departures in Infants" published by Mead Johnson and Co., Evansville, Indiana, 1978.

7. Write the causes and implications of physiologic hyperbilirubinemia of the newborn. What are the nursing actions or responsibilities to prevent complications?

Be sure you know the implication of kernicterus, exchange transfusion, phototherapy, and jaundice. What is the difference between pathologic and physiologic jaundice? How do you assess an infant for jaundice?

8. Define phenylketonuria.

Describe the testing procedure used to diagnose this condition.

What are the implications of a positive test result to the infant? To the parents? To the nurse? What other blood tests are required to be performed on newborn infants in your state?

9. Identify some common parental concerns regarding their newborn. For example, list reasons for having a circumcision performed and reasons that parents may choose not to have a circumcision performed on their newborn.

10. Describe the following reflexes of the newborn:

Moro

Tonic neck

Stepping

Dancing

Rooting

Sucking

Blinking

Babinski

Palmar grasp

Plantar grasp

Sneezing

Bring this descriptive list to your group discussion.

■ B. Putting It into Action!

1. Attend a group discussion on "Characteristics of a Normal Newborn."

To prepare for this group complete the following data and bring your findings to share with the group.

(a) Describe the periods of reactivity that a newborn goes through, especially during the first 6 hours.

(b) What are the major differences between the fetal and newborn circulation?

(c) Name eight major reflexes present at birth and describe how they may be tested.

(d) Name two laboratory tests done on the normal newborn and two medications routinely given in the first 8 hours.

(e) What is the importance of heat production, temperature regulation, and effects of cold stress on the newborn?

2. Write your description of the normal newborn for your instructor to see. Use brief phrases—not an essay. Justify your description.

Comments on Assessment of Newborn

Careful nursing observations will never be replaced by monitors. A thoughtful, alert nurse can see a change in an infant's condition before a monitor will indicate a problem. Don't make the mistake of depending on the

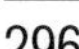

monitors. Many conditions cannot be detected by a monitor. The condition of a normal newborn can change rapidly. Never assume that all is well until you have assessed the situation carefully and frequently.

---

3. Plan for a clinical experience in the nursery.

▲ Repeat your observations of babies a few hours old, 1 day old, several days old. What is their color when crying? When not crying? How does the head feel? Look? How is it shaped? Is the face symmetrical? What is the relationship of the head to the body in size? Look at the eyes. Describe the color and movement. What is the average weight and length? Do you observe any reflexes? How do you take the temperature, pulse, and respirations of a newborn?

▲ Make at least two physical and behavioral assessments of babies in the newborn nursery. Compare your assessments with those of other students and staff.

▲ Observe and make rounds with an experienced nursery nurse. Make your own observations. Ask questions. Continue to be a very careful, alert nurse.

▲ Observe the physical exam of a newborn given by your instructor or a pediatrician.

▲ Give a return demonstration of a physical exam of a newborn for your instructor.

▲ Compare the physical characteristics of the babies in the nursery. How do the fontanels and sutures differ? What color is the skin? Do you see milia, erythema toxicum, Mongolian spot, or molding?

▲ Observe an infant being examined for gestational age.

▲ Compare the babies in the nursery for term characteristics.

Breast and Bottle Feeding

Objectives

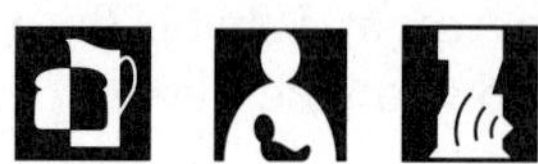

7. Describe in writing and demonstrate teaching and assisting a new mother to breast feed her baby, maintaining comfort of the mother and ability to suck by the infant.

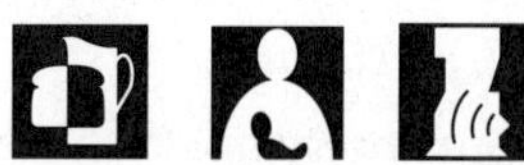

8. Demonstrate teaching and assisting a new mother to feed her baby formula, maintaining comfort during feeding and increasing the infant's ability to suck.

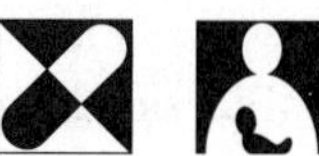

9. Identify medications to suppress lactation and state the route, side effects, and frequency of administration. A list will be provided by your instructor. Describe also a nonmedication method used to suppress lactation.

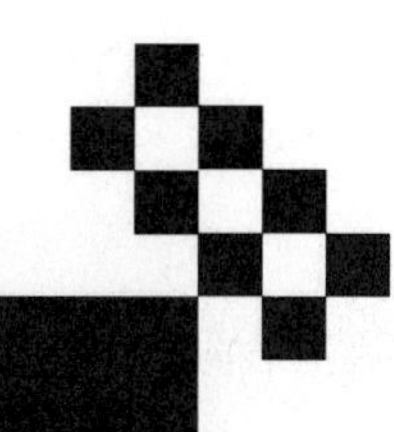

A. What's It All About?

1. Think about the process of lactation. How does the mother learn to nurse her infant if she has never seen anyone nurse a baby? How can a mother be assisted to nurse her infant in the hospital, and what follow-up care should she have after discharge?

Many mothers decide to bottle feed their babies. How can the mother learn the skills she needs to bottle feed her baby? Remember it is important that the nurse support the mother and the method of feeding she has chosen for the baby.

Many nursing students have had no prior experience with breast or bottle feeding. This will be an opportunity for you to assess both methods and assist the mother as you learn yourself. Pay special attention to the influences of attitudes toward methods of feeding. Success in breast feeding may be influenced by attitudes of those surrounding the mother.

2. View audiovisuals and read articles and books on breast or bottle feeding from a list given you by your instructor.

3. Attend a lecture on "Breast and Bottle Feeding" given by your instructor.

4. Write or discuss answers to the following questions. You will need to know the answers to these questions as you help your patients.

(a) What is the La Leche League? How can you find out?

(b) What are the advantages of breast feeding to the mother? To the baby?

(c) What makes a baby sleepy instead of hungry? How can you wake her up? What can the mother do with a sleepy baby? Is this important?

(d) Describe the process of lactation and identify what influences the promotion of successful breast feeding.

What influences the letdown process?

How do attitudes influence maternal tension and the letdown reflex?

(e) What will you do if the baby is screaming when you bring her to the mother?

(f) What if the mother expresses concern that her baby is not getting enough milk? How can you tell if the baby is getting enough fluid?

(g) How do you correctly position the baby on the breast?

(h) How do you break the suction to remove the baby from the breast?

(i) If you needed to give water as a supplement to the breast milk, how would you give it? Why?

(j) What are the advantages of using both breasts for each feeding to the mother? To the baby? Why?

(k) How does positioning of the infant and mother differ for breast and bottle feeding? Why?

What may be the result of giving a breastfeeding baby a bottle? Why?

(l) When will the milk supply be established?

(m) What are the four phases of mother-infant attachment? Why is early contact with the infant important?

(n) Give an example of medication used to suppress lactation. Include:

Route of administration

Side effects

How long the drug is usually given

(o) How can lactation be suppressed by nonmedical means?

(p) How do you burp a baby? Do you need to burp a breast-fed baby?

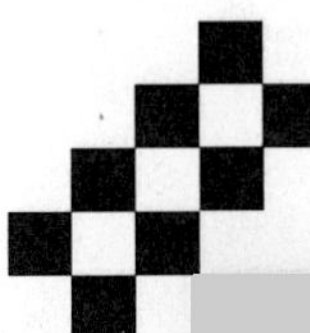

LEG VIII-B

■ B. Putting It into Action!

1. Attend a small group discussion on "Assisting Mothers to Breast Feed."

■ Role play responses to the following patient statements:

"I don't know how to feed my baby."

"Why must I stay in bed to nurse?"

"How will I know when my milk comes in?"

"My breasts are so sore I can hardly stand to nurse him this afternoon."

"My sister said she used a breast shield when she nursed her baby."

■ List and discuss the advantages of allowing the baby to nurse immediately or within 1 hour after delivery, and then on demand. Add more rationales from your readings.

Advantages for the Baby	*Advantages for the Mother*

How does the policy of allowing the baby to nurse on demand affect hospital routines?

2. Practice (in campus lab or at home) teaching a new mother about infant feeding: REMEMBER TO WASH YOUR HANDS.

- Teach a new mother how to grasp her breast (two-finger technique) to form the nipple and then hold the baby's chin extended to keep the nipple against the roof of the mouth. Role play, with another student or yourself, for the two-finger grasp. Borrow a baby to get the feel of extending the chin.
- Feed a baby formula. Try different positions. Burp the baby. Does the baby seem to do better in an upright position or a flat position? Why? Do you find it easy to cuddle the baby while feeding him or her?
- Bathe, diaper, and give care as you role play your teaching.

3. Check on the type of bottle used in your hospital. Compare three or four different types of bottles and nipples. Read the directions and the objectives or rationales for the differences in size and shape. Check the nipple openings: large or small, one or many, slits or pinholes.

4. Plan for a clinical experience.

▲ Check the charts of breastfeeding mothers. Note medication received during labor and date of delivery. How do you expect this medication to affect the babies, if at all?

▲ Observe breast-fed babies. Scrub and gown. Check infants' charts; note Apgar scores; look at these babies. Change diapers; note the type of stools, voiding, rashes; check vital signs.

▲ Observe a nursery nurse assisting a mother to breast feed her baby. Notice the number of times the baby has been taken to breast, the attitude of the mother, how she handles her infant and positions herself, and the baby's sucking ability and interest. Listen to both the nurse and the patient.

▲ Make feeding rounds with your teacher or the staff RN. Observe how the teacher or nurse assesses and intervenes in assisting the mother and infants during feedings.

▲ Observe a new mother who is having problems with breast feeding. What cause do you see? What is the position of the mother? Is the baby sleepy? Is there engorgement? Is the mother tense? Jot down some ideas you would like to try for improving the situation. Discuss these in postconference.

▲ Observe two new mothers, (1) a primipara and (2) a multipara, who have breast fed their babies successfully before. Compare the way these two women approach breast feeding. How can you help? What if the multipara patient has not had a successful breastfeeding experience before?

▲ When doing your postpartum checks each shift, remember to assess the breasts for colostrum, engorgement, filling, and milk. Assess the nipple carefully for redness and fissures or possible signs of skin breakdown. If problems are noted on the nipple, instruct the mother accordingly.

▲ Attend a postconference. Discuss the outreach programs the hospitals or community agencies in your state have for assessing and assisting new mothers with infant feeding problems after they have returned home.

▲ Observe patients feeding their babies formula. Assist them. Listen as they ask questions about the care of their babies.

▲ Read charts for orders of medications to suppress lactation. Observe patients. Look for side effects. Note the method and time of administration of lactation suppressants.

▲ Assist and teach a new mother to breast feed her baby. Document your teaching. Evaluate her progress.

▲ Assist and teach a new mother to bottle feed her baby. Document the mother's ability to handle and hold her baby.

▲ Attend postconference. Evaluate and discuss the following charting:

> Mother tense and unsure of self. Instructed in care of handling baby.
>
> More comfortable in semi-Fowler's position nursing.
>
> Baby nursing well now.
>
> Baby nursed poorly.
>
> Mother expresses fears of inadequacy at home.
>
> Suggested that if problems arise she contact Le Leche League for help.
>
> Baby refuses to use left breast.

Discuss your own charting.

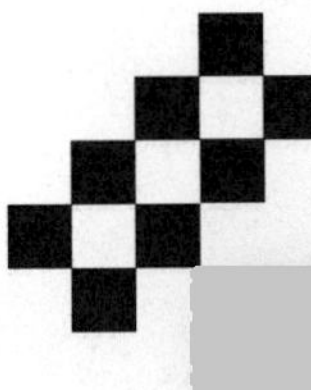

LEG VIII-B

Caring for the Normal Newborn

O b j e c t i v e s

Note: All of the Objectives below are related to care of the neonate from admission to the newborn nursery until discharge from the hospital.

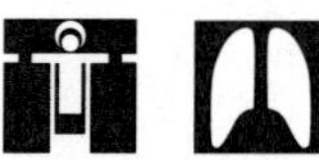

10. Describe, orally or in writing, the Apgar system of evaluation of the newborn.

11. Demonstrate or role play admitting a normal newborn to the nursery, including: giving vitamin K, weighing, assessing condition (skin, cord, vital signs, color), gestational age, assessment, physical assessment, immediate care, and charting.

12. Demonstrate or role play caring for a newborn infant following admission to the nursery.

13. Demonstrate teaching a mother about newborn care by preparing and using a teaching and discharge plan for baby and mother.

LEG VIII-B

■ A. What's It All About?

1. Think about the newborn as he continues to adjust to extrauterine life. How is the hospital nursery designed and used to provide special care to the newborn infant? What guidelines do the nurses use to approach each new baby admitted to the unit? The Apgar scoring method is a major standard guide for initial infant care. You will also learn about several other methods of neonatal assessment that are applied to all babies. Assessment skills are extremely important as it is often the nurse who first examines the newborn after birth.

2. Review newborn resuscitation and immediate care following childbirth in LEG VIII-A. Review infant CPR techniques.

3. Read in references provided by your instructor about the normal newborn: *behavior, characteristics, assessment, nursing care, feeding, PKU, suctioning, circumcision,* and *teaching neonatal care to parents.*

4. View audiovisuals and read additional articles and books from a list provided by your instructor.

5. Preview LEG XI-A to read about neonates who are at risk for problems, are having problems, or have low Apgar scores.

6. List the observations you would expect to see for the infants with the following three Apgar scores:

Sign	Baby 1 Score	Baby 2 Score	Baby 3 Score
Heart	2	1	2
Respiratory	2	1	1
Muscle	2	0	1
Reflex	2	1	1
Color	2/10	0/3	1/6
Observations:			

7. Define the following terms related to weight as well as the physical and neurologic exam characteristics of the newborn:

preterm

term

postterm

AGA

LGA

SGA

(a) Why is it best to assess the estimated gestational age (EGA) within 2 to 8 hours after birth?

(b) How do the Dubowitz or Ballard assessment guidelines help you examine a newborn accurately?

(c) What is the significance of the information gained by formal assessment weight and the EGA as compared with relying on the estimated date of confinement (EDC) and labeling the baby accordingly?

8. Attend lectures and demonstrations conducted by your instructor on the following newborn topics:

Dubowitz or Ballard assessment

Observing the newborn

Vital signs

Basic newborn care

9. Attend a lecture or demonstration on the Brazelton behavioral tool identifying the states of the neonatal period.

■ B. Putting It into Action!

1. Attend a small group discussion on "Helping Mothers with New Babies."

- Find out the most common types of formula used in your hospital. Look at the labels and note the differences. Review breastfeeding techniques and practices. Bring this information to the group to share.
- Demonstrate planning nursing care for the following infants: include bathing, vital signs, observations, need for oxygen, changing diapers, feeding. You are the nursery nurse receiving report on the following babies:

> Baby with phototherapy.
>
> One-day-old boy, lusty cry at birth, Apgar score 9, taking 120 cc q3–4h; to have a circumcision at 1:00 P.M.
>
> Term newborn, SGA.

- Demonstrate admitting the babies described above to the newborn nursery. (Some of these activities can be done in campus lab.)
- Demonstrate a newborn infant exam.
- Role play teaching a small group of new mothers about bathing infants, sterilizing bottles, types of formulas. React to the following questions by these mothers:

> "Which type of bottle do you recommend?"
>
> "I thought it was unnecessary to sterilize bottles if a dishwasher is used."
>
> "I heard that babies aren't washed very often because of the drying effect of soap on the skin."
>
> "Is it O.K. if I give my baby a pacifier?"
>
> "What about the bottles that are shaped like a breast?"
>
> "Why this formula instead of the one (Enfamil) my neighbor uses?"
>
> "What should I do if my baby chokes or spits up?"
>
> "Is it O.K. to put my baby on her stomach in the crib?"
>
> "How do I position my baby in the basinette and in the crib?"
>
> "Can my baby be in a room with air conditioning?"
>
> "How warmly should I dress my baby?"
>
> "Will my baby need a hat and sunscreen when taken out in the sun?"

- List at least five statements that you, as students, might use to find out what knowledge the mother has about caring for her baby after discharge. Make these statements specific, and all members of the group should have suggestions to make. These statements must draw the new mother out so that you really know what she needs to learn before she goes home with her new baby.

2. Create a poster or a sample box with pictures or actual samples of formula, bottles, bath equipment and lotions, diapers, pins, and so on, for showing and teaching the new mother.

As you use this in teaching make notes of the questions mothers ask. Bring these to postconference for discussion.

3. Practice in campus lab.

■ Role play assessing a newborn's condition using a head-to-toe assessment tool. Use the chart on p. 306, or whatever tool is used in your facility.

■ Role play reactions to the following comments or questions by mothers who are receiving their babies for feeding:

> "You handle my baby too roughly, like a football."
>
> "Why isn't the milk heated?"
>
> "Why must I wait so long before I get my baby?"
>
> "Why are her hands covered?" (Some nursery gowns have sleeves closed to cover hands to prevent scratching by long nails.)
>
> "My baby stops and rests a lot during feeding. Should I change position each time she stops to rest?"
>
> "How do you burp a baby, and how often should I do it?"

■ Discuss teaching and discharge plans. Role play teaching a new mother about infant care.

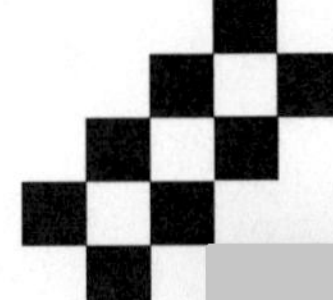

4. Plan for a clinical experience.

▲ Demonstrate proper handling and positioning while caring for an infant under the supervision of your instructor.

▲ Care for babies in the newborn nursery. Large babies, small ones, long, short, weak, strong, and so on. Admit one or more under the supervision of your instructor.

▲ Observe nurses making gestational age assessments. Record your own assessment as you observe. Compare your findings with the nurse's.

▲ Observe the nurse discharging an infant.

▲ Discharge at least one baby. Did the mother seem well prepared to take up the care of the baby? How do you know?

▲ After the RN has initially examined the newborn, follow up with your physical exam of the infant under the supervision of your instructor.

▲ How does the initial physical exam differ from the exam done each shift?

▲ Perform the following nursing measures with supervision after observing them performed in the newborn nursery or on the children's floor.

- ■ Suctioning mucus with a bulb syringe or De Lee mucus trap connected to mechanical suction.
- ■ Heel stick for the PKU/Guthrie, galactosemia and hypothyroidism screening test.
- ■ Giving injections (vitamin K).
- ■ Assisting with a circumcision.
- ■ Dextrostix

Discuss these procedures in postconference.

▲ Observe a neonate with jaundice; list the nursing responsibilities for babies being treated with a bilirubin light.

LEG VIII-B

Nursing Assessment of the Newborn*
Points to Be Noted

I *HEAD*
(a) Circumference
(b) Relationship to rest of body
(c) Size and shape compared with adult
(d) Size and shape of
—anterior fontanel
—posterior fontanel
—sutures
(e) Caput succedaneum
(f) Cephalhematoma

II *EYES*
(a) Epicanthal folds
(b) Pupil reaction
(c) Cornea and iris
(d) Discharge
(e) Movement
(f) Evidence of vision

III *EARS*
(a) Symmetry
(b) Placement
(c) Skin tags
(d) Evidence of hearing

IV *NOSE*
(a) Nares
(b) Bridge
(c) Symmetry

V *MOUTH*
(a) Lips
(b) Palate
(c) Gums
(d) Tongue
(e) Suck, swallow, and rooting reflex

VI *NECK*
(a) Torticollis
(b) Length
(c) Tonic neck reflex

VII *CHEST*
(a) Circumference
(b) Shape
(c) Breasts
(d) Respiration—describe rate
(e) Heartbeat—rate

VIII *ABDOMEN*
(a) Shape
(b) Cord

IX *SPINAL COLUMN*
(a) Pilonidal dimple

X *LEGS AND FEET*
(a) Symmetry
(b) Movement
(c) Toe pressure
(d) Babinski
(e) Plantar grasp
(f) "Stepping"

XI *HIPS*
(a) Abduction of thighs
(b) Gluteal folds
(c) Mongoloid spot

XII *GENITOURINARY*
(a) Patency of anus
(b) Patent vaginal orifice—discharge
(c) Urinary meatus
(d) Labia majora
(e) Labia minora
(f) Scrotum

XIII *POSTURE*
(a) Sleeping
(b) Waking
(c) Moro—how long does this persist?
(d) Muscle tone
(e) Position of comfort

XIV *SKIN*
(a) Color
(b) Differences from adult
(c) Areas of edema, redness
(d) Petechiae
(e) Rashes

XV *TEMPERATURE*

XVI *CRY*
(a) Pitch
(b) Frequency
(c) Behavior

*Reprinted with permission of Brandon General Hospital School of Nursing. Brandon, Manitoba, Canada.

▲ Practice using an estimated gestational age assessment tool on newborns in the nursery. Make notes and share these in postconference. Memorize the weeks of gestation that are defined as term, preterm, and postterm and the physical and neuromuscular characteristics.

▲ Attend a postconference. Discuss the care and supervision of the neonate after discharge until the end of the first month after birth.

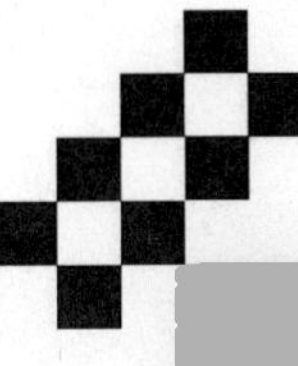

Assessing a New Parent's Feelings and Attitudes

Objectives

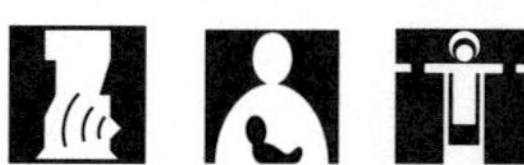

14. Describe the development of mothering, the attainment of the maternal role, and nursing measures that will assist the new mother in the transition.

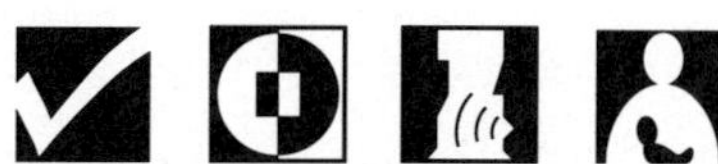

15. Using an assessment tool, and given a patient situation (or actual patient to care for), identify the attitude of the parents toward their new role.

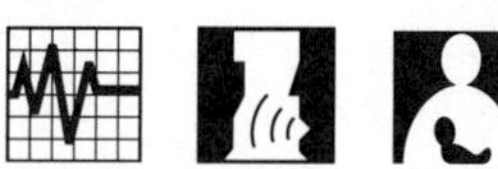

16. Describe emotional needs that might change because of being a new mother and demonstrate or role play helping a new mother recognize these changes.

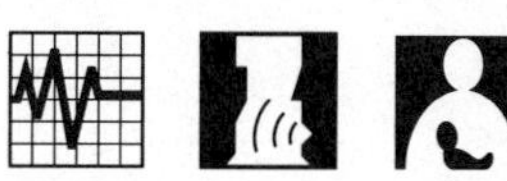

17. Given a list of symptoms, identify which are characteristic of postpartum blues and which are characteristic of psychoses.

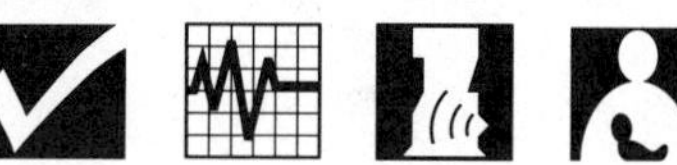

18. Given a patient situation, identify clues that might indicate one or more of the following maternal feelings or attitudes: disinterest, preoccupation with self, complete preoccupation with infant.

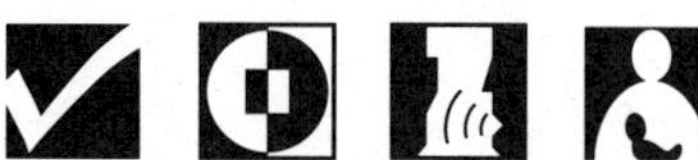

19. Demonstrate planning two nursing actions, before giving care to a postpartum patient, that are aimed at helping the mother to have an early success experience with her infant.

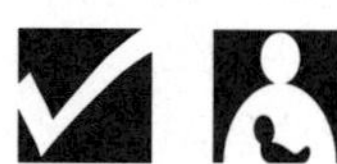

20. Write a nursing care plan on your postpartum patient. Select one positive nursing diagnosis as well as several other nursing diagnoses that focus on physiologic and psychosocial problems.

A. What's It All About?

1. Think about the stereotypical views of the new mother portrayed in the popular literature and in the media. Do all mothers adjust easily to motherhood? Do all mothers feel motherly simply because they gave birth a few moments or days ago? What happens when new mothers do not feel as they think they should toward their new babies? Can they experience a sense of guilt and a feeling that they have failed to meet their own expectations and those of society? How do fatigue, discomfort, and concern affect a patient's mood? What are some of the ways that nurses can help new mothers and fathers as they begin their parenting roles? Families are given a much better start when a broad range of maternity care is provided, and nurses have many more responsibilities for independent nursing actions.

Have you ever had the blues or felt depressed? Do you know the actual cause or the precipitating cause? (Review LEG VI-A.) What are some symptoms of the blues? Think about the contributing factors that can cause depression for a new mother. How do they differ from the causes of the depressions of everyday life?

2. Review:

LEG II-B Psychosocial Concerns of Pregnancy

LEG III-C Anxiety and Defense Mechanisms

3. Read about the development of *mothering, fathering,* and *parenting, maternal role attainment, postpartum blues, postpartum psychosis, maternal-infant bonding,* and *postpartum care* in your maternity textbook and in other resources provided by your instructor.

4. Answer the following questions:

(a) What are the steps of maternal role attainment or attachment?

(b) How do positive nursing diagnoses compare with other standard nursing diagnoses? What are the benefits of each? How do you support maintenance of appropriate maternal actions?

(c) What physical or physiologic and psychologic adjustments must women make during the postpartum period?

(d) For each adjustment identified above give one nursing intervention and its rationale.

(e) What are signs and symptoms of the postpartum blues as compared with those of postpartum psychosis?

(f) How can nurses meet the needs of patients in terms of feelings, attitudes, new roles, and psychologic adjustment when the hospitalization stay is so short?

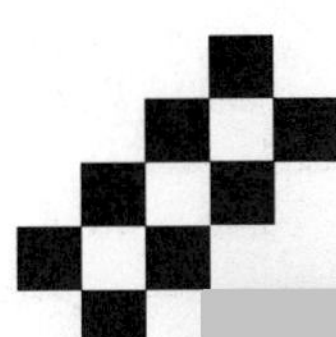

5. List reasons why the new mother may have ambivalent feelings about being a mother.

Comments on Assessing Attitudes

As you read and respond to isolated patient remarks, you must realize that one isolated statement or action is not indicative of abnormal patient reaction. The key word to indicate problems with feelings is *excessive* or overreacting too often (fear, pain, joy, casualness, demands, worry). It is not your responsibility to decide what is excessive. Your role is to recognize *clues* from patients that should alert you to reevaluate the situation, and you must report the clues so that they may be shared with the physician and your other colleagues on the health care team.

6. Attend a series of lectures on postpartum problems featuring the following topics:

postpartum blues

postpartum psychosis

development of mothering and fathering

■ B. Putting It into Action!

1. Describe in your own words the following patient's attitude toward her new role as a mother.

> "I'm so excited about getting my baby home. I have so many clothes to dress her up in, and it will be such fun. My little doll!"

What are your thoughts, and therefore what would be your reply? What is the purpose of your reply?
What is the purpose of the following reply?

> "Yes, babies are fun and they are cute all dressed up. But there is much more to the care of your baby. What changes do you think your baby will make in your home routine?

Compare the following two patient responses:

> (a) "Yes, that's so true, and I have plans all set for a very good sitter, so my husband and I can still get away together, and I'm prepared for baby care, but right now I'm just thinking of the fun part."
>
> (b) "Oh well, my mother said she'd help, so I'm not thinking about anything but the fun of playing with my baby."

What response would you make to each of those statements? Why?

2. List three observations that would indicate that a patient is in the "taking-in phase" and three observations that a patient is in the "taking-hold phase."

3. Select four descriptions of symptoms from list A below (cover column B) that may be characteristic of the blues. Cover column A and circle those in column B characteristic of the blues. Compare your answers. If there is a difference in your answers, how do you explain the difference? Which symptoms may be clues and which symptoms seem normal or expected? Why?

A	*B*
(a) Difficulty in sleeping	(a) Insomnia after visiting hours; sleeps well once she gets to sleep
(b) Talkative about delivery experience	(b) Comments about delivery experience; does not dwell on discomforts or anesthesia
(c) Irritable and tearful	(c) Cries or is irritated once or twice; not daily or even frequently
(d) Good appetite and talks with interest about food	(d) Requests milkshakes and sweets from husband; snacks frequently, eats ravenously

(e) Loses her appetite	(e) Refuses one meal or "picks" at food the first day but gradually, with encouragement, appetite improves
(f) Talks of a "letdown" feeling	(f) "Letdown feeling" lessens after holding and feeding her baby

Here are some ways to get additional information: *ask questions of staff members, talk with patient, make observations, stay with the patient, show support and caring.*

■ Imagine that you are receiving report. To get additional information about the patient who has "difficulty in sleeping" what would you ask the evening nurse?

■ You walk into a patient's room and find the patient irritable and crying. You wonder what this behavior means. What would you look for during the next 8 hours to give you the necessary additional information?

■ In order to get additional information how would you talk to a patient who complains of a "letdown" feeling?

Guidelines to Be Used in Assessment of Maternal Attachment to Infant

Behavior	Yes/No
1. Does the mother talk to the baby?	
2. Does the mother have eye contact with the baby?	
3. Does the mother touch the baby with her fingertips or palms of hand?	
4. Does the mother hold the baby close to her body?	
5. Does the mother respond to and is she sensitive to the baby's needs?	
6. Does the mother smile and show pleasure in the baby?	
7. Does the mother hold the baby in the en face position?	
8. Does the mother look at the baby when you compliment her on the baby?	

Comments on Feeling Maternal

Remember that just having a baby does not arouse maternal feelings. This is normal, and if a new mother expresses this concern and a feeling of guilt, you should help her become aware that many new mothers feel this way. Prenatal classes usually cover this so that parents are aware that by caring and cuddling, love and feelings start. You must be sure that you intervene when needed so that guilt feelings do not arise.

4. List five behaviors of the new mother and father that indicate bonding, and the beginning of parenting.

5. Attend a small group discussion on "Postpartum Problems."

■ Role play what you would do and say to the following patients (see Objectives 15 and 16):

(a) Patient you find crying quietly at night.

(b) Patient who is still alternately wandering around her room and reading at midnight.

(c) Patient who says she can't eat the "terrible food."

(d) Patient who tells you she feels "let down" and appears at loose ends.

(e) Patient who delivered 1 month ago who calls the maternity unit for advice saying she has not slept in 4 weeks.

(f) Patient who says at her postpartum clinic visit that she feels that she cannot control her own thoughts.

■ Examine and respond to the patient comments below. (See Objective 18.) What do you think each patient is saying? What is your responsibility?
Role play your responses for group evaluation. After completion of each, go back and evaluate your thoughts and responses.
Identify factors that contribute to successful and unsuccessful parenting.

Patient 1. "Oh, I just saw Mellie again. She is so beauuutiful—every feature is just perfect. She doesn't resemble any of us, just her precious self. Don't you agree?"

Patient 2. "Let me tell you what happened last night. My baby was brought out with much too much wrapping. His feet were bound down, and the bottle was dripping because the nipple didn't fit right, and the nipple looked DIRTY! I had to ask the head nurse to come and change the whole thing. I'm so afraid little Jack will get sick from a nursery infection—you've heard of nursery infections, haven't you?"

Patient 3. "Here, take her. I'm too tired today. You feed her. I'm here for a rest—why can't I just have her fed in the nursery until I go home?"

Patient 4. "My mother nursed all three of her children and wants me to nurse Joanie. I've tried, but just don't have any luck. Don't you think I've tried long enough?"

Patient 5. "Look, I have another book on child psychology; my best friend sent it. She knows I want to raise Mary just right. I've always admired children with good manners, and I'm going to teach mine right from the start. Look at how she spit up some milk. Hand me that cloth. I'll wash her off. She can't be messy, not *my* baby."

6. Plan for a clinical experience.

▲ Ask multipara patients to identify what worried them after they went home (e.g., baby's care, their own physical condition). What nursing actions helped them most? Least?

▲ Talk with a father; include him in child care instructions. Teach him to diaper, take an axillary temperature, position the baby for feeding, burp the baby, and position the baby in the crib, and also teach the use of the bulb syringe. Demonstrate all these infant care tasks and follow up with a return demonstration from the father.

▲ Read charts of selected obstetric patients who (a) have signs of neurotic mechanisms and/or (b) were discharged following symptoms of blues or psychosis. Think about how you might have assisted these patients.

▲ Make rounds with your instructor to all postpartum patients. Observe how the instructor relates to the patients and assesses them.

▲ Take babies to their mothers. Stay with them during feedings (both breast and bottle feedings for comparisons). Look for maternal attitudes and success experiences. Take time to listen and help the new mothers. You need not wait to be asked!

▲ Identify behaviors that would indicate how a new mother is adjusting to her mothering role, using an assessment tool.

▲ Make rounds with the staff nurse in postpartum or your instructor to assess mother-baby, parents-baby, or family-baby interactions. Observe how the nurse relates to the mother, father, relatives, and siblings. Observe how all people relate to each other and the baby. What nursing assessments were made and what were the nursing interventions? Evaluate the interventions. Discuss your observations in a postconference.

▲ Research the community outreach programs in your locale that will offer support and interventions for problems of postpartum that occur after discharge.

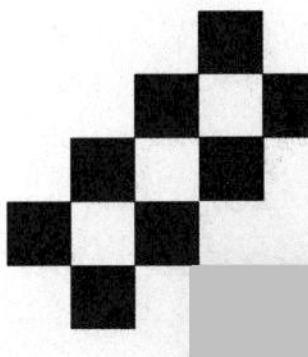

Teenage Pregnancy, Single Mother, Nontraditional Childbearing Couples, and Birth Control

Objectives

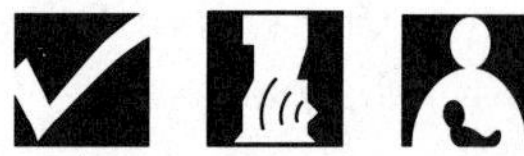

21. Describe the nursing care for single mothers and nontraditional childbearing couples.

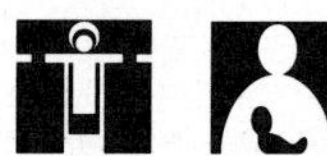

22. Identify the effects that pregnancy and parenthood have on the developmental tasks of a teenager.

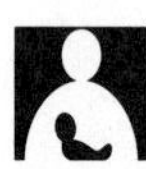

23. Compare contraceptive methods, action, and the advantages and disadvantages of each.

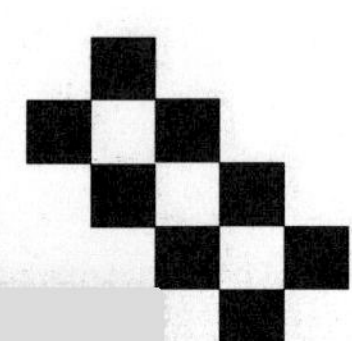

■ A. What's It All About?

1. Think about *your* own attitudes. What do single mothers, teenage mothers, unmarried childbearing couples, surrogate mothers, and mothers who relinquish or keep their infants mean to you? Many unique and complicated situations arise in maternity nursing. It is important that nurses examine their own feelings before they care for patients. The nurse is the patient advocate as well as caregiver and does not judge or give advice to patients. Instead the nursing role is to provide information and clarification, and then to support the patient in her decision.

2. Read about *single mothers, surrogacy, lifestyles, nontraditional childbearing couples, adoption,* and *birth control* in maternity, sociology, psychology, and nurse-patient relationship references.

3. View audiovisuals and read articles and books from a list given you by your instructor.

4. Answer the following questions:

> **(a)** What special needs might the following single mothers have during their pregnancy, labor and delivery, and postpartum period?
>
> **(b)** Where will they find such assistance in your community? Include medical, legal, and psychosocial care.

16-year-old teenager

28-year-old widow

32-year-old lesbian

36-year-old executive

30-year-old divorcée

25-year-old surrogate

22-year-old college student

21-year-old secretary

5. Attend a large group session by a social worker from a child protection agency in your community on "Care of the Single Mother" or a session by a speaker from the Planned Parenthood Association.

■ B. Putting It into Action!

1. Describe the manner in which each of the following measures works as a method of contraception. Then, give one advantage and one disadvantage of each.

Cervical cap
Oral contraceptive
Coitus interruptus
Billing's method
Basal body temperature method
Intrauterine devices (IUD)
Norplant
Rhythm or calendar method
Vasectomy
Vaginal diaphragm with spermatocidal jelly
Vaginal spermicide
Vaginal sponge
Tubal ligation
Condom
Female condom

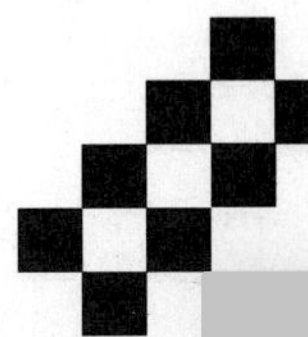

LEG VIII-B

2. Attend a group discussion led by your instructor on the "Resumption of Sexual Intercourse after the Birth of a Baby."

- Discuss anticipatory guidance and teaching that will be helpful for the couple.
- Role play a discussion between the newly delivered mother and the nurse.

3. Attend a small group discussion on "Therapeutic Communication with a Teenage New Mother."

■ Read about the effects of pregnancy on an adolescent. Discuss how pregnancy superimposes a maturational crisis onto the adolescent.

Comments on Being Available

Patients need to talk about their concerns. If they have little or no contact with a social worker, you may be their only professional contact. You must make the most of your time in helping them talk about their concerns.

■ Role play situations between a maternity patient and a nurse or a couple and a nurse with both satisfactory and unsatisfactory outcomes. Develop scenarios in which the nurses have different values or expectations for childbearing and childcare than the patient couples. As you role play, experiment with the following nurses' reactions after the patient leaves an opening for the nurse.

Nurse avoids the opening.

Nurse gives an opinion.

Nurse asks patient to explore the area left open.

Nurse does not explore the area left open.

Nurse judges the patient.

Nurse puts patient at ease.

Nurse makes patient feel guilty by words or mannerisms.

Nurse imposes own values.

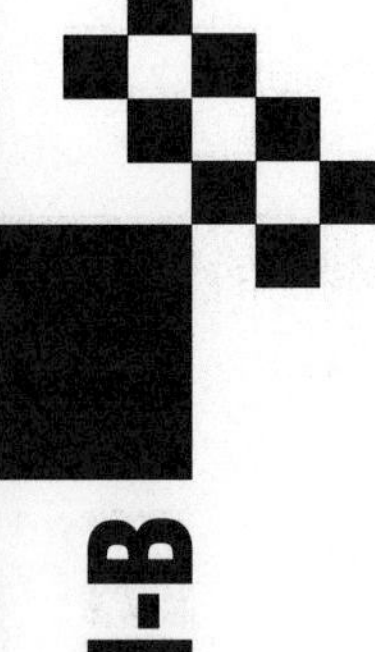

LEG VIII-B

4. Write a thought paper about your attitude, or changes in attitude, about birth control, and changing mores regarding lifestyle and childbearing.

5. Plan for a clinical experience.

▲ Care for one or more single and/or teenage mothers.

▲ Discuss methods of contraception with your patients in postpartum.

▲ Discuss the resumption of intercourse with your patient in postpartum. Listen to the concerns of your patient.

▲ Identify your community resources for social services, home health care, legal assistance, public health management, and other supportive agencies for special childbearing and childcare needs. Visit at least two of these agencies.

▲ Read about Margaret Sanger and her role in the birth control movement. Discuss in postconference the influence of her activities on the lives of women today.

Helping a Family Deal with Loss of Health or Life of Infant

E x t r a A d d e d
O b j e c t i v e

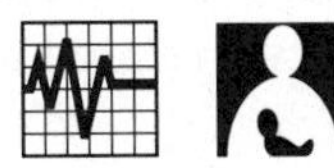

24. Identify the needs of the patient and family when faced with the loss of the newborn, a premature infant, or a newborn with a physical anomaly.

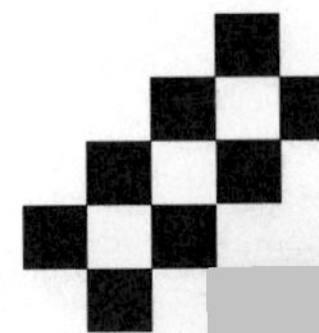

LEG VIII-B

■ A. What's It All About?

1. **Think about** the phases of grief. This time the grief takes place in the maternity unit, where most experiences are very happy. How do nurses care for patients, couples, and their families in grief situations in maternity? You will have an introduction to this very important component of maternity nursing.

2. **Review**:

   LEG IV-C Caring for the Dying Patient
   LEG VI-A Crisis, Grief, and Psychoneurotic Disorders

3. **Read** about *grief, grief in maternity, abortion, stillbirth, preterm infants,* and *infants with physical anomalies,* in maternity references.

4. **View** audiovisuals and read articles and books from a list given you by your instructor.

5. **Preview** LEG XI-A, High-Risk Neonates.

6. **Answer** the following questions:

   (a) How are grief situations in maternity different from those on the medical-surgical unit?

   (b) How can giving birth to a child that was not the desired sex be a grief situation for a particular patient or couple?

   (c) How can the nurse assist the mother and her partner in the early stage of grief experienced in the hospital?

   (d) Can you say something wrong in a maternity grief situation?

7. **Attend** a lecture on "Grief in Maternity" given by your instructor or another expert in the field.

■ B. Putting It into Action!

1. **Attend** a small group discussion "Helping Grieving Parents."

■ Discuss your readings and feelings about maternal reactions to the problems listed in Objective 24. Some of the group members may have had experiences of their own to contribute to the group.
How do men and women work through grief differently?
How does grief work differ for the mother and the father?
How can the couple help each other?

2. Plan for a clinical experience.

▲ Accompany your instructor or an experienced maternity nurse as she cares for a mother in a maternity grief situation.

▲ What are the ways in which patients in grief situations are identified by the staff on the unit? What particular interventions are expected in the policies related to maternity grief situations in your medical facility?

▲ Visit the mother of a premature infant. What are her special worries? Would you consider this a crisis for the mother? Note the Apgar score of the premature infant. Help this mother work through her grief reaction as you give her physical care. Does she deny the problem? How can you bring it up and discuss it with her?

▲ Talk with the mother of a stillborn or a child with a defect. Be available during visiting hours. Talk with the father. What are your own reactions to this situation?

Note: You will have more experiences with parents with complicated pregnancies next semester. Review this LEG then; look ahead now.

Have I Learned?

The following questions are for you to answer in order to find out if you have met the Objectives. All of the Objectives in LEG VIII-B are covered in this series of questions. Pick a quiet time and answer them. Answers are found at the end of this selftest.

No space has been left for answering the questions related to the "doing" Objectives. Use a separate sheet of paper for those answers, and then use the answers in clinical or campus lab for your own evaluation.

Objective	Question
1	**1.** What physiologic changes occur in each of the following systems: reproductive, vascular, endocrine, GI, urinary, and muscular (abdominal)?
2	**2.** Complete a nursing care plan on a normal postpartum patient.
3	**3.** Describe a nursing measure for each: hemorrhoids, engorgement of a lactating mother, episiotomy, urinary retention, constipation.
4	**4.** List the postpartum checks and steps you would take when you give or teach peri care to a new mother according to the criteria in Objective 4; demonstrate this.
5	**5.** Identify two oxytocics that could be given to a woman who delivered a female infant, weight 9 lb 7 oz, 1 hour ago. Her labor was 20 hours long. The mother has no other problems except for the signs and symptoms of beginning postpartum hemorrhage. Add to your answer the possible routes of administration, dosage, and rationale for why these particular drugs would be used in this case.
6	**6.** List at least five physical characteristics of a normal newborn.
6	**7.** How does fetal circulation differ from newborn circulation?
6	**8.** Describe the periods of reactivity.
6	**9.** Describe eight major reflexes of the neonate.
6	**10.** What are normal vital signs for the neonate?
6	**11.** What are the normal blood values for the following lab tests? white blood count platelets hematocrit hemoglobin Dextrostix
6	**12.** What is the importance of heat production, temperature regulation, and the effects of cold stress on the neonate?
7	**13.** List the steps you would take to teach and assist a new mother to nurse her baby.
8	**14.** List the steps you would take to teach and help a new mother to give her baby formula.
9	**15.** Give an example of lactation suppression using a nonmedication method.
10	**16.** Describe the Apgar system of evaluating a newborn.
11	**17.** List the steps you would take to admit a newborn to the nursery.

LEG VIII-B

11 **18.** Billy Jake is a 6-hour-old infant who weighs between the 20th and 40th percentile of weight for babies who have the physical and neurologic characteristics of 39 weeks' gestation. What is Billy's estimated gestational age?

12 **19.** List the steps you would take when giving care to a newborn.

13 **20.** List the steps you would take to teach a parent about infant care.

14 **21.** How does the "taking-in" process begin to prepare the mother for the next step in the development of mothering?

15 **22.** Describe in your own words the following patient's attitude toward her new role as a mother. (Questions 22–25 refer to the following situation.)

> Mrs. N. M. is a college student. She had hoped she would complete the semester before delivery, but the baby came 3 weeks early. She is 2 days postpartum and is to be discharged tomorrow morning. During morning care you overhear these comments to her roommate: "Tom and I won't graduate together now. My folks warned me about this. Tom is so thrilled about the baby; he doesn't understand how hard it's going to be for me. Oh, I guess I shouldn't say that, my baby is so sweet."

15 **23.** Use an assessment tool. What additional information do you need about this situation to be helpful to Mrs. N. M.?

15 **24.** How can you obtain this information?

16 **25.** List several emotional needs of this new mother. Write what you would say to Mrs. N. M. to help her recognize her own changes in needs.

17 **26.** Identify which of the following symptoms are characteristic of (a) psychosis and (b) the blues:

- **(a)** temporary depression
- **(b)** excessive anxiety
- **(c)** fatigue
- **(d)** letdown feeling
- **(e)** discomfort
- **(f)** excessive talkativeness
- **(g)** amnesia about delivery
- **(h)** sleeplessness
- **(i)** crying
- **(j)** irritability

18 **27.** Identify the clues of disinterest, preoccupation with self, and/or complete preoccupation with the infant for patients 1–5 on p. 312.

19 **28.** Plan and write two actions you would take to help the mother in the situation below have an early success experience in caring for her baby. You receive the following report on your patient:

> Mrs. N. S., 2 days postpartum, is to be discharged tomorrow. The baby falls asleep while she is eating, and she usually finishes her bottle in the nursery. Your assignment is "Give A.M. care to Mrs. N. S."

20 **29.** Care for a postpartum patient. Write a nursing care plan on your patient. Select at least one positive nursing diagnosis as well as two nursing diagnoses that focus on physiologic problems and one psychosocial problem.

21 **30.** Care for a single mother in antepartum, intrapartum, or postpartum. Develop a nursing care plan for her with three nursing diagnoses.

22 **31.** What are the effects that pregnancy and parenthood have on the developmental tasks of a teenager?

23 **32.** What is the action of the oral contraceptive pill?

24 **33.** What are the needs of the patient and family when faced with the death of a newborn, a premature baby, or a newborn with a physical anomaly?

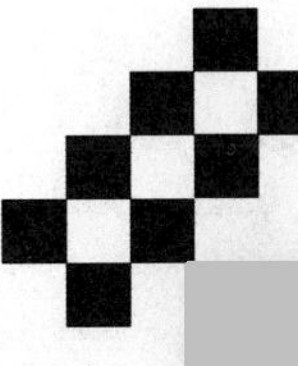

Answers to Have I Learned?

LEG VIII-B

1. *Reproductive system:* Involution; weight of uterus decreases from 500 gm at the end of the first postpartum week to 100 gm at the end of the third week; fundus decreases in size; lochia progresses from rubra to alba in about 10 days; ovarian function begins; cervix and vagina begin to regain their tone, although never to the pregravid state.

Vascular: Declining blood volume with increase in hematocrit; the blood volume is generally back to prenatal amount by third week; blood clotting factors are activated—predisposes to thromboembolism.

Endocrine: Hormones produced by trophoblastic cells are reduced; adrenal function becomes normal soon after delivery; thyroid function returns more slowly.

Gastrointestinal: Patient is usually hungry; bowel function may be delayed several days due to decreased muscle tone, diarrhea before delivery, or fear of pain from episiotomy or hemorrhoids.

Urinary: May be marked diuresis within 12 hours of delivery; kidney function and ureteral dilatation are greatly improved during the first month; bladder may be bruised and edematous; urinary retention must be anticipated and prevented; the bladder is easily distended after birth, and the mother may have decreased sensation that she needs to void.

Abdominal muscles: Regain tone and prenatal length. Laceration (pelvic floor) and overdistention may cause delay.

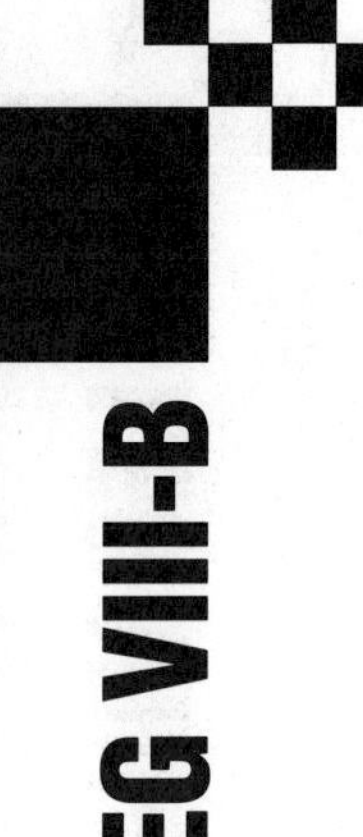

2. Check your plan with another student or with your instructor.

3. *Hemorrhoids:* Cold witch hazel compresses; sitz bath; local anesthetic spray or ointment; hot or cold water.

Engorgement of lactating mother: Massage breasts; put baby to breast often; warm compresses; instruct the mother to wear a proper-fitting and supportive bra throughout the day and night.

Episiotomy: Redness, edema, ecchymosis, discharge, and approximation (REEDA)—the five criteria for assessment; apply heat or cold; sitz baths and showers; cleansing; anesthetic sprays or ointment.

Urinary retention: Check every 2–4 hours, assist to void; keep good records on amount voided; place on intake and output; assess fundal height before and after voiding.

Constipation: Stool softeners and/or laxatives first or second day; exercise; roughage in diet; good fluid intake. Suppository or enema may be needed after third day.

4. Use your list as a checklist as you demonstrate doing a postpartum check.

5. Give your answers concerning postpartum oxytocic choices and rationale to your instructor for evaluation.

6. Healthy color; good strong cry; heart rate 120–160 per min; well-flexed extremities; good muscle tone; irritable reflexes, milia, erythema toxicum, caput succedaneum.

7.

	Fetal	*Newborn*
Umbilical arteries	Patent	Functionally closed
Umbilical vein	Patent	Closed
Ductus venosus	Patent	Closed
Ductus arteriosis	Patent	Closed
Foramen ovale	Valve opening	Functionally closed

8. *First period:* Infant appears alert, eyes open; vigorous cry; sucks fist. Ideal time for being introduced to mother and father and to breastfeeding. After about 30 min the neonate may become less responsive and go to sleep.

Second period: Awakes from deep sleep; alert and responsive. It takes *observation* by the nurse to identify normal and abnormal activity during these periods. Some of the patterns seem erratic. Monitors cannot make judgments. This period lasts 2–5 hours and provides another get-acquainted time for parents and baby.

9. Your answer may include these and others:

Corneal reflex (blinking)	Babinski
Pupillary reaction	Moro
Nose: sneezing	Startle
Mouth: sucking	Tonic neck

10. *Temperature:* Axillary, 36.5–37°C (97.7–98°F).
Heart rate: Apical, 120–140 per minute.
Respirations: 40–60 breaths per minute.
Blood pressure: Systolic, 60–80 mm/Hg; diastolic, 40–50 mm/Hg.

11. *White blood count:* 9,000–30,000.
Platelets: 100,000–300,000.
Hematocrit: 44–64%.
Hemoglobin: 14–20.
Dextrostix: 45 mg% or greater.

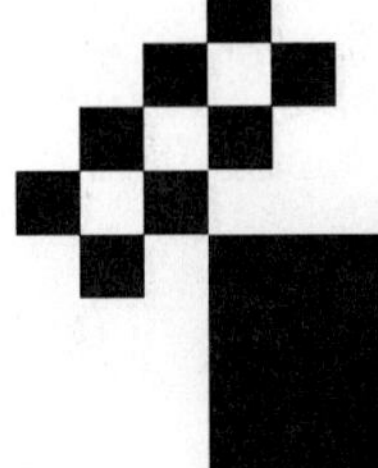

12. *Heat production:* Shivering mechanism is usually not operable. Brown fat (rich vascular and nerve supply) produces almost 100% of the neonate's heat. Brown fat is rapidly depleted by cold stress.

Temperature regulation: Thermal insulation is less in neonate. Blood vessels are closer to skin surface, vasomotor control is not well developed. Sweat function is very little before fourth week. Neonate has a larger body surface per weight ratio. All of the above make temperature regulation precarious at best.

Effects of cold stress: Oxygen consumption and energy are diverted from normal brain cell and cardiac function in order to create heat for the neonate. Vasoconstriction may follow, causing abnormal arterial blood gases. For temperature control the neonate must depend on you to keep an even, optimum environment.

13,14. Evaluate your listed steps with at least one other student. Use them as checklists for helping a new mother.

15. Apply ice packs to the breast. Wear a breast binder or supportive bra, and do not stimulate the breast.

16. The Apgar system is a simple, accurate, and safe means of quickly evaluating the condition of the infant. Five signs, in order of importance, are heart rate, respiratory effort, muscle tone, reflex irritability, and color. Each sign is evaluated according to a score of 0, 1, or 2. This evaluation is done at 1 min and 5 min after birth. Note very carefully low scores on infants and observe the infant so that you can evaluate a newborn accurately.

17. Compare your list with at least one other student. Use it as a checklist to evaluate your nursing actions as you admit an infant to the newborn nursery.

Did you include giving vitamin K, weighing the neonate, assessing the condition of the skin, cord, vital signs, color, gestational age assessment, physical exam, eye prophylaxis?

Did you consider minimizing heat loss from the neonate? Did you chart?

18. Term AGA.

19. Evaluate your steps against your nursing actions with at least one other student.

20. Evaluate your steps of teaching a parent about infant care with at least one other student. Use it as a checklist as you carry out the procedure.

21. The "taking-in" process allows the mother to review her pregnancy and labor and delivery. This is a time for rest and physiologic and emotional nurturing so that the mother will be able to go into the next phase successfully.

22. She is resentful of the interruption of her career goals. She feels her husband can't appreciate her problems or feelings. She feels guilty because of those feelings.

23. Find out how Tom really feels. Find out more on each of the patient's feelings stated in Question 22. Did you use an assessment tool?

24. Talk with Tom and listen to his feelings. Take time to talk with the patient.

25. Acceptance of feelings of resentment, recognition as a new mother, satisfaction and success as a new mother.

"I overheard you talking to your roommate about not being able to finish the term at school. You must have mixed feelings about your baby and school."

and/or

"Do you feel guilty about wishing the baby had arrived a little later?"

and/or

"Are you thinking: 'Lucky ol' Tom, this won't change his life very much'?"

and/or

"Seems like you've been doing all the adapting, and instead of giving *you* the recognition, all he talks about is the baby."

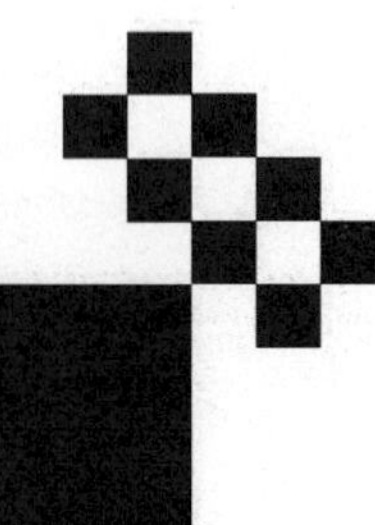

26. *The Blues:* (a), (c), (d), (e), (i). *Psychosis:* (b), (f), (g), (h), (j); all excessive.

27. Clues:

Patient 1: "Every feature is just perfect." Excessive preoccupation with infant? Keep alert; could be natural pride; could be more.

Patient 2: Long list of concerns—remembered in detail. Follow this up to find out validity of concerns.

Patient 3: "... too tired." "I'm here for a rest." Disinterest? What more will you look for? What day postpartum did this occur? Why is this important?

Patient 4: "*My* Mother ... *I've* tried ... " Preoccupation with self? Find out what's behind these comments, may be normal response.

Patient 5: "She can't be messy, not *my* baby." Preoccupation with self? Observe mother-infant relationships.

28. Plan time to talk with Mrs. N. S. about infant feeding to determine her thoughts, feelings, and knowledge about it. Plan to be there when the infants are brought out of the nursery; observe, make some specific suggestions, and give praise. Talk to the nurses in the nursery to encourage them to reinforce the teaching and give support to this mother.

29. Complete your care of the postpartum patient and submit your nursing care plan to your instructor for evaluation.

30. Complete your care of the patient in antepartum, intrapartum, or postpartum. Submit your nursing care plan to your instructor for evaluation.

LEG VIII-B

31. *Teenage tasks:*

Achievement of new and more mature relations with age mates of both sexes: finds herself isolated from peer group.

Achievement of a feminine social role: limits feminine role to one of procreation; becomes overt adult sexuality; opportunities for social development are given up or delayed.

Achievement of independence from parents and other adults: her move toward independence comes to an end, although many teenage mothers do achieve independence with assistance in later years.

Teenage pregnancy tasks:

I am pregnant: The usual response is denial; postponement of medical care.

I am going to have a baby: Happy, cuddly baby is fantasized; baby is not seen as a growing child.

I am going to be a parent: The most difficult task. She has very little life experience to help her toward this reality. She is still growing up herself.

Teenage parenthood tasks:

Reconcile actual child with fantasy child.

Establish the newborn as a being separate from herself.

Needs to become adept in the care of the infant.

Establish a place for the neonate within the family group.

The teenager has many of these needs for herself, and needs more help than she really wants from other adults, including her parents.

32. The oral contraceptives estrogen and progestin inhibit release of the ovum by decreasing the secretion levels of FSH and LH. The cervical mucus is also affected by high levels of progestin and is inhospitable to sperm.

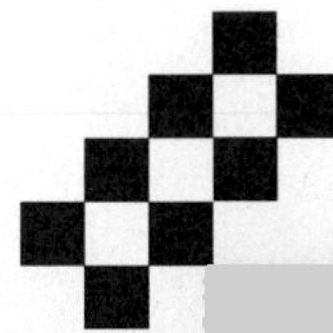

33. Acknowledgment of their grief, support in their grief.
Mourning the loss of the perfect baby.
Immediate diagnosis and management of the neonate.
Clinical evaluation and diagnosis of the causes of the infant's problem.
Preparation and planning for care.
Redefinition of their parental role in their society.
Family planning and genetic counseling.

What Will I Learn?

LEG VIII-C Gastrointestinal Problems

We are what we eat. So the saying goes, and you will soon see that the gastrointestinal body system is very responsive to stress and the regulatory processes. You may need to review the way in which food and diet affect the body. This **Body System** responds to both medical and surgical measures. You will learn how to help with both.

Not only can surgery and hospital admission be seen as a *crisis* situation, but so can certain gastrointestinal problems (e.g., jaundice, colostomy). You will learn what is involved and how to help patients adapt to their limitations and the inevitable body image changes that result.

The ulcer patient and the ulcerative colitis patient have problems of adaptation that may tax the most knowledgeable and empathetic nurse. All of these patients need you, so get involved! Take every spare minute to go in and visit or sit with these patients. Find out how they feel; let them know that you care and are willing to help.

Consider *all age groups.* Many of these patients have a relatively short hospitalization. Don't let yourself fall into the pattern of ignoring the "quiet wheel." The quiet wheel needs oiling to keep it running smoothly just as much as the "squeaky wheel" needs it. You can't wait for your patients to call you; some of them will never call even though they need you, and others will call so often that you'll stop hearing them. The trick is to be so well informed and alert that you can anticipate and give care before you are asked or even if you are not asked!

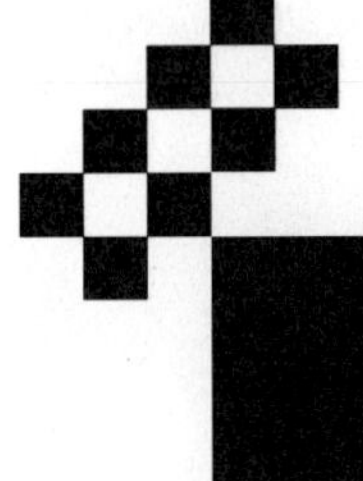

This LEG will give you a chance to review LEGs VII-A and VII-B and apply those Objectives to surgical nursing care and care of patients with fluid and electrolyte disturbances. Some time may have elapsed since you studied those LEGs, so this will be a good refresher before you finish the term.

LEG VIII-C

What's Ahead in Later Legs

In Volume III you will continue to study patients with GI problems.

LEG IX-A	Anorexia and Bulimia
LEG IX-C	Teaching Patients with Ileal-Conduits
LEG X-A	Helping Convalescent Patient after Colostomy
LEG X-B	Care of Patient in Hepatic Coma
LEG XIII-C	Care of Patient with Pancreatitis

Overview of Learning Experiences in LEG VIII-C

Objectives	Campus Lab/ Self-Practice	Group Discussions/Lectures	Clinical Lab Focuses
Admission and Assessment			
1. Admitting patients with alterations in GI function **2.** Physical assessment of patients with GI problems **3.** GI diagnostic tests	**B6.** Physical assessment of abdomen and GI system Admission to short-stay unit	**B1.** Interpreting diagnostic studies **B3.** Admission of patients with alteration in GI functioning GES Objectives 1,2	**B7.** Admit patient with alteration of GI functioning Practice assessment skills Auscultate for bowel sounds Write NCP Observe diagnostic procedures Talk with patients about what diagnostic tests feel like Observe endoscopy Care for babies and young children Collect stool specimens
Nutritional Needs and GI Problems			
4. Diet therapy in GI problems **5.** Caring for a patient receiving hyperalimentation therapy	**B5.** Role play dietary assessment	**B4.** Solving nutritional problems for patients with alterations of GI system	**B6.** Observe special diets Talk with patients about diet Make a dietary assessment Visit diet kitchen Help patients select food from a menu Observe and assist in care of patients with hyperalimentation Observe insertion of central venous line for IV nutrition
Pharmacology			
6,7. Pharmacology			**B4.** Complete drug cards on GI medications Talk with pharmacist Talk with patients about drugs
Nursing Care of GI Patients Receiving Conservative Medical Therapy			
8. Using the nursing process with patients receiving conservative medical therapy **9.** Teaching and discharge planning for patients with GI problems		**B3.** Caring for patients with GI problems	**B4.** Observe patients who show demanding or hostile behaviors Observe and talk with patients with GI problems Observe patients of all ages; pediatric and adolescent units Care for patient with GI alterations Write NCP

■ Overview of Learning Experiences in LEG VIII-C (cont.)

Objectives	Campus Lab/ Self-Practice	Group Discussions/Lectures	Clinical Lab Focuses
Hepatitis and Infection Control Measures **10,11.** Nursing care for patients with hepatitis		**B2.** Care of patients with hepatitis and jaundice.	**B3.** Admit a patient into room set up for infection control. Care for patient Care for a patient with jaundice Write drug cards
The Nursing Process and GI Surgical Patients **12,13.** Caring for patients with GI surgery **14.** Assessing for complications following GI surgery		**B6.** Care of patients having surgery	**B7.** Observe patients after GI surgery Care for patients with GI surgery Write NCP Look for patients with distention Care for pediatric surgical patients
Wound Care **15.** Changing surgical dressings **16.** Irrigating a wound	**B2.** Applying dressings Wet-to-dry dressings Irrigating and packing a wound		**B4.** Assist with or observe a dressing change, wound irrigation, wound culture Change a dressing Evaluate patients' conditions
Ostomy Care **17.** Emotional needs before a colostomy **18.** Caring for a patient with a colostomy		**B1.** Concerns of a patient scheduled for a colostomy	**B4.** Care for patients with colostomies Examine types of colostomy appliances Talk to an enterostomal therapist about colostomy care Talk with patients facing colostomy Review Clinical Performance Expectations

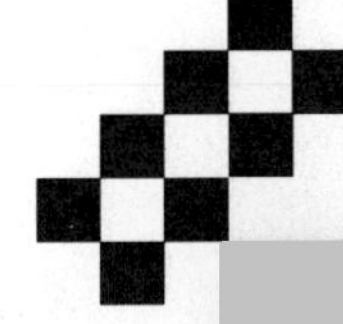

New Terms

adhesions
anastomosis
asterixis
borborygmus
deglutition
enterostomal
extrinsic
flatulence
hematemesis
hematochezia
hepatic
herniation
icterus
idiopathic
ileus
incarceration
intractable
intrinsic
jaundice
lactase
lactose
malabsorption
malaise
mastication
melena
obstipation
occult
organomegaly
steatorrhea
stoma
strangulated
stricture
subphrenic
tympany

Abbreviations

ALT
AST
Anti-HAV
bx
ERCP
GERD
GI
HAV-AB
HBsAg
HBV
HIDA
IBD
NANB
PEG
PPN
TPN

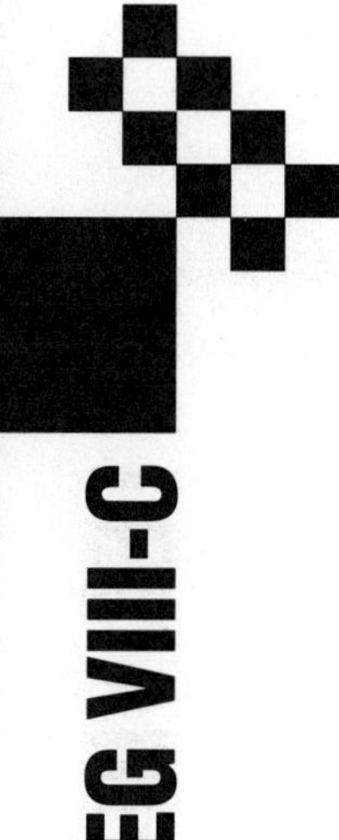

Admission and Assessment

O b j e c t i v e s

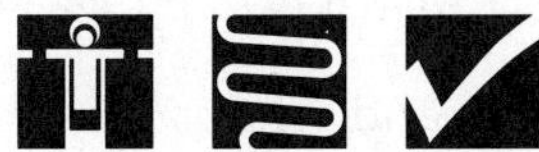

1. Demonstrate admitting a patient with an alteration in gastrointestinal function, completing the orientation and charting as required, and making at least three assessments pertinent to each health problem.

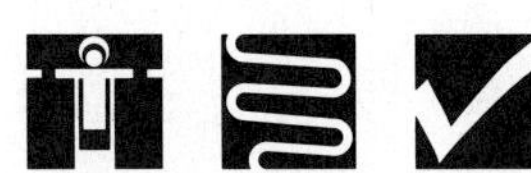

2. Demonstrate doing the physical assessment of a patient admitted with an alteration in gastrointestinal function.

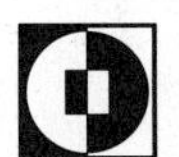 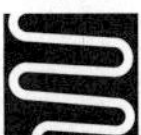

3. Given a list of diagnostic tests of the GI system, explain the purpose, and identify preparation and posttest nursing actions and rationales that are required for each test. (Your instructor will provide the list of tests.)

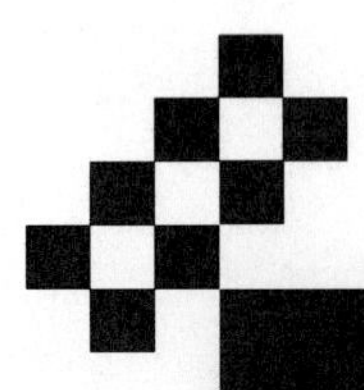

LEG VIII-C

■ A. What's It All About?

1. Think about how you feel when *you* have a disturbance of the gastrointestinal tract. What are your symptoms? Pain? Where and what kind? Nausea, vomiting, distention, excessive gas, diarrhea? Imagine how you would feel with a combination of these symptoms. Now combine those feelings with thoughts of being admitted to the hospital. What can you do to ease the anxiety and stress of the admitting process for your patient? What visual observations can you make about your patients and their condition as you go through the admitting process? How are you going to provide maximum comfort and anticipate your patients' needs?

What if you have to have diagnostic tests? Have you or someone you know waited for results? Have you heard that a test needed to be repeated because the results were not clear? How did it feel? Were you angry at the delay? Anxious that you might not be told the whole story? As a hospital patient, how concerned might you be about delays? Can it mean more money and more worry? Be careful that you don't cause delays for your patient.

How can you find out exactly how to prepare a patient for tests? How dependable do you want to be? What kind of nurse does your patient have?

2. Review:

LEG II-A Nursing Process—Assessment: Observation and Physical Assessment

LEG III-A Patient Admission

3. Read your hospital's procedure manual(s) on the *admission procedure*. List how you will modify or change each of the steps for a patient with a gastrointestinal problem. Note where you find the information that you use to modify the procedure. Make sure that your rationale for each modification is sound!

4. Read about *the anatomy and physiology of the gastrointestinal system* and *physical assessment of the gastrointestinal system* in medical-surgical, pediatrics, anatomy and physiology, and physical assessment references. Read about *GI diagnostic tests* such as *stool specimens, cholangiography, endoscopy, sonography, x-rays, gastric analysis, CT scan,* and *biopsy.*

5. View audiovisuals and read articles and books from a list given you by your instructor or read the following:

Holmgren, C. "Perfecting the Art of Abdominal Assessment." *RN,* March 1992, pp. 28–34.

6. Write what you would *do* if you observed the following stools and what *other problems* might also be present because of the stools.

A patient with ulcerative colitis has a very watery stool with streaks of mucus and a few streaks of blood.

A patient with a duodenal ulcer has a tarry stool.

An infant has severe diarrhea that resembles "currant jelly."

A patient with a possible gastric ulcer who had a GI series and a barium enema 2 days ago has a grayish-whitish, glistening stool.

A patient with a healing gastric ulcer is on Amphojel, a modified bland diet, and ferrous sulfate because of a low Hgb; he has a black, almost tarry stool.

Your patient has a fatty, frothy stool.

A 3-month-old infant has greenish liquid stools.

Your patient has a clay-colored stool.

7. Describe and give examples of problems in the GI tract caused by the following alterations:

	How It Interferes with Function	Major Problems Created
tumors		
strictures		
adhesions		
herniation		
diverticulum		
polyp		
infection		
hypomotility		
hypermotility		
hypersecretion		
hyposecretion		

8. Write the steps you will take in doing the physical assessment of a patient with either an increase or a decrease in gastrointestinal functioning. Remember, when you actually do this assessment you will need to be organized and thorough. Why are you going to listen to bowel sounds before you palpate the abdomen? What questions do you need to ask in your interview? How will your actions change if your patient is connected to NG suction? What would normal bowel sounds sound like? Hyperactive bowel sounds? If obstruction is present?

■ B. Putting It into Action!

1. Attend a small group discussion on "Interpreting Diagnostic Studies."

Come prepared to talk about the diagnostic studies on the list given you by your instructor. Note how different results can have different meanings dependent on other diagnostic study values. Review your answers to the question in B.2.

2. Write the differences in the procedure for collecting these stool specimens:

Type of Specimen	Specific Difference in Procedure
Routine stool	
Stool for parasites	
Stool for bacteria	
Stool for occult blood	

How would you collect a specimen for Cindy Carter (p. 355)? For David Kong (p. 353)? What would you do if they didn't have a stool and you needed to collect a stool culture?

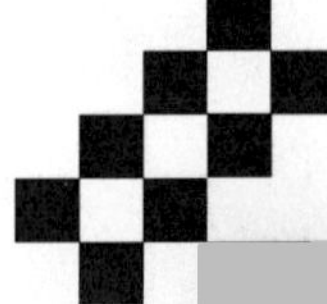

3. Attend a small group discussion on "Admission of Patients with Alteration in GI Functioning."

■ Discuss the admission and initial assessment of the following patients.
What questions would you ask to get more information during your admission assessment? Why?
What observations would you expect to make?
What observations might surprise you?
What observations would be related to fluid and electrolyte imbalance?
What special needs might each one have because of his or her age or condition?
What nursing interventions would you plan to help each of these patients because of the special needs?

LEG VIII-C

Mr. Martin Morris, 29, bleeding peptic ulcer, is admitted from the ED with the following symptoms: vomited bright-red blood just before admission; pale, clammy, nervous, and fidgety.
In ED he received Pitressin, vitamin K, and iced saline gavage.
The doctor's orders are:

I&O q8h
Guiac all stools
Amb with assist
GI series in A.M.
Hbg, Hct IN A.M.
VS q4h
Demerol 50 mg } IM q4h prn pain
Phenergan 25 }
Tagamet 300 mg po tid ac & hs

Mrs. Janet Jetson, 38, is admitted for hemorrhoidectomy. She walks as if she has extreme discomfort; appears shy and ill at ease.
Her postoperative orders are:

Colace 100 mg po bid

Demerol 50–75 mg q4h prn

Vicodin i or ii q3–4h prn

Diet as tol

I&O q8h

Encourage fluids

Sitz bath qid

CBC, PTT

VS q8h

Raj Indira, 1 month old, has been vomiting for 2 days. It is now projectile, and there have been no bowel movements for 12 hours. She is crying and irritable.
Her admitting orders are:

CBC, UA, S. electrolytes

VS q1h til stable then qid

Parents may visit any time

Offer D/5/W orally as desired

Robert Rupsure, 17, is admitted to the same-day care unit for a bilateral herniorraphy this morning. He has a history of asthma and excessive smoking. This is his first time to have surgery and he appears anxious.
His orders are:

Cefotan gm i on call to OR

NPO

Betadine prep to both groins

Hgb, Hct, PTT

Mrs. Helen Horness, 68, admitted with "possible small bowel obstruction." Her comment to you: "I'm so worried, I haven't moved my bowels in over a week, and today I began vomiting the most awful-smelling stuff."
Her orders are:

NG tube to lo intermittent suction

NPO

Permit for explor. lap; release small bowel

D/5/LR with KCl 20 mEq at 150 cc/hr

I&O

VS q4h

CT scan, chem 16

After scan, Golitely 1500 cc in 4 hr/NG tube

Cindy Carter, age 2, admitted with diarrhea, accompanied by her mother. Mother states, "Cindy has had diarrhea since two nights ago."
Her orders are:

Hct, WBC

NPO, ice chips

I&O q8h

Daily wt.

D/5/0.2 saline 90 cc/hr for 8 hr then 70 cc/hr

Add KCl 2 mEq to ea 100 cc

VS q2h

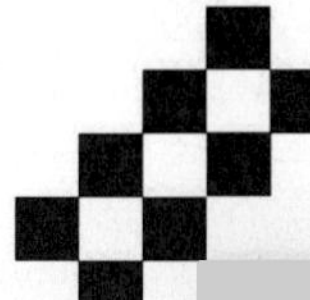

Mr. Gerald Stone, 57, has had repeated gallbladder attacks for the past 5 years. He may have surgery, but tells you, "Only if I'll die otherwise."
His postoperative orders are:

PCA Demerol

Compazine 10 mg IM q4–6h prn N/V

D/5/0.45 Saline with KCl 40 mEq at 150 cc/hr

Ancef gm i IV q8h

NPO, ice chips

NG to lo gomco

Chg dsg prn

tcdb q2h

VS q4h

I&O q8h

Amb qid

LEG VIII-C

4. Write three NCPs: one for a patient with a gallbladder problem, another with a GI problem, and a third with a rectal problem. Include a brief history collected by you when you admitted the patient. Assume that each of the three patients has at least one diagnostic test ordered. (Your instructor will provide the list of tests.) Consider each of the patient's basic needs, and emphasize only the problem areas for each patient. You may use the patients described above.

5. Consider the laboratory tests for the patients below.

Laboratory Reports for Gerald Stone			
	6/16	**6/17**	**6/18**
BUN	67	BUN 70	BUN 62
Cl	99		
Na	137	Pro Time	
K	4.9	Control 11.3	
		Patient 13.9	

Where would you look for these lab reports in the patient's chart? What symptoms would you expect the patient to have?

Laboratory Tests Ordered for Helen Horness
Electrolytes
Urinalysis
Hematology
Chem 16

When and where will you look for the results of these tests?
How can you check the implications of these tests?

Laboratory Test Results for Cindy Carter			
Hgb 12.5 gm	Hct 37	Na 137	Urine pH 5
RBC 6,500,000	WBC 6,900	K 4.4	Ketones 3+
		Bicarb 18	
		Cl 105	

What does this lab report indicate?
What signs and symptoms would you expect to find when you see Cindy?

Laboratory Test Results for Janet Jetson	
Bleeding and clotting time:	6/14 2 min 4 min

What would it mean for a patient scheduled for surgery if the results had been 5 minutes and 10 minutes?

Laboratory Results for Martin Morris			
	6/12	**After 2 Units of Blood 6/13**	**6/14**
Hgb	9.5	12	12.4
Hct	47	43	45
Stool for occult blood	4+	4+	1+

How do lab tests indicate if a patient is still bleeding?
How does dehydration affect Hgb? Hct?

Laboratory Report for David Kong	
Total serum bilirubin 3	PTT 14 sec, 46%
HBsAg +	Platelet count 71,000
Amylase 150	Reticulocyte count 1%
	SGOT 55

What do these lab reports indicate?
How will this affect your nursing care?

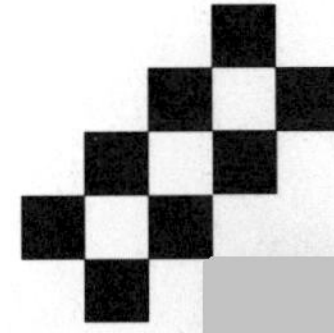

Laboratory Tests Ordered for Robert Rupsure
Routine urinalysis
Routine blood work

You fill in the tests you would want to check before you sign that Robert is ready for surgery.

6. Practice in campus lab.

■ Role play a physical assessment of the abdomen and GI system. Use the guidelines given you by your instructor.
What questions will you ask?
What will you look for when you do each of the following:

inspection
auscultation
percussion
palpation

In what order will you assess the abdomen?
What will you do if you hear no bowel sounds?
What causes hyperactive bowel sounds? Hypoactive bowel sounds?

LEG VIII-C

What is rebound tenderness? What other symptoms would the patient have?
What variations would you make in your assessment of the young child? Of the older adult? What differences will you observe?

■ Role play admitting a patient to the hospital or short-stay unit.

■ Develop a method for completing both the admission process and preoperative care and teaching of a patient in 45 minutes.
Compare each other's plans to see how to be most effective in the use of your time. When patients are admitted the same morning as their surgery, preparing them on time for surgery takes good organization and skill.

7. **Plan** for a clinical experience.

▲ Admit at least one patient who has an alteration in gastrointestinal function. Immediately after admitting the patient, write what you did; evaluate your strengths and weaknesses. Did you try to shift your weaknesses to the strengths column? Write down changes you would make for your next admission. Ask another student to evaluate your next admission.

▲ Practice your assessment skills. Select a patient who is receiving a variety of treatments to observe for 3 minutes. When you leave the room, write down everything you observed. Compare your list with another student's who has done the same thing. What are your strengths and weaknesses in observation? Repeat the experience with another patient and see if you make more accurate observations.

▲ Observe as many diagnostic procedures as possible. When your patient is scheduled for a series of tests, in what order are they to be done? Note what special precautions are taken before you are allowed to watch a radiological procedure. Listen to the explanation given by the technicians. Note how long the patients have to wait, and in what kind of surroundings. Are they comfortable? Warm? Cold? How tasty is barium? How can you tell? How do patients react to the x-ray table? How can you prepare the next patient you send to x-ray?

▲ Talk to patients to find out what it feels like to have diagnostic procedures. What happens when you are NPO several days in a row for tests?

▲ If available, observe endoscopic laser therapy for GI bleeding.

▲ Observe an endoscopy examination as an RN assists a physician. List the actions taken by the nurse before, during, and after the procedure. What medications are used? Why?

▲ Care for babies and young children in both the newborn nursery and pediatrics. Note the color and consistency of stools. Speculate as to the cause. How is stool measured?

▲ Collect stool specimens. If no specimens are ordered, "walk through" how you would have completed the procedure.

▲ Auscultate for bowel sounds.

▲ Write a nursing care plan after you have done a nursing assessment on your patient. After caring for the patient, bring the NCP to postconference to share.

Nutritional Needs and GI Problems

Objectives

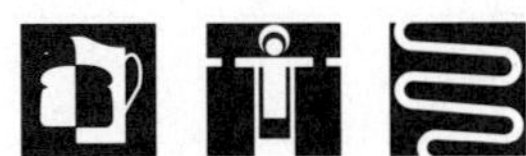

4. Describe the changes in a normal diet that would be needed to meet the nutritional needs of a patient with an alteration in the GI system.

5. Describe, orally or in writing, hyperalimentation including the nutrients administered and at least three nursing implications.

Note: You will learn more about hyperalimentation and give more complete care to patients receiving this therapy in LEG X-B.

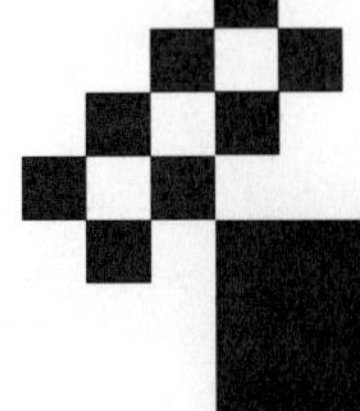

LEG VIII-C

A. What's It All About?

1. Think about how food influences your feeling of well-being (eating after hunger pangs) or feeling of not-so-well-being (overeating a big dinner or eating food that "disagrees"). What is the purpose of food? How does the body use food? When does food become especially satisfying to you? What kinds of food do you think of when you are nervous and upset? What foods are most soothing after an upset stomach? As you find out what dietary regimes are prescribed for patients with gastrointestinal problems, you will see that many common foods are used to soothe and heal the digestive tract. You will need to learn what specific factors are involved and help your patients understand the importance of sticking to their diets.

2. Review:

LEG I-B Nutrition and Nutrients
LEG II-C Nutritional Needs and Basic Diets
Measuring and Recording Intake and Output
LEG IV-C Giving Tube Feedings
Special Diets and Feeding Problems

3. Read about the *diets for GI problems* and about *tube feedings* and *hyperalimentation* in medical-surgical, pediatrics, IV, and diet references.

Look ahead to LEG X-B, Parenteral Hyperalimentation.

4. Compare the diets, desired outcomes, and nursing implications for the GI alterations listed in the following chart.

GI Alteration	Diet Change Required	Desired Output	Nursing Implications
Obesity			
Ulcer			
Celiac disease			
Colostomy			
Ulcerative colitis			
Constipation			
Diarrhea			
Hepatitis			
Cholecystitis			
Dumping syndrome			
Lactase deficiency			
Hiatal hernia			

5. Write the answers to the following questions:

(a) List two reasons a patient might receive parenteral hyperalimentation therapy.

(b) What are the nursing problems associated with parenteral hyperalimentation?

(c) List the assessments you would make on your patient who is receiving TPN.

(d) Compare the nutrients in D/5/0.9 NS, TPN, and PPN.

(e) Will the patient on TPN have normal, regular bowel movements?

■ B. Putting It into Action!

1. Plan and eat a lunch for a bland diet. How appealing do you think this menu would be to Mr. R., who is a goal-oriented man of 35, successful in business, and presently hospitalized for an ulcer? Are there any ideas you have to make the menu and the meal presentation acceptable to Mr. R.?

Plan and eat a low-carbohydrate dinner menu. What foods are suitable for this diet? Which foods did you need to reduce or eliminate from the menu? Is this diet suitable for people trying to lose weight?

What ethnic groups do you care for in your community? Will any of these patients have difficulty with the change in their diet?

What would you include in a dietary assessment?

2. Interview someone who has been hospitalized with an ulcer or gallbladder problem. If you do not know someone who can be interviewed for these problems, interview a person who has been on a weight-reduction regimen because of a physician's recommendation to do so. In your interview, try to obtain information regarding the following:

1. What type of diet was followed?
2. If the diet was served in the hospital, how satisfying was it? Were some foods on the tray ignored?
3. Did the diet include favorite foods?
4. How long was the diet followed?
5. Was there a desire to "cheat" on the diet? If so, what kinds of foods were eaten in addition to the diet?
6. What information about special diet instructions was given to the patient and to the patient's family?
7. If the diet was stopped, what was the main reason from the patient's point of view?

Present a summary of your interview at the group discussion. Look for commonalities in the reports.

Discuss how nurses can help patients and dietitians to meet the nutritional needs of patients on special diets.

3. Describe how you will plan care for the following patient with a nutritional problem, using the steps of the nursing process. You may add facts or assume certain conditions if you include them in your assessment. How will you evaluate your plan? Be specific!

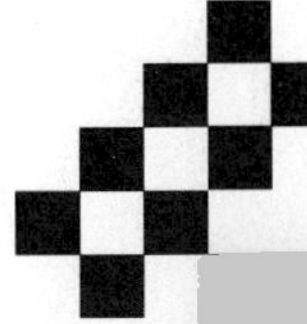

> Mr. Frank Frale, age 76, was brought to the hospital 2 days before you were assigned to give him care. A volunteer community worker had found him sitting motionless on his porch, too weak to care for himself. You note that he is quiet and does not react to his "roommate," Mr. Morris, or to general hospital routines. During report you learn that his admission diagnosis is malnutrition; his admission weight was 151 lb. (You remember he seemed tall in the bed.) The day nurse says, "He has no interest in anything; I can hardly get him to talk."

Take it from here:

Write out other facts that can be found in the admission history and write your assumptions, solutions, rationales, and evaluations.

Develop two possible alternative approaches you could use if your solution does not work.

How will you involve the patient in the decision-making process?

Bring your answers to the group discussion.

4. Attend a small group discussion on "Solving Nutritional Problems for Patients with Alterations of the GI System."

■ Write nursing diagnoses and set goals and interventions for the following patients:

> Mrs. Plum, age 27, with two small children, hospitalized for depression. She is 5'5", weighs 193 lb, and told you, "I'm so tired all I do is eat and sleep."

> Mrs. Nelson, age 51, cholecystitis and obesity; complains of severe colicky pain but just loves pork chops and bacon.

Mr. Morris (see p. 333) is on a bland diet. He hates "diet rules."

Mrs. Jetson (see p. 334), after surgery, is extremely fearful of constipation. "I have always had to take laxatives."

David Kong (see p. 353), age 30, is recovering from a severe bout of hepatitis. He is still jaundiced and has anorexia.

Mr. Ceva, age 73, is recovering from a cerebral vascular accident (stroke) and is on a soft diet. His right side is paralyzed, and he is unable to use his left hand well. His skin and mucous membranes appear dehydrated.

Baby Celia, 9 months, had a viral infection 2 months ago. Since then she has failed to gain weight and shows little interest in eating. She cries a lot and doesn't want to crawl around and play. Her stools are frothy, with a foul odor. She is admitted with possible celiac disease.

■ How and when would you decide that the problem is not solved and needs a different approach? How would you decide on alternatives?

5. **Practice** in campus lab.

■ Role play a dietary assessment on a friend or family member before your clinical experience.

6. **Plan** for a clinical experience.

▲ Observe special diets being served to patients of all ages. If you question any foods on the tray, ask about them in the diet kitchen or check the diet manual.

▲ Talk with patients about their diet. Is it appealing? Soothing? What would they prefer? How can you help?

▲ Make a dietary assessment on one patient and bring it to postconference.

▲ Visit the diet kitchen in your hospital. Look at the trays as they are prepared. Talk with the dietitian about the problems of creating therapeutic diets that appeal to patients with alterations of the GI system.

▲ Observe insertion of central venous line for IV nutrition.

▲ Help patients select foods from daily hospital diet menus.

▲ Obtain daily diet menus from your hospital; practice adapting basic menus to special dietary requirements.

▲ Observe and assist in caring for patients receiving hyperalimentation therapy. What special nursing care is required? Where is the solution prepared? What complications could occur because of the treatment?

Pharmacology

O b j e c t i v e s

 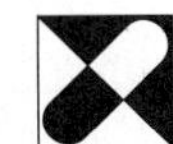

6. Given any of the following classifications—antacid, anticholinergic, anti-infective, antipruritic, hematinic, antiemetic, cathartic, antidiarrheal, digestant, vitamins, and minerals—describe the intended action/use for gastrointestinal alterations, untoward effects, and nursing implications of each.

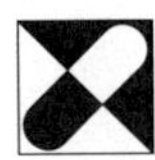

7. Given any of the following classifications—anticholinergic, H^2 receptor antagonist, analgesic, and antacid—describe how each acts differently to relieve pain.

A. What's It All About?

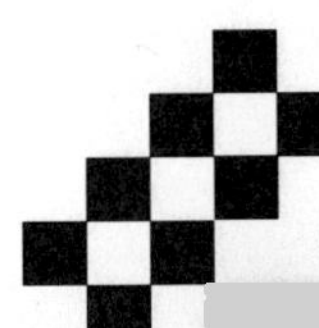

1. Think about drugs used for gastrointestinal problems. These are frequently "home remedies" and can be purchased over the counter without prescription. Look in your own medicine cabinet at home. How many do you see that fit into the classifications listed in the Objectives above? Start with these as you think about how they soothe irritated mucosal linings, curb diarrhea, sweeten "sour stomachs." Note that many of the drugs are the same as those used for other problems. Find out how certain drug classifications can fit into treatment of different types of problems (e.g., preoperative medication, asthma, and gastrointestinal problems). What GI problems can antacids cause?

2. Review:

LEG I-C Introduction to Pharmacology
LEG III-B More Drug Classifications and Calculating Dosages
LEG VI-A Antianxiety Agents
LEG VI-B Actions of Insulin and Glucagon
LEG VI-C Drugs Used for Respiratory Problems

3. Review drug classifications and answer the following questions.

(a) Review drug classifications (and specific drugs) used and discussed in other LEGs of this Volume and list the drugs that are used for more than one type of problem. For an example, see the chart on p. 344 and ask yourself: How does the amount of drug given influence its action? Look for other drugs with a variety of uses.

(b) How do soda bicarb and Alka Seltzer affect the body's buffer system? How do Maalox and milk of magnesia affect the buffer system? How do you explain this effect to a patient? Try it with someone who always takes soda for a "sour stomach."

Name of Drug and/or Classification	GI Use	Other Use
atropine	antispasmodic antisecretory	mydriatic for eye problems
morphine		
prednisone		
Tagamet		
Benadryl		

(c) Can Tagamet and antacids be given together? Can they both be given at mealtime? When should Sucralfate be scheduled?

(d) Write why each of the following drugs might be given.

Immune serum globulin
Vasopressin
Sucralfate
Imferon
Asulfidine
Heptavax B
Golytely

4. Read about the *drugs used for GI alterations* in pharmacology references. Look in the index under the drug classifications and under specific drug names and consult:

Spratto, G., and A. Woods. *RN's NDR-94 Nurse's Drug Reference.* Albany, NY: Delmar Publishers, 1994.

LEG VIII-C

B. Putting It into Action!

1. Look at the over-the-counter vitamin and mineral preparations. Note the amounts and variety included in each product. Which vitamins are stored by the body? Why is it important to note the specific vitamin content in each product? What would you say to a patient (or a child-patient's mother) if asked about taking a vitamin preparation? Which of your patients with altered GI function are likely to need supplemental vitamins and minerals?

2. Write the answers to the following questions:

(a) Which vitamin may need to be given to children who suffer with an interference with fat absorption due to cystic fibrosis?

(b) Which vitamin is found abundantly in orange juice, cabbage, and tomato juice?

(c) Which vitamin is found in abundance in milk and orange juice?

(d) Which vitamin may be lacking in premature infants and may need to be supplemented?

(e) Which vitamin is found in fish and egg yolk?

(f) Does vitamin D come "down on a sunbeam"? Explain your answer.

(g) Why do rickets (↓ vitamin D) occur more frequently in black babies in winter months than in white babies who may be outdoors with only their faces exposed?

(h) What vitamin may need to be supplemented for children who have allergies and are on a milk-free diet? What is the relationship of vitamin D to calcium?

(i) What minerals are of prime importance in ECF and ICF?

(j) Which mineral is necessary for the production of hemoglobin? When giving iron supplements in order not to irritate the gastric mucosa would you give it: after meals? once a day? three times a day? between meals (1 hour before)? Why?

(k) What replacement vitamin must often be taken by the patient who has had a gastrectomy? Why? How is it given?

(l) Name two examples of digestants.
When are these drugs most likely to be used?
Which age group is most likely to need them? Why?
What are some nursing implications when these medications are being given?

(m) List three ways antacids work.
Describe the side effects of antacids that contain:

magnesium

aluminum or calcium

sodium bicarbonate

List some nursing implications for patients taking Amphojel, Tums, Rolaids, Riopan, milk of magnesia, Gelusil, and Maalox.
Which would be better for patients with chronic constipation? Diarrhea?
For ulcer-prone patients?
Which are salt-free? Sugar-free?
Select one or more of the answers and state your rationale.

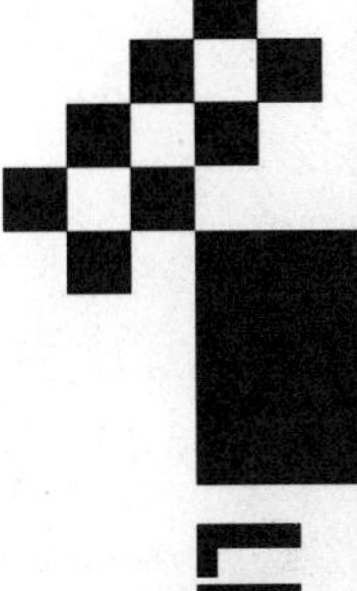

3. Note drugs listed for all patients in this LEG. Look up all of those unfamiliar to you. Be sure you know the classification and action/use in each specific instance. List at least two side effects you would watch for.

4. Plan for a clinical experience.

▲ List drugs being given to patients. Identify classifications, side effects, and expected reactions. Read charts for signs of side effects. Talk with patients. Do they know what they are getting? Should they? Which drugs are kept at the bedside and why?

▲ Give medications to groups of patients. Evaluate and compare your strengths and weaknesses with your performance at Levels Six and Seven. What areas need further practice and work? List them below. What are you doing to improve? Complete a drug card for each medication you give.

▲ Discuss the use of drugs for the GI system with a pharmacist. Find out which drugs are commonly misused by patients at home and what education patients need before being discharged.

▲ Look for patients taking Azathioprine, Vasopressin, Cytotec, Pepcid, Carafate, Prilosec, Flagyl, Hep. B immune globulin.

Nursing Care of GI Patients Receiving Conservative Medical Therapy

O b j e c t i v e s

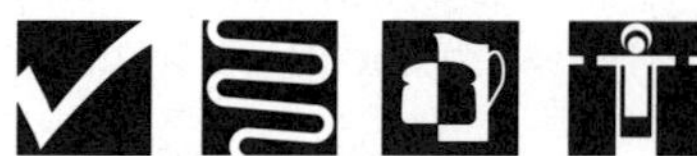

8. Given a patient who is receiving a conservative medical therapy for a problem of ingestion, absorption, and/or elimination, use the nursing process to promote wellness.

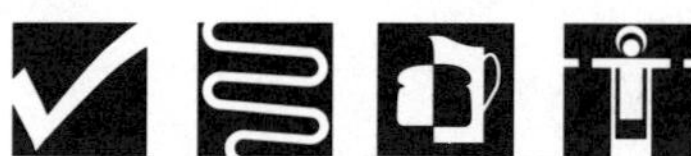

9. Given a patient who is experiencing a problem of ingestion, absorption, and/or elimination, develop a teaching plan and a discharge plan that includes the patient's nutritional needs and considers the patient and family needs and community resources available. 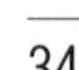

LEG VIII-C

■ A. What's It All About?

1. Think about the whole process of absorption of nutrients. This really is the reason for the process of digestion. The food we eat must be broken down for absorption to occur. What happens to the individual who has an intolerance for certain foods? What if this intolerance is to a basic substance such as *gluten,* which is found in most grains? What happens to babies who have an intolerance to lactose? How can their diet be adjusted to provide the nutrition they need to grow and develop? How would you feel if you could not drink milk or eat bread?

2. Review:

LEG II-B	Nutritional Assessment and Teaching
LEG III-A	Patient Discharge
LEG V-B	Helping a Patient Prepare for Discharge
LEG V-C	Assessment and Teaching Plan before Discharge
LEG VI-B	Diet History, Planning, and Teaching
LEG VII-A	Preoperative Teaching
LEG VIII-B	Teaching Newborn Care to a Mother

3. Read about *ingestion, absorption,* and *elimination problems, ulcerative colitis, peptic and duodenal ulcers, diverticulitis, Crohn's disease, gastroenteritis, lactase deficiency, cholelithiasis, cholecystitis, dumping syndrome,* and *upper GI bleeding* and *fluid volume deficit, metabolic acidosis, metabolic alkalosis, alteration in serum sodium and potassium* in medical-surgical, nutrition and pediatrics textbooks.

4. View audiovisuals and read articles and books from a list given you by your instructor or read from the following:

Johns, J. L. "When the Patient Has an Ulcer." *RN,* November 1991, pp. 44–51.
Meize-Grochowski, A. R. "When the Diagnosis Is Crohn's Disease." *RN,* February 1991, pp. 52–55.

5. Preview:

LEG X-B Liver Disorders
LEG XIII-B Child with Cleft Lip and Palate
Acute GI Problems of Childhood
LEG XIII-C Diabetic Crisis, Pancreatitis

6. Compare the following inflammatory conditions:

Condition	Effect on GI tract	Symptoms	Diet	Teaching Needs
Diverticulitis				
Ulcerative colitis				
Crohn's disease				
Gastroenteritis				

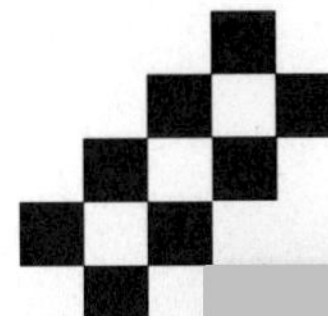

How is irritable bowel syndrome (IBS) different from colitis?

7. Describe lactase deficiency.

(a) What formula preparations would be suitable for babies with lactase deficiency?

(b) Can these babies be breast fed?

(c) List some foods that would supply the calcium needs of patients on lactose-free diets.

8. Explain why the "dumping syndrome" may occur. Describe the symptoms.
What type of diet is prescribed for the dumping syndrome?

Select from the following list those actions and foods that may contribute to the dumping syndrome. State why after each selection.

Drinking a milkshake
High-protein, high-carbohydrate diet
Rest after eating
Eat small, frequent, dry meals
Juice between meals
Consume two glasses of fluid with meals
High-protein, high-fat diet

What other actions might you take to help a patient overcome the dumping-syndrome complications? What health problems can it cause?

Compare Baby Celia's problems (p. 342) with problems of other patients who have had portions of their stomach or bowel removed. Malabsorption is a problem for both. What are the long-term diet implications? How can you help?

9. Prepare to care for patients receiving medical therapy for their gastrointestinal disturbances.

(a) Compare gastric and duodenal ulcers:

Ulcer	Location	Etiology	Symptoms
gastric			
duodenal			

(b) Name three complications of ulcers.

(c) List drugs that can cause ulcers (called ulcerogenic drugs).

(d) Name some other causes of GI bleeding.

(e) What is the nursing responsibility in life-threatening GI bleeding?

(f) To promote healing and wellness and to prevent the need for surgical intervention, it is important for the nurse to assist the patient in accepting, understanding, and adhering to the medical regime prescribed by the doctor. Complete the following chart.

Condition	Medical Regime (Include Meds)	Pain Relief	Diet	Nursing Interventions
ulcer				
diverticulitis				
cholecystitis				
cholelithiasis				

(g) What effect might the medications that patients with the conditions in the chart may be receiving have on their fluid and electrolyte balance?

(h) Name some common causes of metabolic alkalosis in GI patients.
What are the primary symptoms of alkalosis?
What fluids and electrolytes are lost with

vomiting
gastric suctioning
intestinal suctioning
ileostomy
prolonged laxative use

(i) List the normal changes that occur in the GI tract with aging.
What are the most common GI problems found in the elderly adult?

■ B. Putting It into Action!

1. Plan a gluten-free lunch for yourself. How difficult was it to do? How would you share the information you have gained with a patient? What teaching aids would you need to develop?

LEG VIII-C

2. Write a teaching plan for a patient with an alteration in GI function. Use a nutrition book as one of your resources. What type of permanent changes in eating habits must you anticipate your patient is going to have to make? Don't forget to involve other family members who might be doing the cooking. Think about the difficulties a person with celiac disease will have to face when eating in a restaurant. The next time you go grocery shopping spend some time reading labels. How many of the items you buy might contain grain byproducts? How hard is it for you to tell just what might have been added to the basic product? How will you teach your patients what they have to know?

3. Attend a small group discussion on "Caring for Patients with GI Problems."

Use your answers in A.6 through A.9 to make a NCP for each of the following patients. Be sure to include teaching and discharge needs. Compare their symptoms and nursing diagnoses.

Identify the differences in giving nursing care on the basis of their personal preferences or needs. Describe the symptoms you would expect to see and feelings or attitudes that might be displayed by the patients related to their change in body image or ways of coping with stressful situations.

Mr. John Amarillo, age 58, admitted with nausea, vomiting, and ascites.

Mrs. Helen Martin, age 28, admitted because of constant diarrhea for the last 6 months.

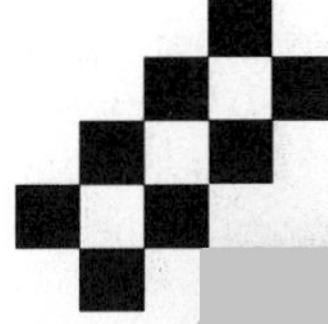

Mr. Jack Speada, age 36, admitted because of "burning, gnawing" pain in epigastric region "between meals."

Martin Morris with diagnosis of bleeding peptic ulcer (p. 333).

Cindy Carter with diagnosis of diarrhea (p. 335).

Comments on Accepting Patients' Behaviors

You have learned that patients with acute heart disease may be uncooperative, and you know you must cope with this kind of behavior because of its negative influence on the patient's recovery.

Respiratory patients are notoriously hostile. Why not, when it is such an effort to take the next breath! Such patients might easily think, "Nobody's doing anything to help me."

Your description of the colitis or ulcer patients will depend on your experiences. These are not easy or "happy" patients. They can be hostile, demanding, uncooperative, and more, all at the same time. They, too, are reacting to a crisis (hospital admission) and threat to health and to a way of life, just as are your cardiac and respiratory patients. Use your "individualized" approach to these patients.

Accept them as they are. Sit down with them when hydrochloric acid begins to shoot into their empty stomachs, and "waves" begin in the jejunum, and they complain of pain, discomfort, lack of service, or care.

Evaluate your patients' reactions to your "involvement." Think about it. Mobilize your forces and try again. Keep involved! Force yourself to go in to the patient who is not "happy" and "good" before the call light goes on. Accept the challenge of these patients to improve and strengthen your nurse-patient relationships and broaden your understanding of human behavior.

4. Plan for a clinical experience.

▲ Seek out patients who are labeled uncooperative, or demanding, making a difficult adjustment to hospital routines. Give care to these patients or just talk! Can you identify the stressors? Defense mechanisms used? What approach do you take toward the patient? List measures you are going to take.

▲ Observe and talk with patients with GI problems. Read charts and look for charting of symptoms, lab reports, and treatments.

▲ Observe patients on the children's unit, adolescents, and each adult age group and take notes on the common GI problems of each age group. Share this information in postconference.

▲ Care for a patient with ingestion, absorption, or elimination alterations or inflammatory or infectious problems. How is your patient coping with the everyday problems associated with the disease? How does the family cope? Can you offer any suggestions that will make the day-to-day coping easier?

▲ Look for patients with common bowel alterations such as constipation, diarrhea, and flatulence.

▲ Look for patients at risk for paralytic ileus, peritonitis, or parotitis.

▲ Care for patients receiving medical therapy for pseudomembranous colitis, gastritis, Crohn's disease, sprue, diverticulitis, stress ulcers, Mallory Weiss tear. Write a NCP.

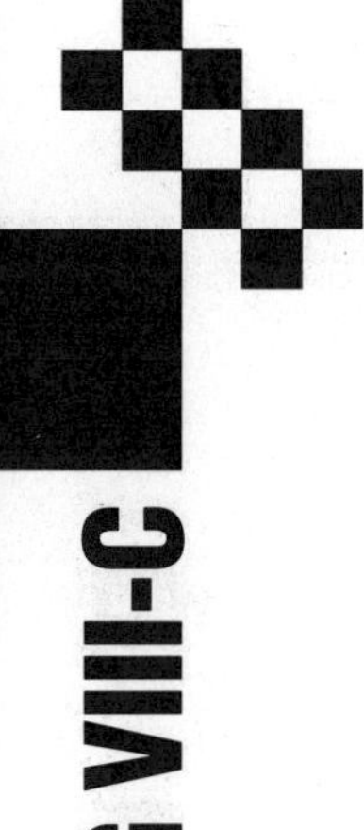

LEG VIII-C

Hepatitis and Infection Control Measures

Objectives

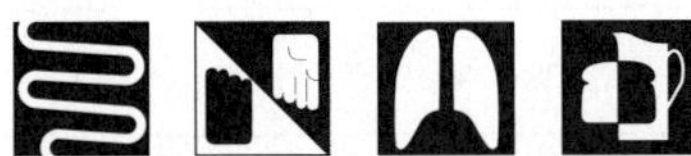

10. Compare the causative factor and nursing implications for hepatitis A, hepatitis B, and non-A, non-B hepatitis.

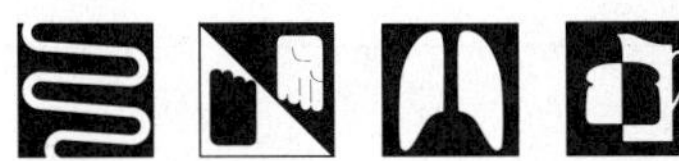

11. Given a list of nursing actions, select those that would be required for infection control of each type of hepatitis.

■ A. What's It All About?

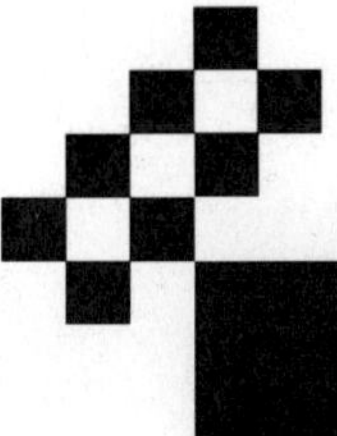

LEG VIII-C

1. Think about how diseases are spread. Refer to LEG VI-C for respiratory infectious diseases. Compare methods of preventing spread of infection from the respiratory route and the gastrointestinal routes. How does serum hepatitis differ from a respiratory infection in its means of spread? You will learn that if you know how a disease is spread and what chemicals kill the infecting organism, you can control the spread of infectious diseases. Remember, if you know the problem and can protect yourself and others from contamination, you are much safer; it is the unknown or careless practice that can harm you. Number-one rule: WASH YOUR HANDS!

2. Review:

LEG I-A Medical Asepsis

LEG III-A Immunizations and Immunity

LEG III-C Infection Control

LEG VI-C Respiratory Problems

3. Read about *types of hepatitis (A, B, C, D, E) and infection control* in medical-surgical textbooks.

4. View audiovisuals and read articles from a list given you by your instructor.

5. Preview LEG X-B, Immunological Disorders.

6. **Answer** the following exercises.

(a) Complete the chart below after you read about viral and serum hepatitis.

Hepatitis			
	Hepatitis A	**Hepatitis B**	**Non-A, Non-B**
Mode of transmission			
Carrier state			
Incubation period			
Preicterus state			
Icterus state			
Convalescent time			
Treatment			
Prevention			
Important markers			

Underline the *similarities* between each type of hepatitis in blue; underline the *differences* in red.

(b) Can hepatitis be transmitted to the unborn child? If so, what precautions are taken?
What information should a carrier receive?
Are any of these diseases reported to your local health department?

(c) Explain the cause of jaundice in the patient with hepatitis. What causes jaundice in the patient with cholecystitis?
Explain how to assess jaundice in patients with light and dark skin tones.

Comments on Jaundice

All patients with jaundice worry about how they look to others. This concern is normal and to be expected. However, the nurse needs not only to deal with the patient's concerns, but also to be alert to signs and symptoms of changes in the patient's condition. One of the best ways is for the nurse—that's you!—to be aware of the significance of the color of various parts of the patient's body and of body secretions.

The skin and sclerae may be of a different color in people of different ethnic origins. The assessment of color is one of the hardest assessments to do in nursing. Color descriptions are very subjective. Check with your classmates about the color yellow after drawing it on white paper, tan paper, and light brown paper. Do you all agree about what to call the resulting color? This is one of the many reasons that whenever possible the same nurse should do assessments on as many consecutive days as possible!

■ B. Putting It into Action!

1. **Write out** the steps you would take to admit the following patients with either hepatitis A or hepatitis B.

Mrs. Serus, age 48, was readmitted 9 weeks after being discharged from your unit after a radical mastectomy. During her previous admission she had received two units of blood in surgery. On admission this time she is quite jaundiced, feels tired, has some abdominal discomfort, and is quite discouraged about her readmission.

Mr. Fekshus, age 26, was admitted with jaundice, temperature of 99.8°, anorexia, and flatulence. The physician asked him if he had received any injections or transfusions during the past 6 months. He replied no. The doctor then asked if he had been in contact with anyone who had had hepatitis recently. He said, "Yes, a man at work about a month ago was put on sick call; come to think of it, he is still out. The rumor is that he has hepatitis."

What type of hepatitis does each patient appear to have? How do you know? How is each type transmitted? Write exactly how you would admit each patient. You may need to research your hospital policy to find out where the equipment is kept and how it is obtained. How would you collect a stool specimen in isolation?

2. Attend a group discussion on "Care of Patients with Hepatitis and Jaundice."

Review your answers to A.6 to determine the probable course of illness for the following patient:

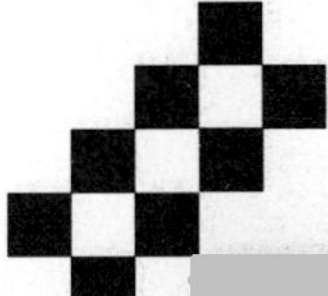

David Kong, age 30, is admitted with chronic hepatitis B. He is drowsy, slightly confused upon awakening, with a faraway look. He looks yellow and has slight asterixis of the hands. His temperature is normal. He c/o anorexia and general malaise.

The doctor orders the following lab tests: S. amylase, hepatitis serology, PTT, platelets, S. bilirubin, SGOT (AST).

David is scheduled for a liver biopsy, a GB sonogram and an ERCP.

The doctor also ordered:

Demerol 50 mg & Phenergan 25 mg q6h prn

Elavil 10 mg po tid

AquaMyphyton 10 mg/da × 6da

Tagamet 300 mg po qid

Multivit i qd

D/5/0.45 with KCl 20 mEq at 125 cc/hr

Enteric & body secretion precautions

Explain the rationale for each of the doctor's orders and for the lab tests above.

Review the isolation precautions necessary to protect the other patients from David Kong.

Identify all the potential health needs of this patient while acutely ill and hospitalized.

Identify the teaching and planning that should be initiated before discharge to prevent complications at home.

3. Plan for a clinical experience.

▲ Admit a patient into a room set up for infection control. Make notes on your feelings and the patient's feelings and behavior. Did you forget anything? How do you know?

▲ Care for a patient in a room set up for infection control. How long has the patient been in isolation? How has isolation affected the patient's morale?

▲ Care for a patient with jaundice. Observe carefully your patient's feelings and attitudes. Record your own feelings and actions. How did you feel when your washcloth "turned yellow"? Why do you think this occurred? What do you think your patient felt? Thought?

▲ Write drug cards in preparation for giving medications to patients with gastrointestinal and hepatic problems.

▲ Talk to your employee health department. Find out how many health care workers in your community have contracted hepatitis. How much disability time is generally used? How many nursing personnel have been vaccinated with the Hepatitis B vaccine? Why do health care workers refuse the vaccine? What are OSHA requirements for health care workers?

LEG VIII-C

The Nursing Process and GI Surgical Patients

O b j e c t i v e s

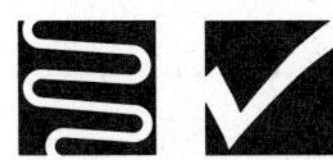

12. Write a nursing care plan for a patient before and after surgery for an obstruction of the bowel due to any of the following: tumors, intussusception, Hirschsprung's disease, pyloric stenosis, ileus, volvulus.

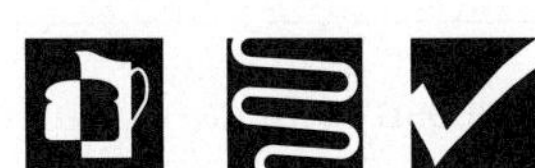

13. Describe how normal function is altered by each of the following surgical procedures, and state the nursing interventions to relieve pain, maintain adequate nutrition, and prevent complications: antrectomy, gastrectomy, Bilroth I, Bilroth II, vagotomy, colostomy, ileostomy, cholecystectomy, hiatal herniorrhaphy.

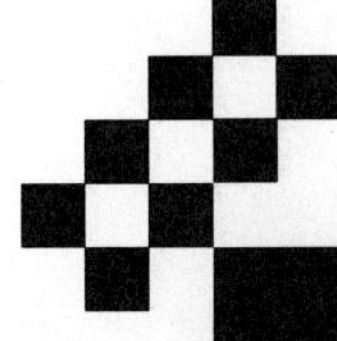

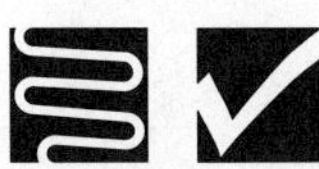

14. Select from a list, signs and symptoms that may indicate complications after GI surgery.

■ A. What's It All About?

1. Think about what surgery means to a patient. Quite a wide spectrum of thoughts and feelings! Until now you have been concerned with general surgical procedures. Now you must apply your knowledge to care of the patient facing gastrointestinal surgery. Most of the principles are the same. At this level, however, you are expected to learn how to find out what is necessary to carry out nursing actions required and to follow through with help needed in the event of emergency problems. Problems short of an emergency you may now be able to solve yourself!

2. Review LEG VII-A, Perioperative Teaching.

3. Read in medical-surgical and pediatrics references about *GI surgery and its complications, abdominal distention,* and *ileus.*

4. View audiovisuals and read articles and books from a list given you by your instructor or read from the following:

Bryant, G. A. "When the Bowel Is Blocked." *RN,* January 1992, pp. 58–67.

Willis, D. A., M. D. Harbit, and L. M. Julius. "Gallstones: Alternatives to Surgery." *RN,* April 1990, pp. 44–56.

5. Preview LEG XIII-B, GI Problems of Childhood.

6. List the common surgical procedures done in each section of the gastrointestinal tract, the changes in function, and the patients' adjustment problems that occur because of the surgery.

	Surgical Procedure	Change in Function	Patient Problems
Mouth			
Esophagus			
Upper duodenum			
Small bowel			
Large bowel			
Rectum, anus			

What does the term *acute abdomen* mean? What nursing assessments can you make?

7. List the predisposing factors, discomforts (symptoms), and/or complications that may result from herniorrhaphy, and some nursing interventions for each.

	Predisposing Factors	Symptoms/ Complications	Nursing Interventions
Hiatal			
Incisional			
Femoral			
Inguinal			
Umbilical			
Ventral			

Would you select carbonated or noncarbonated drinks for a patient with hiatus herniorrhaphy? Why? What other conservative measures are tried before surgery? On the following figure, draw the incisional line you would expect to find for hiatal hernia repair. Why might a thoracotomy be done?

Describe the pre- and postoperative care and emphasis for a patient scheduled for each type of hernia repair. Include all age groups.

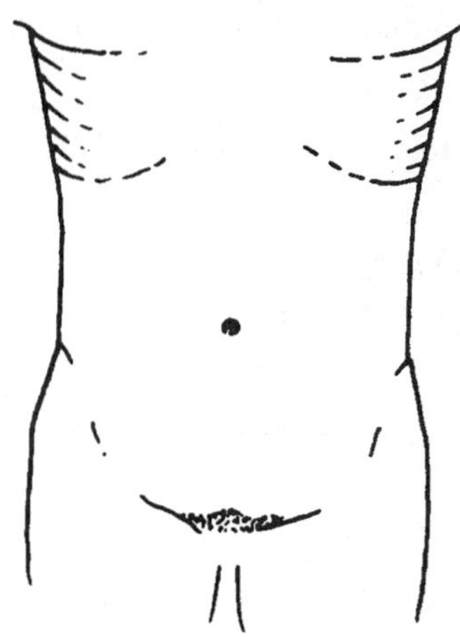

LEG VIII-C

8. Draw a picture that describes the changes made in the GI tract with each of the following surgeries.

vagotomy	antrectomy	gastrectomy	hiatal herniorrhaphy
Bilroth I	Bilroth II	colostomy	ileostomy

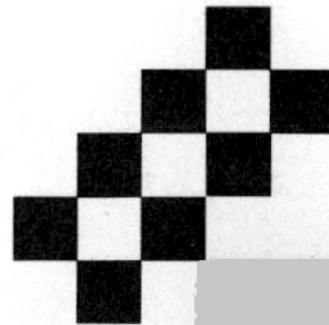

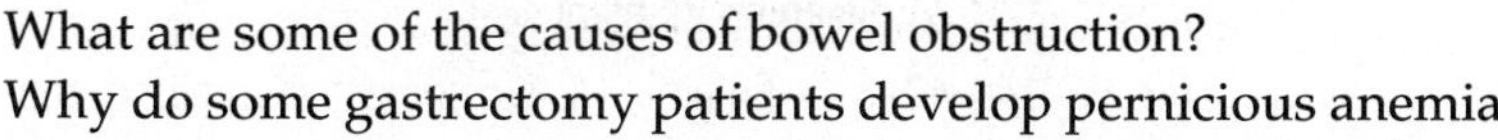

What are some of the causes of bowel obstruction?
Why do some gastrectomy patients develop pernicious anemia?

9. List the steps you could take to prepare your patient for abdominal surgery. (Use the preoperative checklist from your agency.) These steps can be taken from the time of admission until the patient goes to the OR. An example would be preparing a patient for sleep the night before surgery.

How can you best do this? How about a shower or tub bath if allowed? What about a good back rub to aid in relaxation? Fresh water and a fortified drink if allowed, until the NPO order is in effect. All of this gives you time to listen to and assess your patient's emotional state. What would you do if you were the night nurse and the patient couldn't sleep, or became anxious at 3:30 A.M.?

Add more; let yourself go with ideas to help your patient.

■ B. Putting It into Action!

1. Look below at the doctor's orders and notes on Raj Indira. Review the usual preoperative and postoperative care of a baby with pyloric stenosis.

- **(a)** What special needs would the nurse have to know about to plan patient care?
- **(b)** Make a sample chart for this patient.
- **(c)** What observations are related to fluid and electrolyte balance?
- **(d)** Evaluate the care given and identify what information is missing that prevents evaluation.
- **(e)** Did you write some outcomes before you evaluated?

Dr. Orders

3/25	Dx: Intractable vomiting
Admit	CBC, UA, S. electrolytes
	Barium swallow in A.M. R/O pyloric stenosis.
	VS qh if stable qid
	Enfamil formula per usual routine.
	Parents may visit any time.
3/26	NPO.
8:30 A.M.	Empty stomach of barium c̄ NG tube.
	Op consent for pyloromyotomy.
3:30 P.M.	Offer D/5/W orally as desired.
	Begin Enfamil as tol.
3/27	Discharge

Notes Made by Nurses While Caring for Baby Indira

3/25	Baby Indira, 1 month, admitted at 3:45 P.M. with parents. Crying, skin loose and dry; amulet beads on arms. Parents speak East Indian, very little English.
	BP—flush—67; TPR 99^4-140-40 irreg; ht 22 in; wt 8 lb, 6 1/2 oz.
	4—Strapped for urine; sucking thumb; mother here; blood specimen drawn.
	90 cc Enfamil. Projectile emesis 80 cc.
	5—Dr. here. TPR 99^2-132-32. Using pacifier.
	6—TPR 99^2-128-28: Sleeping in infant seat.
	8—TPR 99^2-140-40; 3 oz Enfamil 1/2 str, projectile vomiting, most of feeding.
	10—TPR 99^4-133-32. Awakened, 30 cc emesis.
	11—Diapers wet × 2.
	12—60 cc Enfamil 1/2 str. given slowly, retained.
	NPO for x-ray. Mother left.
	12–6—Sleeping. Diaper wet × 1.
3/26	7—Mother here. Rocking baby.
	8—To x-ray.
	9—#5 Fr feeding tube inserted. Stomach contents aspirated with 10 cc syringe; Dr. here; surg consent signed—pyloromyotomy.
	1—To OR in crib.
3:45	From OR; TPR 98-144-44; dressing dry; sleeping, arouses easily.
	4—Cries occasionally. Comforted by mother.
	6—TPR 98^2-144-42; D/5/W 60 cc retained.
	8—TPR 98^8-140-40; D/5/W 90 cc s̄ problems.
	11—Diaper wet × 2; Sleeping in mother's arms most of P.M.
3/27	12—TPR 98^8-140-40; Enfamil 1/2 str. 90 cc.
	6—Slept all night. Dressing dry. Diaper wet × 2.
	8—Mother here; Dr. here; dressing removed; steri-straps intact; wound clean.
	90 cc Enfamil taken, retained.
	9—Home with parents.

LEG VIII-C

2. Match the following three columns: Be prepared to state your rationale.

Patient Complaint or Discomfort	Medical Measures You Might Anticipate Being Ordered	Nursing Interventions You Might Use
_____ 1. Urinary retention	(a) Rectal tube	(A) Running water in bathroom
_____ 2. Constipation	(b) Stand to void	(B) Walk the patient in hall
_____ 3. Pain	(c) Catheterize prn	(C) Back rub, change position
_____ 4. Distention	(d) Ambulate bid	(D) Provide room deodorant
_____ 5. Vomiting	(e) Take BP and P	(E) Provide privacy
_____ 6. Pneumonia	(f) Demerol 75–100 mg IM prn q4h	(F) Give frequent mouth care
	(g) Ancef 1 gm q6h	(G) Plan alternate periods of nursing care with opportunities for rest
	(h) Dulcolax Supp. h.s.	
	(i) Sips of clear liquid for 4 hr, then light diet	
	(j) Frequent special mouth care	
	(k) Compazine, 10 mg IM q 3–4 h	
	(l) Turn, cough, and deep breathe	
	(m) Harris flush	

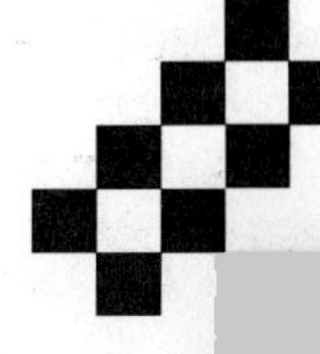

3. Match the following two columns:

Symptoms	Possible Complications
_____ 1. Pallor, drop in BP, rapid P	(a) Wound infection
_____ 2. Cold, moist, clammy skin	(b) Thrombophlebitis
_____ 3. Restlessness and thirst	(c) Dehiscence and/or evisceration
_____ 4. Sudden pinkish drainage on dressing	(d) Bleeding
	(e) Shock
_____ 5. Fever, cough, dyspnea	(f) Aspiration pneumonia
_____ 6. Redness, heat, swelling, pain in lower extremity	(g) Paralytic ileus
_____ 7. Increased pain in incision	(h) Parotitis
_____ 8. Distention and regurgitation of liquids	
_____ 9. Fever, malaise, purulent cough	

LEG VIII-C

4. React to the following (in a small group or individually). Consider that you are the nurse.

> Mr. Hamilton Bord, 56, weight 250 lb, postoperative appendectomy patient of Friday, complained of severe abdominal pain on Sunday morning—"so bad I can't tell you what it's like." Vomiting occurred, but without blood. What additional assessments would you make before notifying the physician on call? (His surgeon is out of town.)
>
> Telephone orders are received from the physician on call, who says to give him Demerol 100 mg IM q4h for pain. Keep him NPO and watch him.
>
> You are on duty. What do you think and what do you do as a concerned student? As a concerned graduate?
>
> Monday morning: You're back; his surgeon is back. After emergency surgery for a perforated bowel and peritonitis Mr. Bord is in shock. He has signs of acute systemic infection and bloody diarrhea.
>
> Three weeks later: Mr. Bord weighs 170 lb and is too weak to turn himself. As you are turning him to change the sheets (bloody diarrhea q 20 min), he shouts, "Don't turn me one more time!" That did it. Three weeks of constant hard work and all you get is abuse. You turn away in tears.
>
> Mr. Bord dies the next evening.

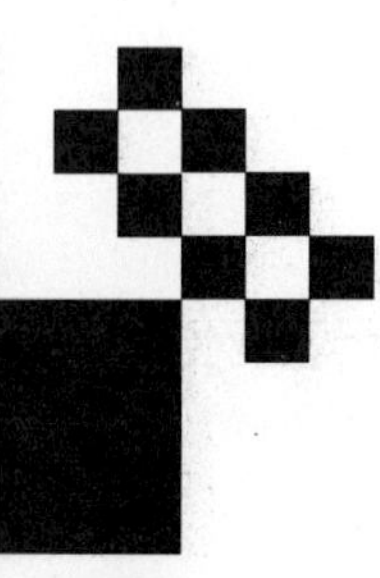

LEG VIII-C

Why did all of this occur? (It is not a make-believe story!)

■ What is the nurse's responsibility in calling the physician? List all the symptoms and nursing actions that you can think of to report in order to give the physician a picture that compels his physical presence to examine the patient:

■ Why did Mr. Bord shout at his nurse? Why did his nurse (you) cry? What could you have done?

■ How does a nurse's failure to react honestly and realistically in such a situation contribute to his final reaction? How much frustration does it take before going over the brink?

5. State what kinds of discomfort occur from distention due to the following causes:

intestinal obstruction

urinary retention

ascites

6. Attend a group discussion on "Care of Patients Having Surgery."

■ Review the care of Baby Indira (B.1) and Mr. Bord (B.4).

■ Compare the preoperative and postoperative care of these patients: Helen Horness, Gerald Stone, Janet Jetson, Robert Rupsure on pp. 334–335).

■ How does the surgical experience differ for the patient who has laparoscopic surgery from that for laparotomy? What is the length of hospital stay?

■ What fluid and electrolyte problems would you suspect when patients are losing GI fluids by tubes or drains?

7. Plan for a clinical experience.

▲ Observe patients who have had GI surgery. Note signs and symptoms of complications.

▲ Look at patient charts. Note those patients who have had complications, treatment, and are out of danger. Talk with them. What symptoms were noted in the chart? What nursing action was taken? Was the patient aware of it? How did the patient feel during the emergency?

▲ Care for patients who have had GI surgery and chart assessments that reveal the presence or absence of complications. Write a NCP. Discuss your nursing care plan in pre- and postconference.

▲ Look for patients with distention. Check the medication orders. If you see that Prostigmin is ordered, you may need to refer to LEG VII-A for review of its use. What other signs and symptoms occur with distention (for example, restlessness, euphoria)? How would you know that distention is increasing?

▲ Care for pediatric surgical patients. How does a pediatric postoperative course differ from that of an adult patient? How did you adapt your nursing care to include the patient's family?

▲ Care for patients who are having any of the following: vagotomy, hemorrhoidectomy, gastrectomy, bowel resection, colostomy, pyloroplasty.

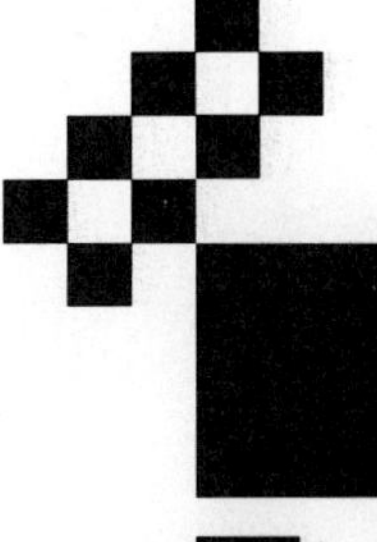

LEG VIII-C

Wound Care

O b j e c t i v e s

15. Demonstrate assisting the physician with a dressing change after abdominal surgery, with minimal direction.

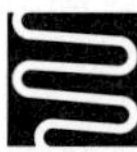 

16. Demonstrate irrigating a wound using sterile technique, and changing a dressing around a T-tube and/or a drain with minimal direction, and record your observations.

■ A. What's It All About?

1. Think about how you would change a dressing. When you prepare to change a dressing, whether assisting a physician or doing it yourself, do you know exactly how you are going to proceed? What if you have 90 seconds before the physician comes into the room? What exactly can and should you do? Can you make adjustments to accommodate your patient or some untoward happening?

2. Review:

LEG V-A Surgical Asepsis Techniques

LEG VII-A Immediate Postoperative Period

Using the Nursing Process for Postoperative Care

LEG VII-B Gastric and Intestinal Tubes and Feeding

3. Read about *dressings, binders, tubes, drains,* and *evaluation of patient's conditions* in medical-surgical and pediatrics references. Look in procedure manuals for types of dressings.

■ B. Putting It into Action!

1. Draw on the figures on p. 363 the types of sterile dressings you think would be best. Shade in the area that requires the thickest dressing. Indicate the various types of dressing beginning with the first and proceeding to the top covering.

Consider that your patient has been on the right side and you plan a turn to the left side. How does this influence your final dressing? Shade this change in red on one of the figures.

■ Here's another problem: You plan to get your patient out of bed to ambulate in the hall after you change the dressing. How does this influence your final dressing? Shade this change in green. Are you sure your dressing and binder will look as smooth after ambulation? You'll find it easy to tell if your dressing is too loose. But how will you know if it is too tight?

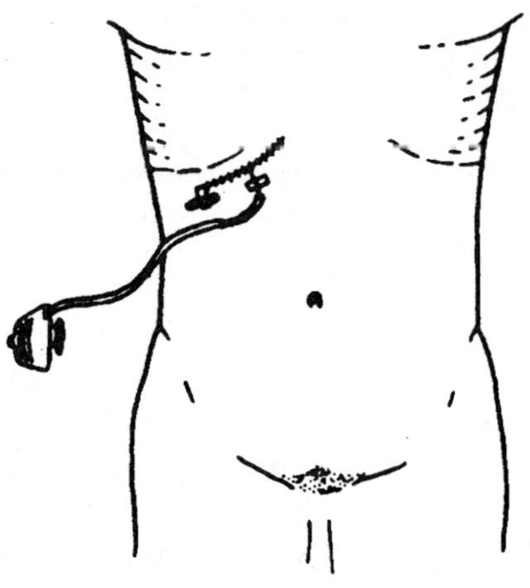

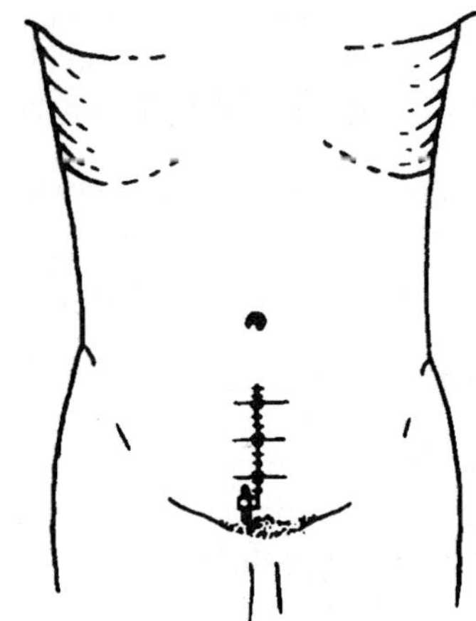

■ What are the advantages of Montgomery straps with dressings over a draining wound? How can you make them?

■ How do you know when to change a dressing or to reinforce it?

■ What are the advantages of using an ostomy appliance over draining wounds?

■ Determine which is the most cost-effective method in terms of supplies and nurses' time.

Place in order the list of nursing actions to change the dressing suggested for the following patient situation. (Hint: Some of the actions may be used more than once.)

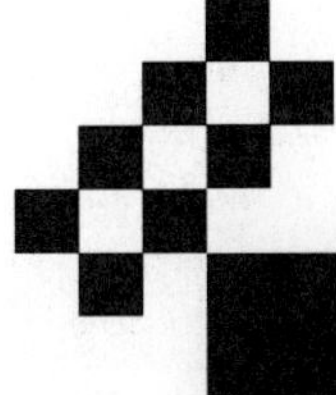

> Mrs. Rock has had a cholecystectomy. In report you learn that Dr. Brown has changed her dressing one time and there is an order to "change dressing prn." You have never seen Mrs. Rock before.

1. Cleanse the wound and remove old tape.
2. Add new Montgomery straps where needed to prevent skin irritation.
3. Check the chart to find out the exact surgical procedure and number of drains.
4. Set up a sterile field.
5. Examine the dressing to note need for change.
6. Explain to Mrs. Rock what you will do and when.
7. Record amount and characteristic of drainage and dressing applied.
8. Apply a sterile dressing positioned for maximum absorption.
9. Remove wet dressings and discard them.
10. Wash your hands.
11. Check on the level of Mrs. Rock's comfort.
12. Assemble all the needed equipment (e.g., instruments, dressing cart).

Answer:

(3), (10), (5), (11), (6), (12), (10), (4), (9), (1), (2), (8), (2), (11), (10), (7).

LEG VIII-C

How would you feel if you went into the room to check a patient's dressing, and when you came out the team leader said: "How is the IV running? How much is left?" You gulp and say: "Well, I didn't look at it. I just went in to check the dressing."

What can you do to avoid this situation in the future?

2. Practice in campus lab.

■ Apply a dressing to a student "patient" and see how well it stays on. Check for tightness and comfort. Reverse roles and you be the patient and react to how it feels and how a patient must feel.

How would the procedure change if the patient had a wound infection and was on infection-control precautions? Practice changing a dressing as if these precautions were in effect.

What observations would make you suspect an infection was present in a wound? What independent nursing actions would you take to investigate further?

■ Why would you use a wet-to-dry dressing? How would it be different from simply applying a dry dressing?

■ Role play packing a wound; practice using 4 × 4s and iodoform gauze. Can you keep the wound dressing from touching the skin?
Figure out how many ways you can do these procedures. What are the advantages and disadvantages of each? Which costs the least and is still safe and effective?

■ Role play irrigating a wound. What solutions could you use? What supplies will you use? How will you prevent soiling or wetting the patient and the bed?

LEG VIII-C

Comments on Dressings

Dressings must be applied according to strict principles of surgical asepsis. Don't fall into the pattern of simply reapplying a new dressing that is exactly like the one you remove. Evaluate the old dressing (e.g., how many layers are dry? Which part is soaked? Where is the drainage seeping through?) and then apply a dressing that is tailored to fit your patient's specific wound.

Many wounds drain excessively and require frequent changes. Take this opportunity to note the drainage; then try different approaches. (For example, cut a slit in a gauze square to fit around a drain; if this is a sterile dressing change, where will you get scissors? Place extra dressings in different places to allow more absorption. Note the body contours; pad the natural crevices well so that the fluid will not drain out under the dressing. As all patients are different (and all nurses), so will all dressings be different and adapted to the individual patient and wound. Don't let dressing changes become routine!

3. List the steps you would take in assessing the following patient on whom you have just received report.

Mrs. Sand, 1 day postoperative, has a Foley catheter, a nasogastric tube to intermittent suction, and a dressing in place following a cholecystectomy and an exploratory laparotomy. You are assigned to give her care this morning. She has orders for NPO and to reinforce dressing, prn; she may have Demerol 50–75 mg q 3–4 h prn for pain.

What questions will you need to ask Mrs. Sand? What will you check on the chart? What signs and symptoms will you look for?

Be prepared to state your rationale for all of the steps listed and for the answers to the preceding questions. Use this list for a checklist when you are actually caring for a patient after a cholecystectomy or other major surgery.

What will be your evaluation criteria?

■ Mrs. Sands's Operative Sheet states "T-tube and drain from stab wound." When you complete her transfer back to her room from the recovery room, what will you check in relation to surgery? List what you will look for. Now, go back and sequence what you will look for beginning with the most important observations.

■ How often will you check the T-tube drainage on the day of surgery? First day after surgery? Third day? Fifth day? What changes in amount of bile drainage would you expect to see on the day of surgery compared with the third day after surgery? Ten days after surgery? Why? Where should most of the bile be draining by the tenth day?

■ What symptoms would alert you to an obstruction? What changes would you expect to note in color of stools as the drainage from the T-tube decreases and the amount of intestinal flow increases? Why?

■ How can you adapt the bile drainage system to allow your patient to ambulate? What do you look for in the system after ambulation? Why?

■ What if you noted blood-stained fluid in the bile drainage bag the day of surgery? The third postoperative day?

4. Plan for a clinical experience.

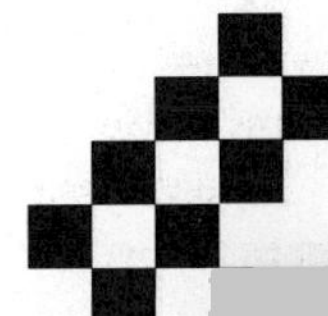

▲ Assist or observe a physician changing a dressing for the first time after surgery. Write down your feelings and the steps you noted as especially important. How did it go? Were you scared? If you answer yes, that's normal. Remember you must have enough anxiety to keep you sharp; practice and know-how will rid you of fear and lead to a successful experience.

▲ Change a sterile dressing with another student as an observer. Evaluate *your* nursing action. Change as many dressings as necessary to meet the Objective.

▲ Evaluate several patients' conditions. Have a student check you with your checklist (B.3). Establish a routine so that you never forget an item. This is not an easy task, so do not get discouraged, or let it be an excuse! Keep at it until you are confident and miss nothing!

▲ Find out what equipment would be needed to irrigate and pack a wound. Examine some iodoform and nu-gauze.

▲ Find out about or observe a wound culture being taken. What equipment is used, where is it sent? What equipment is needed if the physician wants to aspirate an abscess and culture it?

▲ Assist with or irrigate a wound using sterile technique.

Ostomy Care

Objectives

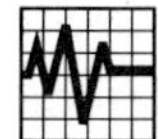

17. State worries or concerns a patient facing surgery for a colostomy may have and how you will help reduce them.

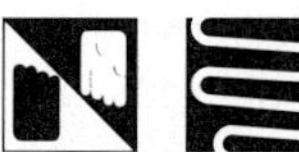

18. Demonstrate caring for a patient with a colostomy including changing a dressing or ostomy appliance and irrigating a colostomy.

■ A. What's It All About?

1. Think about bowel training, bowel habits, and the change a colostomy makes in a patient's life. How do you feel about irrigating a colostomy? How do you think a patient feels about the odors that come from the colostomy when it needs changing? How can you help your patient adjust? Although by now you probably have your own thoughts and feelings well in hand, you may need some reinforcing and modifications of your own attitudes as you help colostomy patients.

2. Talk with people from an ostomy support group in your area. Find out what nursing measures were most helpful. Remember, if your care involves a patient who has an "old" colostomy, you need to allow that patient to use his own routines and supplies. Help the patient adapt the hospital equipment, and use the patient's own routines as nearly as possible.

3. Read about *colostomy* and *ileostomy* and how to *help patients adjust physically and emotionally to living with them* in medical-surgical and mental health references.

4. View audiovisuals and read articles and books from a list given you by your instructor or read the following:

Krasner, D. "What's Wrong with This Stoma?" *AJN,* April 1990, pp. 46–47.

5. Attend an ostomy support group session.

6. Describe the look of a normal stoma. What symptoms would indicate problems?

■ B. Putting It into Action!

1. Attend a small group discussion on "Concerns of a Patient Scheduled for a Colostomy."

■ Discuss how both patients and family members can be helped to accept a change in body image. How is the fear of cancer related to the actual surgery? Share your NCPs from clinical lab.

2. **List** the differences between an enema and a colostomy irrigation.

Enema	**Colostomy Irrigation**

3. **Think** back to an experience in your own life when you were expected to perform some task, such as scheduling yourself for and participating in small group discussions in Volume I, and you just never seemed to do it successfully. Relate this experience to a patient who does not succeed in learning how to irrigate a colostomy after 3 days of instruction. Relate this to the mother who doesn't succeed in feeding her baby comfortably before she and her baby are discharged. How do ambivalent feelings apply to each of these three situations? List two ambivalent feelings for each person: you, the patient with a colostomy, and the new mother.
How does the grief process apply? What loss has occurred to the colostomy patient and the new mother?
What helpful intervention can you provide each person?
What outcomes will show acceptance of the colostomy?

4. **Plan** for a clinical experience.

▲ Care for patients with colostomies, either "old" or "new." What can you learn from a patient with an old colostomy that you can use to help a patient with a new one?

▲ Examine types and styles of colostomy appliances in your central supply department. How is the decision made about what type the patient will use? What happens if meticulous skin care is not maintained?

▲ Talk with patients facing colostomy surgery.

▲ Talk to the enterostomal therapist about care of colostomies. What different methods of skin preparation are used? Make patient rounds and notice the approach to patients and teaching methods. What adaptations are required to meet basic needs?

▲ Review the **Clinical Performance Expectations** for Level Eight on the Why Should I Study page.

Have I Learned?

The following questions are for you to answer in order to find out if you have met the Objectives. All of the Objectives in LEG VIII-C are covered in this series of questions. Pick a quiet time and answer them. Answers are found at the end of this selftest.

No space has been left for answering the questions related to the "doing" Objectives. Use a separate sheet of paper for those answers, and then use the answers in clinical or campus lab for your own evaluation.

Objective	Question
1,2	**1.** Be prepared to demonstrate the admission of a patient and/or make a physical assessment of a patient with altered GI function. Be able to give the rationale for any of your actions when requested.
3	**2.** List the actions you would take if your patient had the following order: "GB & Upper GI Series in A.M."
4	**3.** Match the following GI problems in column 1 with the diet changes in column 2 that would be required to meet nutritional needs of a patient.

Column 1	Column 2
_____ (a) diverticulitis	1. high-calorie diet
_____ (b) ulcer	2. high-protein diet
_____ (c) lactase deficiency	3. gluten-free diet
_____ (d) hiatal hernia	4. high-fiber diet
_____ (e) celiac disease	5. low-fiber diet
_____ (f) hepatitis	6. bland diet
	7. small feedings
	8. eliminate caffeine, alcohol
	9. limit lactose intake

Objective	Question
5	**4.** **(a)** Describe hyperalimentation. **(b)** What nutrients are provided in hyperalimentation? **(c)** Name three nursing implications for patients receiving hyperalimentation.

LEG VIII-C

6 **5.** Fill in the following chart:

Classification	Action/Use	Untoward Effect	Nursing Implications
Anticholinergic			
Antipruritic			
Digestant			
Antidiarrheal			

7 **6.** Describe how each of the following drugs acts to relieve pain:

antacid
analgesic
anticholinergic
H^2 receptor antagonist

8 **7.** The nursing care of the patient with an ulcer includes which of the following:

(a) Noting frequency of pain to determine if gastric acidity is controlled.

(b) Allowing expression of feelings to reduce emotional stress.

(c) Reducing the number of visits to the patient's bedside to reduce environmental distress.

(d) Observing for side effects of anticholinergic drugs.

(e) Observing for the signs and symptoms of the usual complications of infection and obstruction.

9 **8.** Mrs. James is a 35-year-old woman who has just been diagnosed as having ulcerative colitis. Write a teaching and discharge plan for her.

8, 9 **9.** Care for a patient with celiac disease, dumping syndrome, or lactase deficiency. Identify a nutritional need that is unmet, and then develop a teaching plan.

10 **10.** Compare the causative factor and nursing implications for hepatitis A and hepatitis B.

11 **11.** From the list of nursing actions below, select those that you would use for a patient with hepatitis B (write B) and those for a patient with hepatitis A (write A).

_____ (a) Use disposable syringes and needles

_____ (b) No break in skin of hands

_____ (c) Stool precautions

_____ (d) Private room

_____ (e) Provide rest

_____ (f) Encourage nourishing diet

_____ (g) Handle linen separately

_____ (h) Isolation precautions for food service

12 **12.** Care for a patient with a bowel obstruction. Write a NCP for the day before surgery and revise it for the first postoperative day.

13 **13.** Match the surgical procedure in Column 1 with the descriptions in Column 2.

Column 1

_____ (a) Bilroth I

_____ (b) Bilroth II

_____ (c) antrectomy

_____ (d) colostomy

_____ (e) vagotomy

_____ (f) hiatal herniorrhaphy

Column 2

1. Removal of the portion of the stomach where gastric secretion is greatest.

2. A portion of the colon is brought through the abdominal wall to create a temporary or permanent opening.

3. A division of the nerves known to stimulate gastric secretions.

4. Anastomosis of the remaining stomach to the duodenum.

5. Stomach is replaced in the abdomen and the esophageal opening is made smaller.

6. Anastomosis of the remaining stomach to the jejunum.

13 **14.** Choose a nursing intervention from Column 2 to be used in giving postoperative care after the surgical procedure in Column 1.

Column 1

_____ (a) gastrectomy

_____ (b) vagotomy

_____ (c) ileostomy

Column 2

1. Assess for fistulas, peritonitis

2. Observe for diarrhea

3. Prevent B_{12} deficiency

4. Prevent fluid and electrolyte imbalance

5. Assess for symptoms of dumping syndrome

6. Assess for decreased pain

14 **15.** Should any of the complications of GI surgery in Column 1 occur, indicate the signs and symptoms in Column 2 that the nurse would see.

Column 1	**Column 2**
_____ (a) bleeding	1. Shallow, rapid respirations
_____ (b) distention	2. Large amounts of bright red blood in suction drainage
_____ (c) obstruction	3. Hematemesis
	4. Nausea
	5. Feeling of fullness
	6. Tarry stools
	7. NG tube not draining
	8. Cramps in lower abdomen
	9. Boardlike abdomen

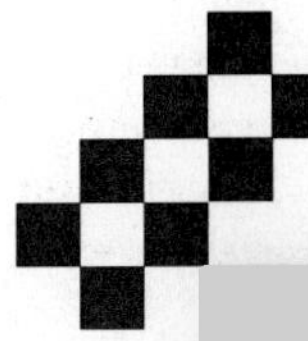

LEG VIII-C

15 **16.** List the actions you would take if the following occurred:

Dr. Brown met you as you came from your patient's room: "I'll be back to change Mrs. Rock's dressing in 5 minutes. Please have her ready."

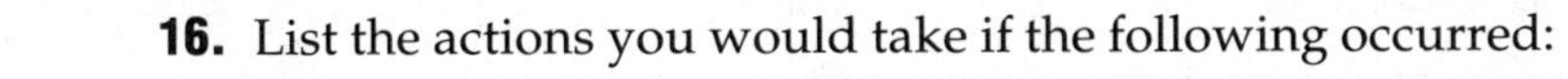

16 **17.** List the steps you would take to do a sterile wound irrigation. Use this list for your observer's checklist as you demonstrate irrigating a wound using sterile technique, changing the dressing, and charting your procedure and observations.

17 **18.** List three worries or concerns a patient may have who is facing surgery for a colostomy, and state how you will help with these concerns.

18 **19.** List the steps you would take in caring for a patient with a colostomy after the stoma is open. Include checking the dressing and preparation and irrigation of the colostomy.

■ Answers to Have I Learned?

LEG VIII-C

1. Attend a GES. Evaluate your performance. Identify your areas of weakness and practice until you are comfortable.

2. Give your list to another student who has agreed to check your list against your nursing actions as you prepare and care for a patient scheduled for both x-rays. Did you actually do everything on your list? Did you do anything more? Were you satisfied with your performance?

3. **(a)** 4; **(b)** 7,8; **(c)** 9; **(d)** 5,6; **(e)** 3; **(f)** 1,2.

4. **(a)** Administration of nutrients by way of a central vein (superior vena cava), called total parenteral nutrition (TPN) or through a peripheral vein, called peripheral parenteral nutrition (PPN). Used when GI tract cannot be used for feedings.

(b) The solution contains a mixture of hypertonic dextrose, amino acids, vitamins, minerals, and electrolytes and differs in tonicity. More hypertonic or more concentrated solutions must be given through the larger central vein.

(c) Assess baseline vital signs and body weight in order to assess changes. VS q4h, daily weight. Maintain careful intake and output records including observing for dehydration and edema. Regular schedule of oral hygiene. Maintain infusion rate. With TPN, bG q6h, assess for hyperglycemia and infection.

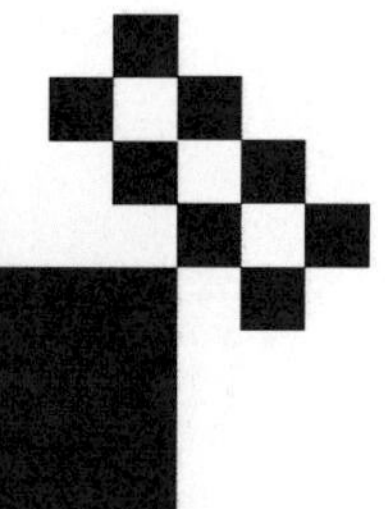

5.

Classification	Action/Use	Untoward Effect	Nursing Implications
Anticholinergic	Relaxes smooth muscles; bilary and renal colic; pylorospasm	Dry mouth, blurred vision, urinary retention	Use candy, gum to relieve dry mouth
Antipruritic	Relieves itching; jaundice/cirrhosis	Drowsiness	Assess safety of activities
Digestant	Increases bile flow	Diarrhea	Assess nutritional status
Antidiarrheal	Inhibits GI propulsion; absorbent and demulcent	Nausea, sedation	Assess for CNS depression, changes in stool

LEG VIII-C

6. *Antacid:* Local coating action to relieve gastric irritation. Insoluble and is not absorbed; buffers gastric secretions.

Analgesic: Acts on the CNS, both depressing and stimulating effects; promotes contraction of smooth muscles; therefore, it may increase discomfort from biliary colic without atropine.

Anticholinergic: Decreases mobility, tone, and peristalsis; mildly antispasmodic on biliary tract. May be combined with morphine to relieve biliary and renal colic.

H^2 receptor antagonist: Inhibits gastric secretions.

7. **(a)**, **(b)**, **(d)** are correct. A decrease in acidity and the reduction of emotional stress are important goals of nursing care. Patients are generally eager to discuss their problems with a nurse, and expression of feelings can reduce emotional stress. Other environmental stresses may need to be reduced. Complications of ulcers include hemorrhage and perforation. Obstruction occurs only when the ulcer is near the pyloric sphincter. Infection is not a complication.

8. Share your teaching and discharge plan during postconference. Your plan should take into consideration the patient's needs for rest, diet, elimination, medications (antispasmodics, anti-infectives, sedatives), mental rest, knowledge of the disease process, and signs to report.

9. Share your teaching plan with your instructor. It should include some of the following:

Celiac disease: knowledge to allow planning gluten-free meals of adequate calorie content, iron supplements.

Dumping syndrome: regular, relaxed meals; rest after meals; decreased concentrated sugar intake, schedule for fluid intake.

Lactase deficiency: knowledge to allow meal planning to limit intake of lactose.

10. Hepatitis A is caused by hepatitis virus A; it has a brief incubation period of 14–40 days, and is transmitted by body secretions such as fecal-oral route, or through contaminated water. Good handwashing techniques by nurses will prevent its spread in the hospital. Hepatitis B is caused by hepatitis virus B; it has a long incubation period of 43–160 days and is present in the serum of affected patients. It can be passed by blood transfusion, blood products, inoculation equipment, and mother-to-infant transmission.

11. *Hepatitis B:* **(a)**, **(b)**, **(e)**, **(f)**. *Hepatitis A:* **(b)**, **(c)**, **(e)**, **(f)**, **(g)**, **(h)**. Because of the difficulty in making a differential diagnosis early, both diseases may require infection control measures; check your hospital policy.

12. Discuss your NCP in a postconference. Note similarities and differences on other students' care plans for different diagnoses.

13. **(a)** 4; **(b)** 6; **(c)** 1; **(d)** 2; **(e)** 3; **(f)** 5.

14. **(a)** 3, 5; **(b)** 2, 6; **(c)** 1, 4.

15. **(a)** 2, 3, 4, 6, 9; **(b)** 4, 5, 7; **(c)** 4, 5, 8.

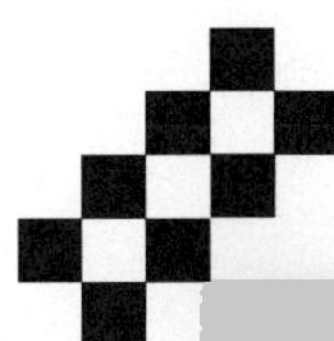

16. Evaluate your list with at least one other student.

17. Evaluate your procedure with your observer.
Practice this until you are not only safe but also at ease with all aspects of wound care.

18. *Change in bowel habits:* Explain that after a few weeks the patient will learn what foods can be eaten, and that a bowel movement once a day will probably become routine. May feel a loss of control or a decreased level of independence. Request a visit from a member of the ostomy support group.

Change in body image: Help the patient talk about decreased self-esteem, effect on sexuality; keep the conversation open to help the patient go through the phases of grief.

Loss of place in family or community; fear of malignancy: Keep conversation open and listen for anticipated problems with social and work life. An ostomy support group member may help with this. Teach both patient and at least one family member about caring for a colostomy after surgery. Preoperative preparation is vitally important.

19. Evaluate your own performance according to the list or ask a student observer to assist you with the checklist. Remember that a patient who has had a colostomy of long standing and has had a repair of the stoma probably knows much more about how to irrigate his own colostomy than you do. Let the patient tell you how to do it. This will help you both. Ask for help if you are unsure about this procedure. It can be a traumatizing experience for a patient with a new colostomy. Your own fears and concerns may be visible to your patient!

INDEX

Abdominal assessment, 337
Abdominal distention, 355, 360
Abortion, 317
  problems with, 346
Acid-base imbalance, 188–94, 204, 207
Acidosis, 62, 91, 189
Activities of daily living, 231
Acute abdomen, 356
Acute respiratory distress, 99
Adaptation, 42–48
  in cardiac patients, 216
Adaptive coping, 74
Admission procedure, 135
  for gastrointestinal problems, 331–38
  for labor patient, 251–58
Adoption, 314
Adrenergic blocking agents, 148
Aged:
  cardiovascular changes in, 216
  dehydration in, 178–79
  GI tract in, 348
  postoperative care of, 160
  respiratory tract alterations in, 99, 122
Airway obstruction, 115–16, 124
Alarm reaction stage, 42–43, 70, 74
Alkalosis, 91, 189
Allergy, 119
American Diabetes Association, 69, 73
Amnion, 248, 272
Analgesia, 264–68, 369, 372
Anesthesia, 152–53, 165, 264, 267–68
  caudal, 265
  general, 266
  inhalation, 266
  lumbar epidural, 266, 280
  paracervical block, 280
  pudendal block, 280
  saddle block, 266, 280
Angina pectoris, 215–16, 236, 240
Anorexia, 105
Antacids, 345, 369, 372
Antianginal, 237, 240
Antiarrhythmic, 237, 240
Anticholinergics, 369, 372
Anticoagulant, 237, 240
Antidepressants, 21, 22, 37
Antihypertensive, 237, 240
Antrectomy, 357, 370, 373
Anxiety, 25–28, 37, 42, 123
Apgar score, 274, 284, 303, 319, 323
Apical-radial pulse, 217, 219–20, 237
Arterial blood gases, 91, 121
Asepsis, 168, 291, 362
Assessment:
  of cardiac patient, 220, 237, 239
  of diabetic patient, 53–54
  of gastrointestinal patient, 331–38, 368, 372
  of labor patient, 256, 277
  of maternal attachment to infant, 308–13, 320, 324
  of newborn, 281, 284, 295–97, 306
  of postoperative patient, 157
  of respiratory problems, 81–89
Asthma, 95
Asulfidine, 344
Atelectasis, 171
Atropine, 224
Auscultation, 86
Autoimmune disease, 49
Autonomic nervous system, 147, 148

Ballard assessment, 303
Barrier technique, 85
Behavioral therapy, 26
Beta-adrenergic blocker, 224
Bicarbonate, 91, 190
Bilroth I and II, 357, 370, 373
Binders, 362
Biopsy, 332
Birth control, 314–16
Blood specimens, 55–56, 72
Blood sugar tests, 55
Blood type, 253
Body fluids, 179
Body image, 11, 15, 135, 163
Bottle feeding, 298–301
Bowel obstruction, 357, 370, 373
Bowel sounds, 337
Breast feeding, 298–301, 319, 323
Breathing exercises, 96–97
Breathing techniques, 282
Breath sounds, 82, 87
Bronchitis, 95
Bronchodilators, 97, 99, 122, 126
Bronchoscopy, 91, 121
Buffer system, 343

Index

Calcium, 224
Calcium channel blocker, 224
Carbon dioxide excess, 82, 91
Carbon dioxide narcosis, 191
Carbonic acid, 190
Cardiac arrest, 219
Cardiac function alterations, 213–16
Cardiac glycoside, 237, 240
Cardiac heart failure, 233, 237
Cardiac hypertrophy, 216
Cardiac monitor, 220
Cardiac rehabilitation, 230
Cardiovascular problems, 214
Catecholamine release, 216
Celiac disease, 368, 369, 372, 373
Cervical dilation, 260–61, 269
Change in body image, 11, 15, 163
Charting, 42, 44, 45
  cardiac medications, 223
  fluid and electrolyte imbalances, 185
  respiratory problems, 101
Chest assessment, 87
Childbirth preparation, 253
Children:
  dehydration in, 178–79
  diarrhea in, 182
  dosages for, 147–48
  oxygen therapy and, 112–13
Cholangiography, 332
Cholecystectomy, 365
Cholecystitis, 346
Cholelithiasis, 346
Cholinergic blocking agents, 148
Chorion, 248, 272
Chronic heart failure, 214
Chronic obstructive pulmonary disease (COPD), 95, 96, 98, 102, 122, 123, 127, 139
Circumcision, 302
Clotting time, 224
Codeine, 168
Colitis, 347
Colostomy, 357, 366, 370, 371, 373
  irrigation of, 367
Community resources, 69
Compazine, 167
Conflict, 26
Congenital heart defects, 215, 236, 239
Congestive heart failure, 214, 215–16
Coping, 230
Coping behaviors, 36–37
Cotyledons, 272
Cough, 105, 123, 125, 139
Coumadin, 224
CPR, 219
Crisis, 2, 35, 130
Crisis intervention, 10–13
Crohn's disease, 346
Croupette, 111, 114, 124
CT scan, 332
Cystic fibrosis, 95

Defense mechanisms, 26
Deficient coping, 74
Dehydration, 173, 176, 178–79, 203, 206
Delivery care, 269
Demerol, 168
Denial, 11, 15
Depression, 21–24, 37
Diabetes mellitus, 39
  community resources for, 69
  complications of, 62–68, 73
  diagnostic tests for, 55–56
  diet for, 51–52, 75
  insulin-dependent, 49, 71, 72
  non-insulin-dependent, 49, 71, 72
  patient assessment, 53–54
  pharmacology for, 57–61, 75
  symptoms of, 50
  teaching patients, 52–53
Diabetic coma, 62
Diagnostic tests:
  for cardiac patient, 217–20, 236
  for diabetes, 55–56, 72
  for gastrointestinal patient, 332
  for respiratory problems, 90–94, 121
Diarrhea, 180, 182, 204, 207
Diastolic blood pressure, 216
Diet:
  for cardiac patient, 224–25, 237
  for diabetic patient, 51–52, 72, 75
  for gastrointestinal patient, 340–41, 368, 372
  for surgical patient, 142–43
Digitalis toxicity, 223
Digitalizing dose, 223
Digoxin, 220, 223
Dilation, 278–79, 283
Dissociative disorder, 38
Disturbed coping patterns, 25–28
Diuretics, 223, 237, 240
Diverticulitis, 346, 368, 372
Dosages, 149
Drainage, 362, 365
Dressings, 362–64
DSM III-R, 25
Dubowitz assessment, 303
Dumping syndrome, 346, 347, 369, 373
Duncan placenta, 272

Duodenal ulcers, 346, 348
Dying patient, 14–20
Dyspnea, 105, 106, 122

Early shock, 152
ECF (extracellular fluid), 176–78
ECS (extracellular space), 196
Effacement, 278, 283
EKG, 218, 236–37
Electrolyte balance, 173, 176, 180–87, 203–204, 206–207
Elimination problems, 346
Embryo, 249
Emphysema, 95
Endoscopy, 332
Enema, 367
Enteral feedings, 199
Episiotomy, 290
Ergotrate maleate, 293
Estimated gestational age (EGA), 303, 320, 324
Estrogen, 325
Exercise, 238, 240
Expected date of confinement (EDC), 257, 303

Fasting blood sugar, 72, 75
Fathering, 309
Fatigue, 105
Fat-restricted diet, 224–25
Fear, 135, 163, 169, 253
Fetal circulation, 248, 249–50, 319, 322
Fetal development, 248–50, 277, 282
Fetal distress, 260
Fetal heart rate (FHR), 259–63
  deceleration of, 278, 283
Fetal monitoring, 260
Fetal presentation, 250
First trimester, 249, 282
Fluid balance, 173, 176–87, 203–204, 206–207
Fluid excess, 233–35, 238, 240
Fluid volume deficit, 346
Fourth stage of labor, 273–76
Frank-Starling mechanism, 216
Friedman graph, 260
Fundus, 274, 281, 284, 290

Gas pressures, 83
Gastrectomy, 357, 370, 373
Gastric analysis, 332
Gastric tubes, 199
Gastric ulcers, 348
Gastroenteritis, 346
Gastrointestinal intubation, 199–202, 205
Gastrointestinal problems, 327
  admission and assessment, 331–38, 368, 372
  conservative medical therapy for, 346–50
  nutritional needs and, 339–42, 368, 372
  pharmacology for, 343–45
Gastrointestinal surgery, 355–61
  complications of, 371, 373
Gastroparesis, 62
Gastrostomy tube, 202, 205
General adaptation syndrome, 42
Glucagon, 58, 70–71, 72, 74, 75
Glucose tolerance test, 55, 72, 75
Gluten, 346
Glycosylated hemoglobin test (GHb), 55
Golytely, 344
Grief, 11, 15–17, 22, 37, 317–18
  in maternity, 317–18, 321, 325

H2 receptor antagonists, 369, 372
Healthy lifestyles, 214
Heart, 213–16
Heart defects, 214
Heart rate, 224
Helplessness, 22, 230
Hematocrit, 253
Hemoglobin, 84, 253
Hemorrhage, 180
Heparin, 224
Hepatitis, 351, 353–54
  diet for, 368, 372
  type A, 352, 369, 373
  type B, 352, 369, 373
  type Non-A, Non-B, 352
Heptavax B, 344
Herniorrhaphy, 356
HHNC (hyperosmolar hyperglycemic nonketotic coma), 62, 64
Hiatal hernia, 357, 368, 370, 372, 373
Homeostasis, 42, 47, 176
Hopelessness, 22
Hospice, 15
Hostility, 105, 106, 123, 127, 349
Humidity, 96, 111–14
Hydrogen, 189
Hyperalimentation, 339, 368, 372
Hypercapnea, 81, 82, 84, 85–86, 120, 125
Hyperglycemia, 49, 62, 63–64, 72–73, 75
Hypernatremia, 180
Hypertension, 214, 236, 237, 239
  step-care approach to, 223
Hyperventilation, 83, 87, 207
Hypoglycemia, 49, 62, 63–64, 72–73, 75
Hypokalemia, 180

Hypomagnesemia, 180
Hyponatremia, 180
Hypotension, 166
Hypoventilation, 83, 87, 153, 207
Hypovolemia, 153, 178
Hypoxemia, 81, 82, 84, 85–86, 120, 214
Hypoxia, 82, 125, 153

ICF (intracellular fluid), 176–77
IDDM (insulin-dependent diabetes), 49, 71, 72
Ileostomy, 357, 366, 370, 373
Ileus, 355
Imferon, 344
Immune serum globulin, 344
Incentive spirometer, 139
Infants with physical anomalities, 317
Ingestion problems, 346
Injections, intradermal, 119, 124
Inspiratory stridor, 116
Insulin, 49, 57–61, 70–71, 72, 74, 75
Interdependence, 7
Intermittent positive pressure breathing (IPPB), 96, 126
Intestinal tubes, 199
Intradermal injections, 119, 124
Intraoperative nursing, 152
Intravenous therapy, 195–98, 204–205, 207–208
Irritable bowel syndrome, 347
Isolation techniques, 82, 84–85
Isolette, 111, 114
Isuprel, 224

Jaundice, 296, 352, 353
Jejunostomy tube, 202, 205

Ketoacidosis, 64, 73
Ketones, 55
Kidneys, 91, 190

Labor, 277–80, 282
- admission and assessment of patients, 251–58
- anesthesia and analgesia for, 264–68
- fourth stage of, 273–76
- monitoring patient in, 259–63
- placental separation, 272
- second and third stages of, 269–71, 284

Lab reports, 164, 192, 217, 319, 323, 336–37
Lactase deficiency, 346, 347, 368, 369, 372, 373
Lactation, 298
- suppression of, 319, 323

Laryngotracheobronchitis, 116, 123
Leopold's maneuvers, 250
Letdown reflex, 299
Lifestyle changes, 230
Lightening, 253
LOA presentation, 280, 283
Lochia, 281, 284, 290
Loss, 17–18, 22
- of infant, 317–18

Loss of body function, 11, 15
Lumen, 200, 205
Lungs, 190, 193–94
Lung scan, 121

Magnesium, 204, 207
Maternal-infant bonding, 309
Maternal role attainment, 289, 309, 320, 324
Medications:
- in fourth labor stage, 274, 283
- gastrointestinal, 343–45, 369, 372
- in postpartum period, 293–94
- preoperative, 147–50, 165

Mental health, 26
Mental illness, 26
Mental maturity, 26
Metabolic acidosis, 173, 188, 190, 192, 204, 207, 346
Metabolic alkalosis, 188, 190–92, 204, 207, 346, 348
Methergine, 293
Microdrip, 204–205, 207–208
Micromists, 114
Miller-Abbott tube, 205
Mineral supplements, 344–45
Moniliasis, 62
Morphine, 167
Mourning, 11, 15
Myocardial infarction, 215–16, 229–32, 238, 240

Nasogastric tubes, 202, 205
Nausea, 180, 204
Nebulizers, 97, 114
Need deprivation, 42
Neonate. *See* Newborn
Nephropathy, 62
Neuropathy, 62
Newborn:
- assessment and care of, 281, 284, 285, 289–92, 320, 324

Newborn (*cont.*)
circulation in, 319, 322
normal, 295–97, 302–307, 319, 322
periods of reactivity in, 319, 323
reflexes of, 319, 323
NIDDM (non-insulin-dependent diabetes), 49, 71, 72
Nitroglycerine paste, 224
Nontraditional childbearing couples, 314–16
Normal blood values, 319, 323
Nurse-patient relationship, 22, 252
Nursing care plan:
for cardiac patient, 221–28, 238, 241
for diabetes, 73
for gastrointestinal patient, 335, 369, 372
for GI surgical patient, 355–61
for labor patient, 280
for postoperative patient, 160
for postpartum patient, 319, 321, 322, 324
for respiratory disorders, 122, 126
for two to four patients, 161–62
Nutrition:
for cardiac patient, 224–25
for diabetic patient, 51–52, 72, 75
for gastrointestinal patient, 339–42, 368, 372
for surgical patient, 142–43

Obstetrical positions and presentations, 248, 250
Obstructed airway, 115–16, 124
Oral contraceptives, 321, 325
Oral hypoglycemic agents, 58, 72, 75
Osmolarity, 177
Ostomy care, 366–67
Ovum, 249
Oxygen, 152
Oxygen equipment, 112–14
Oxygen insufficiency, 82, 84, 86
Oxygen therapy, 111–14, 123, 127
Oxytocics, 293–94, 319, 322

Pain, 216
Palpation, 87
Panic, 26
Parasympathetic nervous system, 148
Parenteral solutions, 195–98, 204, 207
Parenting, 309
Pediatric dosages, 147, 148
Pediatrician, 253
Peptic ulcers, 346, 348
Percussion, 87
Perineal care, 290–91
Peripheral parenteral nutrition (PPN), 372
Peripheral vascular disease, 216
pH, 91, 189
Pharmacology:
for diabetes, 57–61, 75
for gastrointestinal problems, 343–45
Phenylketonuria (PKU), 296, 302
Physiologic behaviors, 74
Pitocin, 293
Placenta, 248, 249
separation of, 272
Play therapy, 135
Positions:
for airway obstruction, 115
obstetrical, 248, 250
Postmortem care, 15
Postoperative period:
complications of, 138, 139, 167
immediate, 151–55
nursing process for, 156–60
Postpartum blues, 309, 320, 324
Postpartum period:
assessment and care, 285, 289–92
check during, 275, 281, 319, 322
oxytocics in, 293–94, 319, 322
parental feelings and attitudes, 308–13, 320, 324
physiologic changes during, 319, 322
Postpartum psychosis, 309
Postprandial blood sugar, 72, 75
Potassium, 204, 207, 224
Preoperative period:
emotional preparation for, 163
medications for, 147–50, 165
physical preparation for, 135
teaching, 138–40
Preterm infants, 317, 321, 325
Progestin, 325
Prothrombin time, 224, 236, 239
Psychologic behaviors, 74
Psychologic stress, 42
Psychoneuroses, 26
Psychophysiologic disorders, 25–28
Psychosis, 320, 324
Psychosocial assessment, 7–9
Psychosomatic illness, 26
PTT, 236, 239
Pulmonary function test, 94, 121
Pulse oximetry, 121
Pyloric stenosis, 357–58

Reality therapy, 26
Rebound tenderness, 338
Recovery room nursing, 152
Reflexes of newborn, 296, 319, 323
Relaxation techniques, 230, 277
Respiratory acidosis, 91, 121, 125, 173, 188, 190, 192, 204, 207
Respiratory alkalosis, 121, 173, 188, 190, 204, 207
Respiratory diagnostic tests, 90–94
Respiratory obstruction, 115
Respiratory problems, 77
  assessing and preventing, 81–89
  diagnostic tests for, 90–94
  relieving distress from, 95–97
Respiratory tract alterations, 98–103, 122
  nursing process for, 104–10
Retinopathy, 62
Reverse protection technique, 85
Rh, 253
Ritualistic behavior, 26
Role function, 7
Rotating tourniquets, 233–34
Ruptured membranes, 253

Schultz placenta, 272
Scopolamine, 167
Second stage of labor, 269–71
Second trimester, 282
Self-concept, 7, 8
Serum potassium, 224, 346
Sexuality, 230
SGOT, 236, 239
Shock, 152
Show, 253
Single mothers, 314–16
Skin color assessment, 87
Skin testing, 119
Smoking, 91
Sodium, 204, 207
Sodium-restricted diet, 224–25, 239
Somatoform disorder, 37
Sonography, 332
Specimen collection and testing, 55–56
Spirometry, 91, 139
Sputum specimen, 93, 105, 121, 123, 125, 127
Stage of exhaustion, 42–43, 70, 74
Stage of resistance, 42–43, 70, 74
Station, 278, 283
Sterile dressings, 168
Sterile wound irrigation, 371, 373
Stillbirth, 317
Stool specimen, 332, 333
Stress, 214, 236
  adaptation to, 42–48
  long-term effects of, 215
  preoperative, 135, 136
Stressors, 10, 39
  illness and, 43
Stress reduction, 214, 230
Sucralfate, 344
Suctioning, 117–18, 124, 152, 165, 171, 302
Sugar, 55
Suicide, 22
Surgery, 130
  emotional preparation for, 134–37
  gastrointestinal, 355–61
  physical preparation for, 141–46
  postoperative, 138, 139
  preoperative, 135, 138–40, 147–50
Surrogacy, 314
Sympathetic nervous system, 148
Systolic blood pressure, 216

Taking-in process, 320, 324
Teaching:
  bottle and breast feeding, 300
  diabetic patient, 52–53
  GI function alteration, 349
  high blood pressure patient, 225
  labor patient, 269
  neonatal care to parents, 302–307
  perineal care, 291
  preoperative, 138–40
Teenage pregnancy, 314–16, 321, 325
Terminal illness, 15
Therapeutic relationship, 7–9
Third stage of labor, 269–71
Third trimester, 282
Three-lumen tube, 205, 208
Throat irrigations, 117
Thrombophlebitis, 171
Total parenteral nutrition (TPN), 372
Tourniquets, 233–34
Tracheostomy care, 117–18, 124
Tube feedings, 339
Two-lumen tube, 205, 208
Type A behavior, 216

Ulcer, 368, 369, 372
Ulcerative colitis, 346, 369, 373
Umbilical cord, 272
Unconscious patient care, 152
Upper GI bleeding, 346
Urine specimens, 55–56, 72
Uterine contractions, 280, 283

Vagotomy, 357, 370, 373
Vagus nerve, 224
Vasopressin, 344
Vital signs, 166
Vitamin supplements, 344–45
Vomiting, 166, 171, 180, 182, 204, 207

Wound care, 168, 362–65, 371, 373
Wound infection, 171

X-rays, 332

Index